A Lacanian Reading of Anorexia

This book presents a Lacanian perspective on the understanding and treatment of anorexia, supported by case material, research and theoretical insight from the author's 25 years of clinical practice.

Domenico Cosenza explains how anorexia constitutes a challenge for contemporary psychoanalytic clinicians, assesses previous theoretical understandings and examines clinical contributions from other schools of psychoanalysis. Cosenza argues that anorexia cannot be treated by following a classical psychoanalytic path, and here draws on numerous clinical cases to articulate a Lacanian approach which addresses core concerns not resolved elsewhere. Elaborating on Lacanian concepts including refusal and the object nothing, Cosenza offers a new approach for all psychoanalytically-informed clinicians working with anorexia.

A Lacanian Reading of Anorexia will be of great interest to psychoanalysts, psychiatrists, clinical psychologists and psychotherapists interested in Lacanian perspectives and the dynamic-analytical approach in the treatment of anorexia.

Domenico Cosenza is a psychoanalyst in private practice in Milan, Italy. He is an Analyst Member and past President of the Lacanian School of Psychoanalysis (SLP) and a member of the World Association of Psychoanalysis (WAP).

A Lacanian Reading of Anorexia

By Domenico Cosenza

Translated by Jonathan West and revised by Fernando Castrillon

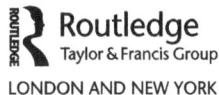
Routledge
Taylor & Francis Group

LONDON AND NEW YORK

Designed cover image: © Getty Image

First published in English 2024
by Routledge
4 Park Square, Milton Park, Abingdon, Oxon OX14 4RN

and by Routledge
605 Third Avenue, New York, NY 10158

Routledge is an imprint of the Taylor & Francis Group, an informa business

© 2014 Rennes University Press

Translated by Jonathan West

The right of Domenico Cosenza to be identified as author of this work has
been asserted in accordance with sections 77 and 78 of the Copyright,
Designs and Patents Act 1988.

The first edition of this work was published in French by the Rennes University
Press in the "Clinique psychanalytique et psychopathologie" series (2014). All
rights reserved. The English translation is published with the agreement of the
University of Rennes Press, copyright holders of the original work.

British Library Cataloguing-in-Publication Data
A catalogue record for this book is available from the British Library

Library of Congress Cataloguing-in-Publication Data
Names: Cosenza, Domenico, author.
Title: A Lacanian reading of anorexia / by Domenico Cosenza ; translated by
Jonathan West and revised by Fernando Castrillon.
Description: Milton Park, Abingdon, Oxon ; New York, NY : Routledge, 2024.|
"The first edition of this work was published in French by the Rennes University
Press in the "Clinique psychanalytique et psychopathologie" series (2014)."--Title
page verso. | Includes bibliographical references and index. |
Identifiers: LCCN 2023008597 (print) | LCCN 2023008598 (ebook) |
ISBN 9781032331539 (hardback) | ISBN 9781032331522 (paperback) |
ISBN 9781003318439 (ebook)
Subjects: LCSH: Anorexia--Treatment.
Classification: LCC RB150.A65 C67 2024 (print) | LCC RB150.A65
(ebook) | DDC 616.85/262--dc23/eng/20230605
LC record available at https://lccn.loc.gov/2023008597
LC ebook record available at https://lccn.loc.gov/2023008598

ISBN: 978-1-032-33153-9 (hbk)
ISBN: 978-1-032-33152-2 (pbk)
ISBN: 978-1-003-31843-9 (ebk)

DOI: 10.4324/9781003318439

Typeset in Times New Roman
by MPS Limited, Dehradun

'Cosenza addresses eating disorders without getting stuck in Lacanian jargon for initiated ones, in a way that is both fresh but at the same time rigorous. An excellent clinical approach, which always involves theoretical interrogations.'

Sergio Benvenuto, *psychoanalyst, founder of the*
European Journal of Psychoanalysis

'Domenico Cosenza's book will be helpful to clinicians for treating "the psychological wall" that anorexic patients build, brick by brick, to detach themselves from the Other. In according to a Lacanian perspective, Cosenza emphasizes a clinical work focused on the role of "the word" in order to develop in these patients their "desire" to go beyond the wall of anorexia. It is a must-read book.'

Giuseppe Craparo, *psychoanalyst and professor of Clinical Psychology at the Kore University of Enna, Italy*

Contents

Author's note to the English edition

This book, published in France in its original edition in 2014, and translated into Brazilian Portuguese in 2018, is now being published in English. Its main contents are known in Italian and Spanish thanks to other publications we have done in these languages over the last 15 years on the subject of anorexia. It is a real pleasure for us that English-speaking readers can now have direct access in their own language of reference to our work on anorexia read in the light of the Lacanian orientation, without necessarily having to go through one of the Romance languages in which we have so far published our books and most of our articles on the subject. In fact, this book is undoubtedly the most comprehensive and systematic work we have written on the subject so far.

In this English edition, however, we have not limited ourselves to translating the original 2014 book. We felt the need to introduce some minor additions that seemed necessary as updates, given that almost a decade has passed since its original publication in French. In particular, we felt it necessary to refer to the revisions of the diagnostic classification systems in psychiatry that have taken place in this decade, which have partly modified the descriptive diagnostic frames of reference.

As we reviewed the work for this edition, we realized that, despite the many years since their original formulation, the strength of Lacan's reading of anorexia remains fruitful, and in our opinion constitutes the perspective most capable of grasping the central enigma of the anorexic position and guiding clinical practice.

My hope is that the English language edition of this book may, in its own small way, contribute to the dissemination of Jacques Lacan's clinical orientation of psychoanalysis in Anglophone countries and especially in the United States, where a more cultural reception of his teaching has prevailed for many years. In this sense, this work follows the orientation offered by Jacques-Alain Miller of the reading of Lacan, in continuity of inspiration with the initiatives of the Freudian Field and the New Lacanian School in the English-speaking world.

We would like to extend special thanks to all those who helped make this English edition of the book possible. In particular, we undoubtedly want to warmly thank Fernando Castrillón, who inspired this idea in the beginning and who generously agreed to do a final revision of the text. Equally affectionately, we would like to thank the book's translator Jonathan West for translating from French to English and for his expertise and constant presence at my side throughout the work.

Our heartfelt thanks also go to François Ansermet, author of the "Preface", Thomas Svolos, Sergio Benvenuto and Giuseppe Craparo, who have wholeheartedly supported our desire for this English edition of the book from the beginning.

Domenico Cosenza
Milan, 30 November 2022

Preface

The fantasy of one's own death, of one's disappearance, of one's loss, is at the heart of the anorexic's problems (Lacan, 1973, pp. 194–195). As a counterpoint, the anorexic refusal, which is at the heart of the anorexic impasse, paradoxically appears as a solution. Through her refusal, the anorexic tries to save her desire (Lacan, 2006, p. 524). It is from this paradoxical role of refusal that Domenico Cosenza makes the lever of a possible treatment of anorexia.

Anorexia is to be situated beyond the pleasure principle, caught in the frozen enjoyment of a behavior that appears to have no exit. We are no longer in the conflictual logic of the symptom: as Domenico Cosenza shows, anorexia proceeds, rather, from a failure of the constitution of a symptom in adolescence that goes hand in hand with a denial of all unconscious knowledge. Thus, the anorexic clinic is also a way to explore the impasses of jouissance. The other jouissance – which could be one of the names of the anorexic jouissance – occupies all the space, overflows in both the subject and her family.

Anorexia can indeed be seen as a primordial defense against an invading jouissance. This is how we can think of anorexia from the early passive infantile anorexia. Everything revolves around the key moment of weaning. As Lacan shows, it is the baby who weans him/herself and not the mother who weans the baby (Lacan, 2004, p. 379). We can measure to what extent this crucial moment can lead to an impasse, bringing into play an appetite for death. Who is weaning whom? The child can propose him/herself to the parental desire, whose object remains enigmatic for him/herself even if he/she proposes his/her own loss.

"Does he/she want to lose me?" For Lacan (1973, pp. 194–195), this is the question of the anorexic faced with parental desire, whose object remains unknown. This question can strike those who are committed to treating the anorexic as well as those who are led to revisit their desire to treat in the face of what systematically puts them in check.

How to get out of the impasse of enjoyment, the beyond of the pleasure principle, this displeasure which comes into play at the same time as pleasure. The anorexic cannot want what she desires: which also means that desire is not far away. It is a question of banking on these potentialities buried under the anorexic pressures.

Rather than as a disorder, we should perhaps take anorexia as a response of the subject, as a solution, even if this solution turns out to be a trap. This is the position of Domenico Cosenza, who at the same time derives from it reference points in the way of treating the anorexic. Did Lasègue not already say that anorexics were doctors of themselves? They treat themselves with anorexia, for lack of anything better.

This is how Domenico Cosenza's position opens a way out by making anorexic refusal a lever to get out of the compulsive confinement in repetition. There would be two paths for the anorexic refusal: on the one hand toward death, with an appetite for death, jouissance, the death drive; on the other hand toward life, with a desire that paradoxically saves itself in its impasse. The refusal toward life makes anorexia shows the hysterical side. The refusal toward death makes it look more like a psychosis, an ordinary psychosis. But above all, this tension reintroduces the possibility of a way out, following the edge of its paradoxical necessity, of anorexia seen at first as a solution. The trapping solution that was at the origin of anorexia perhaps also offers the way out. This is, in any case, the clinical challenge of Domenico Cosenza's thoughts, which is also the challenge of psychoanalysis in the face of anorexia.

François Ansermet

References

Lacan, J. (1973), *Le Séminaire de Jacques Lacan: Livre XI. Les quatre concepts fondamentaux de la psychanalyse 1964*. Paris: Édition du Seuil.

Lacan, J. (2004), *Le Séminaire de Jacques Lacan: Livre X. L'angoisse 1962–1963*. Paris: Édition du Seuil.

Lacan, J. (2006), *The direction of the Treatment. Écrits: The First Complete Edition in English*. New York & London: Norton.

Acknowledgments

This book, taken from my doctoral thesis in psychoanalysis, would not have been possible without the help of a series of encounters that led me to develop a particular desire toward the clinic of anorexia nervosa, based on the teaching of Jacques Lacan. The first approaches to this teaching took place more than 20 years ago; I was enlightened and won over by it and since then it has never ceased to orient me in my work as an analyst and in my clinical practice. It was above all the encounter with the lively teaching of Jacques-Alain Miller, when I was a young philosophy student in Milan, that was unforgettable for me, as was his enlightening and rigorous reading of the texts of Freud and Lacan and his commentary on clinical cases, always aiming to show the singular key point within each of them. This is why my first thanks are addressed to him: without the Lacanian orientation, which he developed from the beginning of his course at the University of Paris 8, this thesis on anorexia nervosa would lose its own foundation, as any reader will be able to easily notice.

I would like to thank Pierre-Gilles Guéguen for having, from the beginning, accepted to direct my thesis and for having followed, with patience and availability, its progress. I would also like to express my gratitude to Éric Laurent, who supported me in the idea of this doctoral work, and to François Ansermet who particularly appreciated it and who did me the honor of writing the preface to this book. I am also grateful to Carole Dewambrechies La Sagna, Pierre Naveau and Hebe Tizio, who kindly agreed to be part of my doctoral commission. And to Gérard Miller, director of the psychoanalysis department at the University of Paris 8, for having supported the publication of this book.

My thanks also go to the various psychoanalytical colleagues of the World Association of Psychoanalysis, to which I belong and to which I refer extensively and explicitly throughout my research. They have made an important contribution to the study of anorexia nervosa from the perspective of Lacanian psychoanalysis, where my work is situated. And, more generally, I thank all those colleagues whose names I cannot mention here and who have contributed and still contribute to my training in the field of psychoanalysis.

In the context of this thesis, I can only thank the many anorexic patients I have met over the last fifteen years in institutions and in my practice. I also owe a lot to the institutional experience with the ABA (Association for the Study and Research on Anorexia, Bulimia and Eating Disorders) of which I was the scientific director from 2002 to 2006, and to the exciting work in the therapeutic community La Vela in Moncrivello (Vercelli, Italy) where I had various encounters with anorexic patients, which proved to be of fundamental importance for me.

I would also like to thank Katy Boidin for her constant support during the various stages of writing the work in French.

Paris, 2014

Introduction

The research objective

In this work, we have approached the problem of refusal in the clinic of anorexia nervosa. The choice of this theme, dictated in part by our clinical experience in this field, is oriented to the point that we consider the fundamental core of the anorexic question, on the basis of the psychoanalytical elucidations of Lacan and the Lacanian orientation of Jacques-Alain Miller in particular. Indeed, the core of the refusal in anorexia radically affects the relationship of the subject to food; to the other of the intersubjective relationship; to the Other of speech and language; and of the subject to his body and his enjoyment.

But what is refusal, precisely, in anorexia nervosa? Is it possible to distinguish the most obvious phenomenological manifestations from a structural dimension? And if so, what characterizes the structure of anorexic refusal? What does its specific modality of jouissance and the real of the drive that govern its economy of satisfaction consist of? These are the fundamental questions that we will ask ourselves in this work.

The function and the field of refusal in the clinic of anorexia nervosa could well be considered, in this sense, as the fundamental axis of this research.

This work, like the formulation of the questions that are at its center, would not have been possible without encountering, on our way, the enlightening indications of Lacan on anorexia nervosa. In this sense, this research can be considered as a systematic attempt, within the limits of the possible, to clarify Lacan's teaching on the basis of anorexia. And we consider this in the light of the contributions on anorexia coming from the psychoanalytical literature and especially from the writings of authors within the Lacanian orientation, combined with the data from the clinical experience of cases of anorexic patients, followed by us in analysis or in institutions.

From our reading, there should emerge a fruitful discontinuity of the Lacanian approach to the theme of anorexia nervosa, not only in relation to cognitive-behavioral and systemic-relational psychotherapeutic approaches, but also in relation to contemporary post-Freudian analytical orientations on

DOI: 10.4324/9781003318439-1

anorexia. Above all, compared to cognitive-behavioral approaches, anorexia nervosa will be thought of as a solution embodying a particular position of the subject; not only, therefore, as a specific syndrome of a constellation of behavioral and cognitive disorders. Compared to systemic-relational approaches, we will highlight the singular irreducibility of the position of the anorexic subject vis-à-vis his status as a symptom of the system of family transactions.

But, concerning the theme of anorexia, it is important to underline its difference from contemporary post-Freudian analytical approaches. In this respect, it seems essential here to emphasize an essential point: with regard to anorexia, Lacan's perspective, as we have already affirmed, marks a distance from all the analytical perspectives that focus the heart of the anorexic question around an essentially narcissistic issue. It is not because, in the Lacanian clinical perspective, we do not recognize the importance of the narcissistic function, but rather because we avoid reducing it to the egological frameworks of a theory of anorexia nervosa, based on the thesis of the centrality of the Ego's fragility and the narcissistic deficit of the anorexic subject. It is a theory that supports and justifies a healing praxis aiming to strengthen the fragile ego on the model of Ego-Psychology, or to support the narcissistic deficits of an unstructured Self (modeled on Kohut's approach in The Psychology of the Self).

In the field of anorexia nervosa, the same crucial problem is posed again which the post-Freudian orientations of psychoanalysis display with regard to the adolescent and the reading of their crisis and which distances them from Freud's lesson: is narcissism a necessary means to reinforce, according to the position of the post-Freudians, or an obstacle in the orientation of the treatment? As Philippe La Sagna has clearly pointed out, there are therefore two ways of envisaging the treatment in adolescence: either the accent is placed on the identification, always too fragile, of the adolescent, or it is put on desire. [...] Either one chooses identification, or else one chooses the value of dis-identification and desire (La Sagna, 2009, p. 21).

This post-Freudian reference model, which has its deep roots in the teaching of Hilde Bruch on anorexia, is widely disseminated in the post-Freudian analytical matrix approaches applied to the treatment of anorexia and bulimia in institutions. The Lacanian approach is not at all insensitive to the importance of the narcissistic issue in anorexia nervosa. It is also true that Lacan, in his references to anorexia nervosa, never refers to the narcissistic question.

Other authors who refer to the work of Lacan, and recently also in a systematic way (Malaguarnera, 2010, pp. 91–130), have pointed out several times that the coordinates provided by Lacan, through the theory of the stage of the mirror and its developments in the diagram of the optical model, allow a clinically important reading of the phenomena of a narcissistic nature, such as, first of all, the distortion of body image in anorexia nervosa. But this is valid on condition that the reading of the narcissistic question of anorexia is

framed by the knotting of the register of the imaginary in its structural relationships to the symbolic and the real, around the devastating link of the
anorexic subject to their own body.

In the Lacanian perspective, the narcissistic issue of the anorexic subject
finds its foundation in the symbolic relationship of the subject to the Other
and to his real economy of enjoyment (*jouissance*). Indeed, it is by having the
subject work in the treatment on their relationship to the Other and to
jouissance, that the narcissistic dimension of his functioning can also succeed
in restructuring itself in a less deadly way for them.

As we will show in detail, in relation to anorexia nervosa, the two structural pillars on which the position of the subject is supported are represented
by a fundamental refusal of the Other and by an economy of jouissance
without loss, which revolves around what Lacan defined the object nothing.

At the same time, in this work we will seek to show how anorexia nervosa
challenges psychoanalysis in its classical functioning, forcing it to rethink the
foundations of its own clinic. This is what Lacan will do, several times in his
teaching, by referring to anorexia nervosa as a paradigmatic clinical exemplification of an internal turning point in his reading of the foundations of
psychoanalysis.

In the 1950s, in antithesis to the biologism of Ego-Psychology, he asserted
that anorexia is the extreme incarnation of the impossibility of reducing the
desire and the demand for love to the dimension of need and the level of
reality. In the 1960s and 1970s, in antithesis to an all-meaning and all-
signifying reductionism, he asserted the anorexic jouissance of the nothing as
irreducible to the field of the symbolic Other, as jouissance which is not lost
and which refuses alienation.

More generally and in the light of the difficulties that the clinic, not only
analytical but above all medical, clearly manifests (both in its psychiatric and
nutritional aspects), anorexia nervosa presents itself as a challenge to the
foundations of contemporary medical and psychopathological knowledge. In
this sense, the parallel with hysteria does not seem incongruous to us, in the
context of the clinical knowledge of medicine and psychiatry at the end of the
19th century, before the Freudian discovery of psychoanalysis.

We know that Freud owes to the encounter with the hysteric the invention
of psychoanalysis as a talking cure and that, originally, Freudian practice was
the result of a good encounter between the words of the hysteric on one side,
and the psychoanalyst's listening and interpretation on the other. The fundamental reason for this success, which is added to the effect of novelty
introduced by Freudian practice, is linked to the original structure of the
hysterical symptom and, more generally, of the neurotic symptom: it functions, for the subject itself, as symbolic substitution manifesting itself in the
somatic conversion of the hysteric or in the obsessive's rumination of the
obsessive of an unconscious and repressed desire. The hysteric produces their
own symptom as a phenomenon to which they attribute an enigmatic

meaning; they then ask the analyst to interpret it in the transference, that is, by assuming that the latter has knowledge of the truth of this enigma. It is up to the analyst, apart from a few rare cases, not to satisfy the hysteric's demand for meaning, so that the analyst can relaunch the work of interpretation around the enigma of their own symptom.

We do not encounter any of this in clinical practice, when we have been concerned with anorexia nervosa, apart from those forms where, apparently as the anorexic symptom, it is hysteria which manifests itself. The anorexic does not see their condition as a problem. On the contrary, they have an egosyntonic relationship, of full identification, and devoid of enigmatic questioning about their own symptom. This is why they ask no one anything about it, they have nothing to say about it, and they do not develop any transference or show the slightest intention of getting rid of their symptom, which, on the contrary, has more of value to them than their own life. This is the radical difficulty that the clinician encounters when they find a subject with anorexia nervosa on their path. The anorexic poses between the Other and themselves an impermeable barrier of division, and remains insensitive to the siren of meaning and interpretation. In this sense, the anorexic does not limit themselves to turning medicine upside down, reducing it to impotence, creating difficulty for clinical nutrition and making the effectiveness of psychopharmacology marginal. Its most radical, new challenge is precisely addressed to the heritage of care practices of Freudian origin, to talking cures, to dynamic psychotherapies and, lastly, to the noble mother of all these practices: psychoanalysis.

For this reason, our work has the dual objective of clarifying a new kind of symptomatic structure, the "anorexic symptom", by highlighting its difference with respect to the classic form of the neurotic symptom, and of rethinking the psychoanalytic clinic of anorexia nervosa in the light of the specificity of its functioning. This leads us to seriously consider the criticisms voiced in the 1960s by Bruch and Selvini Palazzoli of the classical analytic treatment of anorexia nervosa, conceived and practiced as a semantic interpretation of the unconscious psychosexual fantasy world. In our perspective, following Lacan, this leads us to orient the analytical approach toward the real beyond meaning, which is at the heart of anorexic jouissance. In relation to this jouissance, it seems to us more effective to use speech in its characteristic of act rather than of semantic interpretation.

The cardinal theses

Our research is structured around a few cardinal theses on anorexia nervosa, which organize and guide development and which we have tried to articulate theoretically and clinically.

First of all, from the perspective we have chosen, anorexia is not a disorder or a syndromic constellation of disorders but, on the contrary, it reveals itself, above all, as a "solution". This is the first key thesis that we would like to put forward, the one that draws a line of demarcation between the analytical approach and the cognitive-behavioral perspective. This is, of course, a pathological solution. But clinical experience shows us, on a regular basis, the specific "treatment" effect that the onset and development of anorexia have on subjects affected by this form of psychic disorder which involves the body so radically. Indeed, and this is our second thesis, the anorexic solution provides the subject with an unconscious response to something unbearable that they have experienced in their relationship to the Other.

The third thesis, which is the real thread running through all our work, asserts that at the heart of the anorexic response we find denial. Thus, our objective will be to demonstrate that there is a centrality of refusal in the clinic of anorexia nervosa.

This formula must be completed by this specification, which the psycho-analytical clinic of anorexia makes it possible to approach and which structures a fourth thesis: anorexia, and in particular the anorexic refusal, represents for us its cardinal core and function as a response of the subject, in its relation to the Other, to something unbearable which is played out at the level of desire and enjoyment. This thesis means that, in accordance with Lacan's perspective and that of the Lacanian orientation, the essential condition for being able to shed light on the clinical status of anorexic refusal consists in updating the structural relationships between refusal, desire and enjoyment of the subject.

It is clear, in this perspective, that the status of refusal undergoes a trans-formation and a displacement with respect to the currently dominant position in the field of psychopathology: it passes from the status of a (more or less) altered behavior – according to the orientation of the *DSM-IV* and *DSM-5* and of cognitive-behavioral therapies – to the status of a response that is rooted in the singular structure of the subject. In this sense, the analytical orientation also moves away from the orientation of classical systemic-relational psycho-therapy, which is highly developed and used in this clinical field. For psycho-analysis, and this is the fifth thesis, a singular solution comes into play in the production of anorexia. In this solution, the unconscious choice of the subject occupies an essential place, which is not entirely reducible to the demands for stability of the family system.

The deepening of the question of refusal in anorexia nervosa has led us to develop some later theses, which distinguish the Lacanian analytical approach, not only from cognitive-behavioral and systemic-relational psychotherapies, but also from the currently dominant perspectives in the field of post-Freudian psychoanalysis.

First of all, we must distinguish the real depth of the anorexic refusal from the secondary negativism, acted out by the patients once the symptom has been triggered, without reducing the first to the second. This is a fundamental thesis: the refusal, which is at the heart of anorexia nervosa, cannot be reduced to a secondary negativism of the anorexic response. This is a crucial point, since it reverses the perspective developed by Bruch, according to which anorexic refusal is a secondary effect of a fundamental deficit of the ego. As we will try to demonstrate in this work, and in particular in the second chapter, the perspective that we advance, from Lacan, around the theme of refusal in anorexia, subverts the perspective of Bruch. Indeed, Lacan's perspective places at the heart of anorexia a more radical refusal in which there are grafted, in equal measure, the phenomenology of anorexic negativism and the complacent and conformist adhesiveness that we find in the history of the subject, especially before the onset of anorexia nervosa. Anorexic negativism and complacent and conformist clinginess to the demand of the Other are only two sides of the same coin; we also find them in the phenomenology and in the historico-clinical anamnesis of each of our patients, although always in a singular version.

Our idea of the cure for anorexia nervosa, and this is our seventh thesis, in line with an analytical orientation, does not correspond to the idea of a normalizing and adaptive orthopedics of anorexic negativism. This normalizing therapeutic perspective enters into collusion, at the moment of its realization, with the other phenomenological side of the anorexic symptom, that of the superego ideal of the conformity of a false Self where the subject is suppressed by the obligation to respond in an adhesive way. at the request of the Other, whether parent or caregiver. This work is presented as a psychoanalytical study of the clinical foundations of anorexic refusal which first highlights, beyond the negativism of the response, the different modes of functioning brought into play by the subject from one case to another. This allows us to advance our eighth thesis, articulated extensively in chapter 6, according to which it is possible to determine four functions of refusal in anorexia nervosa. These bring into play different levels of its functioning and can guide us in relation to diagnosis and treatment: refusal as a metaphor for a request (predominant in hysterical and neurotic forms of anorexia); refusal as a defense of the drive; refusal as a mode of separation from the Other; and finally refusal as a mode of enjoyment.

The fact of taking into account these different modalities of refusal, to be identified in the relationship of the subject to the Other and to jouissance, allows us to articulate a differential clinic of anorexia which is analytically grounded, as we will be able to verify using different clinical cases.

In reversing Bruch's perspective, it seemed essential to us to highlight a structural dimension of refusal in anorexia nervosa, on which the secondary negativism of the anorexic response is based. This is our ninth thesis, which tries to translate and argue the formula used by Miller, according to which "what is in the foreground in anorexia is the 'refusal of the Other'".

This thesis could be expressed as follows: there is not, underlying anorexia nervosa, a deficit of the Ego but rather a fundamental refusal of the Other.

How should we understand this constitutive dimension of the refusal of the Other in anorexia nervosa? Our thesis is that the structure of this primary refusal, which is at the heart of anorexia nervosa, must be identified in the two grammatical levels of the expression "refusal of the Other". First, in the subjective sense of the genitive, it is a refusal on the part of the Other, which comes from the Other. It is in the symbolic structure of the Other that one can identify a point of unconscious blindness, a fundamental confusion, as Lacan says in "The direction of the treatment and the principles of its power", which does not allow parents to recognize, despite all the love they generally pour out on their daughter, the singular space of her emerging subjectivity. There is something "too full" in this parental Other, something that misses the lack, that does not allow the release of an empty space that the subject can occupy without being filled by their excessive investment on the narcissistic level. In this sense, the refusal of the Other is the unconscious refusal of the singularity of the subject as an other, different and irreducible to the frameworks of the predominant narcissism, internal to the unconscious parental investment in their daughter. And it is also, if you will, the rejection of messages from the anorexic subject within the family system, which Selvini Palazzoli acutely highlighted, in the systemic phase of his research. In our opinion, it is on this basis that one can frame both the maternal difficulty of positioning in the primary feedback relationships with their daughter, and her incongruous responses which, according to Bruch, subsequently produce the main altered-perception symptoms of anorexia nervosa.

Second, in the objective sense of the genitive, it is the anorexic subject who refuses the Other, who puts a wall and a fundamental "no" between himself and the Other. This "no" is not generally, in anorexia nervosa, that of hysterical anorexia where the refusal has, in reality, the essential function of a request based on an original "yes", produced by its meeting with the desire of the Other. This refusal is primary and occurs, in the subject, in the first phase of their encounter with the Other, in the interaction with the mother, where the future anorexic does not find in the maternal position the space of a lack to find a place without having to fill it and be absorbed by it. To find a place in this overfilled Other, the future anorexic is called upon to die as a singular subject, to become uniform with the Other and become its appendage. The anorexic solution that the subject finds will be that of adhering to the aberrant law of his family Other, opposing to it, at the same time, a fundamental refusal which will find, in the symptom and in the treatment of the body that characterizes it, its manifestation bursting at puberty.

The clinic of anorexia nervosa presents itself, therefore, in the Lacanian perspective, as a clinic of refusal and, more radically, of the refusal of the Other. One could say, following Lacan in the Note on the Child of 1969, that the somatic symptom of anorexia embodies, starting from the anorexia of the child, "a primordial refusal" (Lacan, 2001a, p. 374).

But, at the same time, the clinic of anorexia nervosa presents itself as a clinic of the object nothing. This is the central thesis that Lacan elaborates on anorexia nervosa, starting from the references of the 1950s to the Seminar, Book IV and to "La direction de la cure". This is the tenth thesis that we will try to articulate: the Lacanian clinic of anorexia nervosa is a clinic of the object nothing. Indeed, Lacan introduced and clarified the special function of the object in the clinic of anorexia. In our book, we have tried to shed epistemological light on the concept of object nothing in Lacan, by highlighting the double status which makes it, on the one hand, a symbolic object, a key signifier which supports the metonymic structure of desire, and on the other, a real object, the embodiment of a full enjoyment, without loss, around which the life of the anorexic subject revolves.

Put in relation to the refusal of the Other, the object nothing as an object of full jouissance, intact in relation to the lethal action of the signifier, presents itself in anorexia nervosa as its structural complement: the anorexic refuses the Other so as not to give in to the limitless jouissance that the object nothing, encysted in his body, allows him. The clarification of this point allowed us to emphasize the logical welding of the two pillars governing the Lacanian reading of anorexia nervosa: the refusal and the object nothing.

Without canceling the duplicity of its status which turns out to be very useful, above all to illuminate important aspects of the clinic of hysterical and more generally neurotic anorexia, we have highlighted, at the same time, the dimension of the nothing as an object of real enjoyment in anorexia. This vision of nothing tends to impose itself in the teaching of Lacan, from the 1960s, to leave in the shadows the definition of nothing as a signifying key. In chapter 7, we set out to probe the function of the object nothing in the clinic of anorexia nervosa by developing this trajectory in relation, also, to the question of infantile anorexia (chapter 8) and anorexia in young girls (chapter 9).

The research method

The method we have used in our work, in accordance with knowledge and analytical work, cannot be separated, abstractly and previously, from the object of its research. On the contrary, it implies, beyond any technicist and formalist perspective, that it is always necessary to start from a determinate signifying material, and that the work of reading, while respecting the scientific rigor of punctual reference and logical coherence, is already oriented by a direction to which the researcher themselves refers.

In this sense, our work is located above all within the Lacanian orientation which is based on the reading of the text of Lacan elaborated by Miller. Starting from this inscription means above all constructing, from the text of Lacan and his followers, the field of the Lacanian problems relating to anorexia nervosa. This includes work on the text of Lacan and analysts of Lacanian orientation, both theoretically and on the basis of published clinical cases. The comparison of the Lacanian orientation with the other current positions of the field of psychoanalysis constitutes an important node of the research aimed at clarifying the paradigmatic differences between the various approaches and their clinical consequences.

At the same time, to support our argument, after several years of intense clinical activity in this field, we refer extensively, throughout the development of the research, to our clinical experience concerning anorexic subjects treated in institutions or in analysis. In an open dialectic, the theoretical theses developed during this research journey include both the lines of orientation resulting from the reading of the clinical cases and the result of this reading, corroborated, however, by the necessary rectifications. Therapeutic devices and the problematic conditions of the treatment of anorexia nervosa are widely represented in this work: from individual analysis to the small monosymptomatic group conducted analytically, to teamwork in a therapeutic community, to the problems inherent in the intervention in hospital, very often essential within the framework of a general treatment of an anorexic subject. The conditions for the effectiveness of hospitalization which takes these patients to clinical nutrition services (because of the aggravation of the eating symptom) or psychiatry (frequently at issue, because of psychotic decompensation, triggering, radical refusal of food or medicine) will in turn be probed on the basis of the singularity of the cases, as a contribution to advancing the theoretical-clinical elaboration.

Although we have indicated, in the last chapter, lines of orientation in the cure of anorexia, in reality, in accordance with the non-formalistic outline of the work, we have avoided dividing the research according to a clear distinction between theory and treatment. For this reason, contrary to the formalist position identifiable in the majority of psychopathology textbooks, references to cases and treatments are used widely and directly for the construction and demonstration of clinical theses, just as in references to the texts of psychoanalytic theory on anorexia.

Articulation

This work consists of ten chapters each addressing the general problem of the refoundation of the psychoanalytic clinic of anorexia nervosa in the light of a specific question.

The first chapter raises the question of the reduction of the status of anorexia to a disorder or, more precisely, to a syndromic constellation of behavioral and cognitive disorders, which is the basis of the psychiatric descriptive and diagnostic classification system of the last three editions of the *DSM*. This reduction is also the logical-operational presupposition on which cognitive-behavioral therapies and their way of theorizing and treating eating disorders are based. On the other hand, from the perspective of psychoanalysis, anorexia is presented rather as a solution found by the subject, especially during adolescence, to deal with an impasse encountered in the relationship to the Other and to jouissance, in this delicate moment of existence which begins at puberty. The notion of "anorexic solution" is developed and put in relation with the psychoanalytical concept of symptom, while highlighting the difficulty of this comparison and the requirement to elaborate, with regard to anorexia, a non-classic notion of the symptom, different from the analytical paradigm of the hysterico-neurotic symptom. This non-classical notion of symptom is more easily identifiable in Lacan's last teaching, in particular in the light of his elaboration of the sinthome and his conception of the "real unconscious", highlighted by Miller through the reading of the last writings and Seminars of Lacan. The accent is no longer placed, in fact, on the symbolic dimension of the symptom as a metaphor for the subject, but rather on its status as a condenser of jouissance outside meaning, in line with the difficulties that the clinic of anorexia nervosa presents from the start of the treatment: absence of subjectivation of his own pathological condition, non-enigmatic character for the subject of the anorexic condition, consequent tendency to avoid treatment, not to formulate a demand and not to develop any transfer other than one distinctly imaginary-specular in nature.

It is in this frame of reference that we take up and critically rearticulate the inclusion of anorexia, alongside drug addiction, in the paradigm of "new forms of the symptom"; and we do this while taking special care not to reduce the question to the historical-diachronic terms of the social symptom alone.

In the second chapter, we pose the historical and theoretical premises for a refoundation of the current psychoanalytical clinic of anorexia, starting from a careful reading of the criticisms made, in the 1960s, of the classic analytical treatment of anorexia by the "founding mothers" of the contemporary dynamic psychotherapy of anorexia nervosa: the psychiatrists and psychoanalysts Bruch and Selvini Palazzoli. From the observation of the inefficacy of semantic interpretation, placed at the center of the treatment of anorexia by psychoanalysis at least until the 1960s, the authors manage to deconstruct in an autonomous way the framework for reading the dominant anorexic problem in that era. This framework appeared to be anchored in a codified sclerosis of the revolutionary discoveries of Freud and Abraham around the centrality of early oral drive fixation in the clinic of anorexia and, more generally, in eating psychopathologies. Indeed, within the framework of a systematization of the theory of the stages of the development of the libido, operated by the post-Freudian orthodoxy and identifiable in the Treatise of Fenichel, this approach gave life, in the work of the analysts, to a standardized practice of interpretation, centered around the foundation of a psychosexual fantasy universe, of oral matrix, to be unveiled. The anorexic patient is deaf, as Bruch and Selvini had indicated on several occasions, to this interpretation which produces no therapeutic effect in the treatment.

In this chapter, we first highlight the point of intersection between the structuralist orientation of Lacan in the 1950s and the approach of the two great specialists in anorexia, around a systemic-structural epistemological position in the clinic, influenced by linguistics and cybernetics and in opposition to the biological orientation, predominant in post-Freudian psychoanalysis. Indeed, it is around the primacy of language, the symbolic and systemic-communicative-relational transactions, that a new reading of the clinic and more specifically of the clinic of anorexia nervosa is produced.

Internal variants of this new cybernetic approach, with which Lacan comes into contact explicitly in his first Seminars and in his writings of the 1950s, through the mediation of the structuralism of Saussure and Lévi-Strauss, animate the refoundation of the clinic of the anorexia nervosa of the two "founding mothers" of contemporary psychotherapy. Lacan's theses of the 1950s on the primacy of the symbolic, which aim to de-biologize psychoanalysis and the function of the Freudian unconscious, are reflected in his reading of anorexia nervosa of this period. In this reading, in fact, anorexia is placed in a clinical position, paradigmatic of the radical irreducibility of desire to the field of need and of the irreducibility of the register of the symbolic both to the imaginary and to the field of reality.

At the same time, it is appropriate to highlight the impossibility of reducing Lacan's position on anorexia to a symbolic-structural paradigm, in particular when he introduces, within the framework of his teaching, the centrality of the drive in its symbolic status and especially in its real core, as we will see in chapter 4.

In the third chapter, we review two orientations of the psychodynamic-psychoanalytical current, which we currently consider more interesting, alongside the Lacanian orientation, for the reading and treatment of anorexia and bulimia. The first, older, orientation, beginning in the 1960s, is represented by French psychodynamic child psychiatry (of which Evelyne and Jean Kestemberg, Bernard Brusset, Philippe Jeammet and Maurice Corcos are, in chronological succession, the main representatives).

The second, of more recent formation, is represented by the working group, of Kleinian-Bionian influence, coordinated at the Tavistock Clinic in London, from the second half of the 1980s, by Gianna Polacco Williams. These two orientations, located in the same furrow of the post-Freudian orientation of the psychoanalysis of object relations and sharing the common reference to the Kleinian approach, are however differentiated by the importance attributed to the Kleinian matrix. The French niche, which also presents considerable internal differences, among which a stronger rooting in Freud's theses in Brusset, dialectizes the Kleinian matrix with the instances of Ego-Psychology and the psychology of the Self of the Kohut matrix. Starting from these presuppositions, he particularly accentuates the centrality of the narcissistic dimension and of the additive-dependent circuit, by a special highlighting of the thesis of anorexia as the result of the impasse of the process of adolescence.

From a different perspective, internal to the tradition of Anglo-Saxon psychoanalysis but sensitive to the lesson of Lacan, the Tavistockian approach of Polacco Williams accentuates the Kleinian-Bionian side of his reading of anorexia. At the base of the process of constitution of anorexia, one identifies a particular failure, defined as "inversion of the relations between the container and the contained"; it is about the failure of the function of container to "think the thoughts" and of the work of reverie, specific to the mother.

In this process, the mother not only fails to improve the child's anxiety through its symbolic metabolization and its restitution in an "edible" form, but she also projects her own anxiety onto her child who becomes its receptacle and who thus develops the anorexic symptom as a way of defense allowing him to support this condition (Williams, 1997, pp. 927–941).

The fourth chapter is devoted to a reconstruction of Jacques Lacan's thought on anorexia nervosa. He presents four paradigms, identifiable in four historically different phases of his psychoanalytic teaching and research.

In The Family Complexes of 1938, he offers his first significant contribution to the reading of anorexia nervosa. According to a conceptuality influenced by Melanie Klein, the young Lacan develops, from a psychogenetic perspective, his theory of anorexia nervosa rooted in the "refusal of weaning" of early childhood which is regressively reactivated in the passage to adolescence. It is from here that the crucial knot, the common thread of the Lacanian reading of anorexia, will begin to take shape. In this sense, the antiseparative variation of anorexic refusal, which aims to preserve a condition of mythical fusion with the primary maternal object, seems obvious to us. It is in this perspective that, in this text, Lacan brings anorexia closer to drug addiction and gastric neuroses, developing the thesis of an "appetite for death" in anorexia.

In the texts of the second half of the 1950s, at the height of the culminating phase of Lacan's structuralism, when the dialogue with structural linguistics and the thesis of the primacy of the symbolic reached their peak, Lacan developed a hysterical-dialectical paradigm of anorexia. In the text of 1958, "The direction of the treatment and the principles of its power"; as well as in the Seminars, *La relation d'objet* and *Les formations de l'inconscient*, the anorexic question is taken up by Lacan starting from a new perspective: that of the de-biologization of psychoanalysis, which shows the irreducibility of desire to the field of need and the autonomy of the symbolic in relation to the register of the imaginary and to the level of reality. In this context, anorexia nervosa becomes the radical clinical incarnation of this irreducibility, anorexic refusal becomes a metaphor for desire and the demand for love, the anorexic position is valued in its declination closest to hysteria. Here the anorexic refusal, rather than with the characteristics of the refusal of weaning, indicated in the 1938 text, presents itself under the features of the hysterical refusal which is a dialectical refusal. In this conceptual framework, for the first time we see the emergence of the centrality of the object nothing, attributed by Lacan to anorexia nervosa. However, it is important to emphasize that the nothing that takes shape in Lacan in the 1950s is a purely symbolic object, a pure object of desire, signifying the structural inability of each object in the world to occupy the place of the object proper to desire. In this period, the nothing of anorexia nervosa is forged from its reference to nothing as the object of hysteria. In other words, it is the hysterical anorexic who dominates the framework of the Lacanian theory on anorexia of the 1950s.

A real epistemological break is present, in our opinion, in the Seminars, *Anxiety* (1962–1963) and *The four fundamental concepts of psychoanalysis* (1964). Lacan here takes up the theme of anorexia nervosa and includes it in his refoundation of psychoanalytic theory around the new centrality given to the register of the real, which had remained in the shadows throughout the elaboration of the 1950s. It will include, for Lacan, the reformulation of the very concept of the unconscious as not entirely reducible to the signifying structure and the resumption of the drive theory, reinvented on the basis of the conceptualization of the object (a), placed at the very center of the new notion of drive and drive unconscious. In this new framework, Lacan's thesis "the anorexic child eats nothing" emphasizes the no longer symbolic but real dimension of the object nothing which embodies, in an extreme way, an irreducibility of jouissance to submitting to the law of the symbolic Other. By recalling, in a way, the thesis of the 1938 text, anorexia nervosa embodies here a position where the subject does not want to yield to the Other the object of their own enjoyment and prefers to put their life in danger rather than to accept the symbolic law of castration. In the Seminar, Book XI, this (a)dialectic and out-of-discourse jouissance is matched, in anorexia nervosa, by the threat of disappearance as a typical modality of the anorexic of opening up a lack that provokes anxiety in the parental Other.

Finally, in the Unpublished Seminar "Les non dupes errent" of 1973–1974, we find a formalization of the anorexic position which accentuates, in an even more radical way, the character of enjoyment of the anorexic symptom and which highlights its radical refusal of unconscious knowledge. It is the horror of unconscious knowledge that pushes young anorexic girls to constantly ruminate on weight, body and calories. In this Seminar, Lacan indicates in anorexia, in the most radical way, a movement completely opposed to that which tends to open up a lack in the Other, a maneuver of avoidance and denial of castration which marks it, if you will, as the constitutive trait of perversion. This is, in our opinion, the formulation of Lacan closest to the thesis formulated by Miller, of a refusal of the Other in anorexia nervosa.

In the fifth chapter, we have tried to illustrate the main developments of the Lacanian orientation on the subject of anorexia, after the death of Lacan. We have favored the work of Lacanian psychoanalysts who, in addition to their significant contributions on the subject, have combined theoretical contributions with constant clinical practice with anorexic patients, both in their offices and in therapeutic institutions; And this, in the light of the methodological reasons that are the basis of our work, according to which only the experience of the clinical practice of anorexia can make it possible to clarify Lacan's references, enlightening but fragmentary in this regard. All this is combined with the study of the literature concerning the anorexic problem and with a thorough knowledge of Lacanian teaching.

From these presuppositions, we can consider Augustin Ménard as the true initiator of a unitary reading of anorexia nervosa, based on the benchmarks given by Lacan. Supported by his practice as a psychiatrist in a hospital with anorexic patients and as an analyst in his office, he had the merit of articulating for the first time Lacan's references to anorexia nervosa in a unitary reading. He was, at the same time, the first forcefully to emphasize the need to go beyond a reading, widespread in the Lacanian field, which tended to reduce anorexia to the framework of the hysterical structure. He thus put forward the idea of a differential clinic of anorexia which highlights the presence of anorexic frameworks of a psychotic structure, to be carefully distinguished, in the treatment, from the frameworks of hysterical-neurotic anorexia. The most original point of his reading concerns the thesis of anorexia as an elision of the logical time of castration, at the crucial moment when, in puberty, the question of object loss is reactivated as a condition of access to the path of desire. Through the reading of Lacan, Ménard emphasizes that the future anorexic subject responds, in this situation, by rejecting castration and choosing the path of privation by developing the symptom.

From the 1990s, in Italy and Argentina, two clinical research experiments developed in parallel with a Lacanian orientation on anorexia and bulimia. The Italian experience occurred within a mono-symptomatic therapeutic institution, the ABA, dedicated to the treatment of eating disorders. Many Lacanian analysts of the AMP have worked in this institution, and it is to the research work of Massimo Recalcati, the first scientific director of the ABA, that we owe the most interesting theoretical-clinical contribution. Recalcati has contributed, in a specific way, to highlighting a "fruitful antinomy" in Lacan's teaching on anorexia nervosa. This antinomy was represented by the double status of refusal (of which he distinguishes a dialectical side and a second autistic side), of nothing as a lack (in the hysterical-neurotic forms) and as an emptiness (in the psychotic forms). Among the authors of Lacanian orientation, Recalcati is the one who has most valued Brusset's thesis on anorexia-bulimia as a unitary circuit of functioning oriented by the same logic. His work would gradually take the direction of a theoretical and clinical research of new forms of the symptom where anorexia and bulimia find their place; it would also accentuate the social side of psychoanalysis in its applied version, both in terms of therapy and in terms of the reading of social phenomena.

The contribution on anorexia and bulimia, proposed by Nieves Soria and her colleagues (in particular Fabian Schejtman and Alejandra Eidelberg) from the Department of the Clinical Institute of Buenos Aires, aims at a re-reading of the anorexic question in the light of the latest teaching of Lacan. Soria especially highlights, in anorexia nervosa, the issues relating to the female question, the failure of the equation body = phallus and the refusal of the semblance (semblant), thus managing to deconstruct, very effectively, the identification of anorexia and hysteria in vogue in the Lacanian world, at least until the early 1990s. In our opinion, it is to the latter that we owe the most original reading of the altered-perception of body image and the complex relationship with the mirror in anorexia. This relationship was understood as the return to the real of the gaze as drive object, without mediation by the signifier.

For a few years, a contribution which introduces, on several levels, a change of perspective on anorexia has been proposed by Carole Dewambrechies-La Sagna. In the light of her experience as a psychoanalyst and psychiatrist in an institution with anorexic patients, she brought, first of all, a broad clarification of the function of anxiety in the clinic of anorexia nervosa, a clarification which proved to be valuable for the logic of the treatment. A decisive passage in the treatment of anorexia occurs, in fact, when the anorexic subject finds a relationship to anxiety which is no longer reduced only to arousing anxiety by their symptom in the person who takes care of them. The indications relating to the impracticability of a talking cure, when anorexia is radicalized in the loss of weight, and to the absolute necessity of hospitalization, are also essential and in conformity with the indications of the psychiatric tradition. This is a way to set a limit to the anorexic limitless.

Dewambrechies also proposes an autonomous framework for mental or "true" anorexia, which cannot be reduced, in her opinion, to the framework of Freudian clinical structures and which must be limited to the field of anorexia in young girls.

The sixth chapter is devoted to an exposition on the theme of anorexic refusal and its fundamental functions in the clinic, identified in this work.

The four functions of refusal are formulated in the light of clinical situations: as demand, as defense, as modality of separation and as enjoyment (jouissance).

The refusal as a request belongs specifically to the framework of hysterical-neurotic anorexia and is characterized by the symbolic status of the refusal as a metaphor for the request for love, that is to say by its character as an unconscious message addressed to the Other to ask them for the sign of their love.

The refusal in its function of defense of the real is always present in anorexia but takes different forms in the neuroses (where the subject defends themself fundamentally from their own drive) and in the psychoses (where the anorexic refusal becomes a barrier against the invasive enjoyment of the Other).

Refusal as an attempt to separate from the Other constitutes the imaginary modality through which subjects with anorexia try to constitute themselves as autonomous subjects and distance themselves from others. This attempt reveals all its limits in the subject's difficulty in accessing the symbolic dimension of castration as a path allowing separation, starting from the assumption of its own structural dependence vis-à-vis the Other.

Finally, refusal as jouissance constitutes the erogenous-drive dimension at the bottom of anorexic refusal, the libidinal root of egosyntonia symptomatic of anorexia nervosa and of the typical phenomena that characterize it: from euphoria to hyper activism, passing through the autonomic-hypertrophic ideal.

The seventh chapter concerns the object nothing in the clinic of anorexia nervosa and represents an attempt to shed light on this enigmatic notion that Lacan poses at the very heart of his reading of anorexia. Beyond the attempt to clarify epistemologically the Lacanian notion of the object nothing, by iden-tifying its specificity within the Lacanian doctrine of drive objects, we have attempted to clarify its dual status as it appears in Lacan's text (as correlated, on the one hand, to the dialectic of desire and to the field of the Other and, on the other hand, as an object of limitless enjoyment, disconnected from the dialectic with the Other).

In the light of these considerations and from clinical cases treated in practice or in institutions, we try, in this chapter, to highlight some structural modalities of the emergence of nothing in the differential clinic of anorexia.

The eighth chapter concerns the question of child anorexia and all that it can teach us about the status of the object and of anorexic jouissance.

Indeed, while there is no doubt that the framework of anorexia nervosa presents irreducible differences compared to child anorexia, it is, however, important for us, as François Ansermet has rightly underlined, to make a detour via early anorexia (Ansermet, 1999, pp. 161–164), thus following the same theoretical path followed by Lacan in the Seminar, Book XI, where he asserts that the anorexic child eats nothing.

After reviewing the current descriptive frameworks of child psychiatry clas-sification systems for anorexia (DSM-IV-TR and DSM-5-TR, CD: 0-3-R, PDM and PDM-2), we develop the analytical approach of the child anorexia of Bernard Brusset in order to succeed in isolating the more recent Lacanian contributions on this subject: those of Ansermet and Manuel Férnandez Blanco.

In the light of their experience in hospitals, in the neonatology and pedi-atric departments, Férnandez Blanco, as a clinical psychologist in La Coruña, and François Ansermet, as a child psychiatrist in Lausanne and Geneva, were able to offer us interesting contributions, in an area of the clinic where Lacanian literature is scarce.

Emphasis is placed in particular on two irreducible forms of child ano-rexia, already distinct phenomenologically and described by the child psy-chiatric tradition, and which make it possible to verify, from a Lacanian perspective, the irreducible functioning of the object nothing and of refusal in early passive anorexia (close to the autism spectrum) and in child "opposi-tional" anorexia.

Based on their considerations, the hypothesis put forward in the context of this research is that, in oppositional anorexia, corresponding strictly to the nosographic framework of child anorexia, four functions of refusal are at work, whereas in the early passive anorexia of the infant, the subject is one with the object nothing and the refusal functions only in the fundamental modality of pure jouissance without the Other.

The ninth chapter concerns adolescent anorexia nervosa. In this chapter we develop the thesis of adolescent anorexia nervosa as a failure (and attempt at repair) of the process of symptomatization of puberty – with reference to the definition of adolescence provided by Alexandre Stevens. According to Freud's psychoanalysis, reread by Lacan, this process would represent the fundamental task of adolescence: the production, from the effects of the transition to puberty, of a singular solution of the subject's relationship to the Other and to their enjoyment.

Through a rereading, based on Lacan's indications, of the status of contemporary adolescence, we first try to understand the reasons for the spread of the anorexic symptom in contemporary society and to articulate a hypothesis on the reason for its preponderant distribution among young girls. Lacan's landmarks, notably in his "Preface" to Wedekind's *Spring Awakening* (Lacan, 2001b, pp. 561–563), allow us to lay the foundations for a differential clinic of the symptom in adolescence and, especially for our purposes, a differential clinic of the anorexia nervosa in adolescence.

Our hypothesis, already articulated elsewhere (Cosenza, 2009, pp. 46–50), aims to show that in the text of the "Preface" it is possible to find two logical phases of the process of the sexual initiation of the adolescent, essential to situate the position of the subject. The first logical time (T1), which we wanted to define as the time of the veil, is relative to the subject's entry into adolescence and presupposes the construction of an unconscious fantasizing around the sexual relationship which includes the young person and of which he has evidence, on waking, in his dreams concerning sex. The second logical time (T2) that we have defined as the time of the trauma constitutes, for Lacan, a real principle of initiation and is represented by the discovery, on the part of the young person, of the fact that "the sexual relationship does not exist" and that, behind the veil covering the mystery of sex, there is nothing.

In the light of these cardinal points, we have distinguished the anorexias in adolescence which respond to a difficulty of subjectivation of the T2 of the trauma but testify to an accomplished crossing of the T1 of the veil, from anorexias in which, in the encounter with the drive, the T1 of the process of fantasy construction has not yet structured itself effectively and has left the subject without a veil and without the fantasmatic framework around sex which is capable of orienting its functioning. Hysterical-neurotic anorexias in adolescence begin as a response to the impasse of T2, as a difficulty in fully accepting the effects of symbolic castration. The forms of anorexia nervosa beyond neurosis are characterized, on the other hand, by the passage inactive or deficient in T1, although the true beginnings are often identifiable in a situation which exposes the subject to the trauma of castration (T2).

These coordinates also allow us to answer the question: why currently is it mainly young girls who develop this symptom? Also in the "Preface", Lacan recommended that the loss of the veil around the mystery of sex, typical of contemporary society, would not take long to show its effects.

Our hypothesis here determines that these effects occur with more frequency for young girls, because the veil is in a more structural relationship with the feminine position which allows the girl, through the masquerade, to enter into the dialectic of love life. Unlike hysterical anorexia, for which the function of the veil is operative in the form of an extreme phallicization of thinness, in anorexia nervosa we witness a failure of the equation body = phallus and a rupture, even a real absence, of marriage with the veil. Furthermore, our subsequent hypothesis, in the light of Lacan's elaboration in the Seminar *Encore* on the female jouissance, is that the anorexic response, where in the girl the equation body = phallus is not effectively established, implements, on the side of jouissance, a perversion of the feminine not-all (*pas-tout*) which takes the path of the "limitless" typical of the anorexic symptom.

To conclude, the last chapter traces the lines of orientation for the treatment of anorexia nervosa, drawn from clinical experience in institutions and in the office with anorexic patients, as well as the indications of the critical study of analytical orientation by authors, especially Lacanian, who devoted themselves to it with more interest.

References

Ansermet, F. (1999), *Clinique de l'origine. L'enfant entre medicine et psychanalyse*. Paris: Payot.

Cosenza, D. (2009), L'initiation à l'adolescence: entre mythe et structure. *Mental. Revue Internationale de Pssychanalyse*, no. 23, pp. 46–50.

Lacan, J. (2001a), Note sur l'enfant (1969). *Autres écrits*. Paris: Éditions du Seuil, pp. 373–374; "Initiation in adolescence: between myth and structure", Lacunae. Journal for Lcanian Psychoanalysis, Vol. 4 (Issue 1), 2014, pp. 24–30.

Lacan, J. (2001b), Préface à L'éveil du Printemps (1974). *Autres écrits*, pp. 561–563.

La Sagna, P. (2009), L'adolescence prolongée, hier, aujourd'hui et demain. *Mental. Revue Internationale de Psychanalyse*, no. 23, pp. 17–28.

Malaguarnera, S. (2010), *L'anorexique face au miroir. Le déclin de la fonction paternelle*. Paris: L'Harmattan.

Williams, G. (1997), Reflections on some dynamics of eating disorders: "no entry" defenses and foreign bodies. *International Journal of Psycho-Analysis*, vol. 78, no. 5, pp. 927–941.

Chapter 1

The anorexic solution

From trouble to symptom

The contemporary psychopathological clinic is traversed by a constitutive gap between two main guidelines, which goes back to its historical origin, and which is also clearly expressed in the field of anorexia nervosa. Today, the first of these lines finds its most systematic expression on the nosographic level in the descriptive-classifying approach of the DSM-IV and DSM-5 (APA, 2022, pp. 371–397) and on the therapeutic level in the cognitive-behavioral approaches. Such a neo-Kraepelinian perspective, precisely defined by different authors, finds in the bio-medical approach to psychic suffering, to which Kraepelin gave the most consistent clinical systematization in the history of psychiatry, the key to accessing the etiology and therapy. These are the general guidelines that mark such an approach: to bring psychopathology and psychiatry back to medicine and its biological foundations, to place at the center of psychiatric work the universality of mental illness disembodied from the singularity of the subject who suffers from it, and to construct the treatment through standardized procedures of the pharmacological type and restitutive-rehabilitation, the objective of which is to bring the disorder in question back to "cognitive-behavioral normality". At the same time, this is particularly close to the requirements of quantitative evaluation and social control that characterize the power mechanisms of advanced societies (Laurent, 2005; Guéguen, 2005, pp. 15–17; Brousse, 2006, pp. 21–25; Cliniques Mediterraneénnes, 2005). This is the dominant perspective today, both at the theoretical level – the one that is most taught in the most important developed capitalistic countries' universities – and at the therapeutic level – the one that is most used in treatment institutions – in the field of eating disorders.

The other psychopathological guideline, irreducible to the bio-medical approach, is constituted by psychoanalysis, and by the operation that Freud laid at the foundation of the psychoanalytical clinic: the subject of the unconscious and its singularity as a structuring factor of the human being's relationship with what he suffers from. In cognitive-behavioral approaches, the subject has no place in the treatment, which in the end results in a

DOI: 10.4324/9781003318439-2

restitutive rehabilitation of the patient's sick behavior in relation to reality and statistically assessed normality. In fact, the notion of "disorder" and the therapy prescribed in accordance with normalizing such an alteration in behavior can only be constructed on the condition of eliding the subject bearing such suffering. On the contrary, a psychopathology oriented by the teaching of Freud cannot fail to bring back psychic suffering or excess behaviors to the relationship of the subject who adopted them and to their history. For this reason, from the perspective of psychoanalysis, cognitive-behavioral therapies are blind because they focus on the effects (behavioral disorders and cognitive errors), without relating them to the cause immanent to their production, the only operation that makes it possible, in the first place, to read it.

The Freudian operation is therefore the opposite of the Kraepelinian one: while for the latter the subject is detached from the disease of which they are the carrier and in one way or another relieved of responsibility in relation to the problem of its cause, Freud puts the subject at the heart of the "disease" of which they are the bearer by making it their enigma, by making them responsible in their words for what caused it. The notion of symptom taken from the medical lexicon by Freud, but reinvented in the light of psychoanalysis, expresses this operation of involving the subject in the malaise from which they suffer and whose cause is enigmatic to them. In this sense, the Freudian notion of symptom becomes the alternative, in the psychopathological field, to the notion of disorder.

Anorexia as a symptom

This brief preliminary section allows us to shed light on the contemporary horizon in which the clinic of anorexia nervosa is located: between a clinic of the disorder (at the different levels that make up the syndrome: the disorder in eating, in the perception of the bodily image …) and its restitutive normalization, which is that practiced by cognitive-behavioral therapies, and a clinic of the symptom as a singular construction and subjectivation on the part of the one who suffers from it, which is specific to the discourse and practice of psychoanalysis.

Choosing the path of psychoanalysis in the reading and in the treatment of anorexia means, in the first place, starting from the thesis, formulated by Augustin Ménard, that "anorexia is a symptom, not an entity" (Ménard, 1992, p. 3). This means affirming, in other words, first, that the function of the subject of the unconscious is inscribed in the anorexic condition, and that the latter depends on it as much in its own genesis as in its reading and treatment. Second, this perspective revolves around the thesis according to which it is necessary to find and highlight the "subjective position" (Ménard, 1988, p. 23) immanent to the patient's anorexia in order to be able to read and treat their disorder, from their statement of their own condition. If these two axioms are not taken firmly into account, it is the very idea of a psychic causality, as it could emerge in the discovery of the unconscious, which dissolves, leaving a field free to biological determinism and to limitless social conditioning. But the axiomatic solidity of these theses is the sedimented fruit of decades of experience of analytical treatments on anorexic subjects. These theses consist of three corollaries which flow from them and in relation to which the analytical orientations converge. First of all, the affirmation of the singularity of the anorexic symptom, in contrast with the universality of the disease: anorexia can only be understood in relation to the subject who is the bearer and to his singular history, irreducible in relation to the others. Then, the affirmation of the differential plurality of forms of the anorexic symptom. Finally, the highlighting of the enigmatic dimension of anorexia as a subjective symptom, a factor that contrasts with the spontaneous phenomenology of the anorexic condition and its tendency to deny the unconscious and subjective division.

It is no coincidence that the transition of anorexia from a disease and disorder to a symptom, in which the subject is unknowingly involved, is already a result of treatment, and rarely a starting point. Indeed, the symptomatization (Laurent, 2004, p. 58) of their condition is, in the patient's discourse, one of the first important effects of the analytic treatment in its preliminary phase.

Anorexia and the classic form of the neurotic symptom

This kind of consideration enables us to understand what the affirmation of the symptomatic status of anorexia entails as a problematic tension between the phenomenology of the anorexic disorder and the classical status of the Freudian symptom. Indeed, while the latter, for example in the form of the hysterical symptom, presents itself as a condition which divides the subject, of which the hysteric complains and in relation to which it is traversed by an enigmatic obscure point as its cause, the anorexic condition, rather, most often presents itself in the form of an egosyntonic state which does not engender either the patient's complaint or an enigmatic questioning (Kestemberg, Kestemberg, Decobert, 1981, p. 221). This is strikingly noticeable in the form of "*restricter*" anorexia where the patient, renouncing food and satisfying their appetite, experiences themselves as master of their own symptom, deceiving themselves to exercise total control over it and narcissistically enjoying such a mastery in relation to their own drive toward the object. But also in anorexic forms with "purging" vomiting as in bulimia, despite the often obvious emergence of a depressive condition of malaise which leads to the complaint, we most often find at the start of treatment a disincorporated complaint of the enigma that struggles to turn into an enigmatic demand to know about the cause of one's condition. This clinical observation has led various authors involved in the clinic of anorexia and bulimia to speak on this subject of a desubjectivized symptom, disjointed from the unconscious, without demand and disconnected from the dynamics of transference (Recalcati, 1998, p. 188). These character-istics have led, in recent decades, to a questioning of the classic relationship of continuity, going back to the theses of Charles Lasègue (who was with Gull at the origin of the discovery of the medico-psychiatric syndrome of anorexia), between anorexia and hysteria. We have also seen the development, according to the various orientations of the psychoanalytical field, of a framework for anorexia-bulimia beyond neurosis in its classic forms. In particular in the Anglo-American matrix psychoanalysis, strongly oriented in line of continuity with the tradition of "Ego-Psychology" and with the exigences of university psychiatry, the framework of eating disorders prevails with regard to so-called borderline personalities; in the tradition of French psycho-dynamic psychiatry, in addition to the borderline personality, reference is made extensively to bor-derline states and non-delusional or cold psychoses, according to the definition proposed by Evelyne Kestemberg (2001).

Anorexia and new forms of the symptom (NFS)

The Lacanian psychoanalytical perspective, which has faced the problem of the anorexia/hysteria relationship in the context of a lively and far from concluded debate, over 30 years ago introduced a new matrix of psycho-pathological research condensed in the formula "new forms of the symptom". This definition introduced by Hugo Freda and Bernard Lecœur with special reference to clinical experience in the field of drug addiction (Freda, 1989, pp. 115–120; Freda, 1992, p. 85; Freda, Lecoeur, 1997, pp. 139–148) was particularly revived in the course given by Jacques-Alain Miller with the assistance of Éric Laurent, *L'Autre qui n'existe pas et ses comités d'ethyque* (1996–1997). This course offered a reading of the contemporary Other and new forms of malaise in Civilization in the light of Lacan's last teaching. Among the new forms of the symptom, alongside drug addiction, new depressive forms and panic attacks, we also find anorexia and bulimia. The purpose of such a formulation is not so much to introduce, alongside neu-roses and psychoses, a new diagnostic-nosographic structure or category, as to highlight the transformations that the contemporary Other has produced in the formation of socially diffuse symptoms in the present day. The major drug addiction epidemics of the 1960s and 1970s, just like the widespread anorexia epidemic in the 1970s, and especially the bulimia epidemic among young people in the 1980s and 1990s, become legible in the context of these transformations of the status of the Other. It is in particular in the passage from a capitalist society of the disciplinary type – the paradigm is Victorian England in the second half of the nineteenth century – centered on the pro-hibition of enjoyment, to a postdisciplinary society like that of the advanced capitalism, based on the centrality of the consumption of the object and the right to enjoyment, as Miller (2003, p. 17) has pointed out, in which in our opinion the relationship becomes more legible between the so-called new

forms of the symptom and the classic forms of the neurotic symptom analyzed by Freud.

Indeed, while in these last forms, the subject suffers from the prohibiting
effects of a symbolic law which is inscribed at the cost of a considerable loss of
enjoyment prolonged in the life of the neurotic in the form of repetition, the
new forms of the symptom are presented as formations within which the
symbolic law is not inscribed (and we are here in the field of psychoses) or it has
taken hold in a weak way without being able to stem a push to immediate and
disordered enjoyment. This is what Lacan had argued in his 1970 text,
Radiophonie, when he spoke of an ascent of the object *a* to the social zenith
(Lacan, 2001b, p. 414), and which Miller interpreted as a positioning of *a* at
the place as an agent of ultramodern discourse (Miller, 2005, pp. 9–27).[1] This
means that within this discourse, above all, the subject is commanded to enjoy,
and that the drive to enjoy has become an imperative to enjoy which pervades
the functioning of the social bond. Lacan had already predicted, in his 1938 text
Family complexes in the formation of the individual, the decline of the paternal
imago in capitalist societies, and associated with this decline the development of
pathologies linked to a failed separation from the maternal object. These
pathologies are characterized by the search for a full and nostalgic enjoyment
which reconstitutes the primary experience of rediscovery of the maternal
imago. It is within the framework of these pathological forms that Lacan had
inscribed anorexia nervosa alongside drug addictions and gastric neuroses
(Lacan, 2001a, p. 35).

Indeed, the crisis of the paternal function in contemporary social discourse is
the reverse side, the other side of the coin, of the thrust to limitless enjoyment
that this discourse continually promulgates. And the so-called new forms of the
symptom are presented as symptomatic constructions that unite the search
for limitless jouissance, a precariousness, when it is not a real rejection of the
symbolic function in existence. In Freudian terms, this can be formulated as a
partial or total failure of the crossing of the Oedipus complex and of the
constitution of the Ego Ideal, an effect of the subjectivating separation from the
maternal Other as an omnipotent mythical object, without loss.

Indeed, if we disregard a reading of anorexia centered on its enjoyment it
involves in relation to the maternal Other, phenomenology could mislead us
radically disjoin it from drug-addictive behaviors such as, in the first place,
bulimia. These positions highlight on the descriptive level a push to enjoyment characterized by an unregulated dependence on a substance. Indeed the
substance that makes the anorexic enjoy presents itself as invisible, as non-
objectifiable, but not for that reason less irresistible. And it is really this point
that the clinical genius of Lacan centered more than any other in relation to
the strategic core of anorexia nervosa, when he affirms that the anorexic
refusal of food is not a refusal to eat, but is rather to eat the nothing. On the
other hand, if the anorexic does not show the driving object which makes
them enjoy in a particular fashion, they reveal in a radical way what, beyond

the phenomenology of substances in flesh and blood, is ardently desired in the pathologies of dependence: this object nothing whose loss is at the origin of the constitution of the subject as a subject of desire, as a lack of being. At the same time, what the anorexic radically shows in his position of refusal, by analogy with the drug addict, is this rejection of the Other which crosses the NFS like a matrix and which totally adheres to the spasmodic search for a "jouissance" without the Other (Miller, Laurent, 2005, pp. 373–379) which is autistic, outside of phallic significance.

It is in the light of this refusal of the Other and of its structural particularity that it is possible to situate the contemporary clinic of NFS, in the perspective of Lacanian psychoanalysis as a clinic of narcissism and at the same time as a clinic of disordered compulsivity – "of the discharge by the act" (Ansermet, 1999 p. 164), as Ansermet sums it up in an effective formula.

Indeed, what the anorexic refuses to eat is not, in the first place, food, beyond all descriptive evidence. Nor is what it ultimately feeds on identification with the narcissistic image of the skinny body. It is rather, as it has effectively been written, "the refusal to eat the signifier in question" (Ménard, 1988, p. 25). It is to the symbolic-metaphorizing grasp of the Other that the anorexic opposes their refusal in order to preserve the mythical integrity of a full jouissance uncontaminated by the trace of the signifier. It is in the light of this dual operation, of refusal toward the Other and of unlimited preservation of a full jouissance to which Lacan refers us when he affirms that the anorexic eats the nothing, that the anorexia nervosa is fully in NFS.

A new epidemiology

To shed more light on the current status of the anorexic question, it is important to take into account the transformations that have occurred, in half a century, regarding the distribution and epidemiological characteristics of the symptom. For this, we need to distinguish four historical-temporal phases which offer us a clear vision of this rapid metamorphosis.

A first phase that could be called the "epoch of the white flies" is still clearly identifiable in Selvini Palazzoli's 1963 text, *L'anoressia mentale*. In an Italy that had recently entered the era of the economic boom and was one of the economic powers of the capitalist world, one rarely encountered anorexic patients in hospitals and even less in the offices of psychoanalysts and psychotherapists; it was a moment of transition, after the hard years of post-war and reconstruction, and a moment of transformation of economic-social structures (from agricultural to industrial) and family (from patriarchal to nuclear family).

The patients were overwhelmingly women and adolescents who presented an anorexia of an almost exclusively restrictive nature, without any evacuative practice.

A second phase may correspond to the popular text *The golden cage*, written by Bruch in 1978. We are here at the time of anorexia as the disease chosen by young girls from well-off families in the Western world. Indeed, in the United States, particularly in university colleges and high schools, the 1970s marked the spread of the phenomenon of anorexia nervosa at an almost epidemic level. The American psychiatrist underlines the social connotation of this phenomenon and its non-fortuitous distribution: a disease of this kind strikes the girls of wealthy, cultured and prosperous families, not only in the United States, but in many other rich countries (Bruch, 1978, p. 5).

It is a widespread syndrome among the emerging bourgeois classes in the capitalist world, not only in North America and Europe but also in Japan. "Rarely or perhaps never", wrote the author, "does it strike the poor and it has not been described in underdeveloped countries" (Bruch, 1978, p. 12). In nine out of ten cases, it affects women, especially when going through puberty and it is configured as a feminine pathology. According to Bruch, "the spread of the disease must be attributed to socio-psychological factors", among which the pervasive influence of the media; in particular fashion and television seem to have considerable importance on the relationship of young women with their body, in relation to the ideal of female thinness as an icon of desirability, emphasized by mass-media communication.

The 1980s and 1990s would mark the beginning of a new era in the history of the spread of the anorexic symptom, which would radically transform the characteristics of the symptom and the coordinates of its spread. Its structure began to become more complex at exactly the same time when anorexia would be recognized by official psychiatry as a syndrome characterized culturally (culture-bound); it would find a place in the DSM-IV (1998, pp. 918–919) alongside more exotic syndromes such as the amok syndrome, in the Far East (Malaysia, Laos), or the attack of *nervios* (among the Latins of the Caribbean). First of all, the forms that include practices of evacuation, with or without vomiting, took over from pure restrictive anorexias and bulimia became the true epidemic clinical phenomenon of those years. A fourth stage, typical of the beginning of the twenty-first century and in which we are still immersed today, is characterized, in my opinion, by phenomena which we have now begun to identify and study at the clinical and epidemiological level. First, we are witnessing a weakening of the mono-symptom paradigm and a gradual spread of the phenomenon of comorbidity, poly-substance abuse and correlated pathologies. It is more and more frequent, for example, to meet bulimic patients who abuse, at the same time, drugs and alcohol and who no longer find in food pathology alone a compensatory mooring, sufficient to treat their anguish and their discomfort. Second, apart from a few specific exceptions, it appears more clearly that, in the past, there was an unfounded idealization of the intelligence of the anorexic patient, today more easily identifiable, and which is still found in the pages of *The Golden Cage*. The stickiness of the intellectual performance of the anorexic is generally translated, in the clinic, into an operation devoid of adequacy at the request of the Other and not the manifestation of a true intellectual intentionality and a personal search. It is no coincidence that the anorexic patient, often very diligent and studious from childhood, abruptly interrupts their studies, at some point, to devote themselves entirely to the cultivation of their symptom. The myth of the intelligence of the anorexic is therefore in crisis.

Third, we are witnessing a process of globalization of the anorexic-bulimic symptom that goes beyond the borders of the advanced capitalist world to take root also in developing areas, which are subject to a progressive process of Westernization. This is the case, for example, in its (non-homogeneous) distribution in the Mediterranean basin (not only in Europe but also in North Africa and in part of the Middle East, notably in Turkey and Israel): recent studies have shown that in all probability it is not lower than that quantified in the countries of northern Europe (Ruggiero, 2004).

Finally, we are witnessing a transformation that affects the relationship between anorexia and virtual reality and that is developing through the use of the Internet. It is a politico-social phenomenon, in line with the most advanced developments in technologies applied to new media and which poses new problems not only at the clinical level but, first of all, at the political and social level: the birth of virtual communities of anorexics and bulimics. This new phenomenon is giving birth, in my opinion, to a politicization of anorexia-bulimia as a collective phenomenon very different from the feminist frame of reference in which certain authors had tried to read and situate it in previous years. In fact, we are not at all confronted here with the phenomenon of the dissemination of pro-ANA websites which praise anorexia and bulimia as a symptom of the irreducibility of the position of the female struggle in a phallocentric world dominated by masculine power and values.

The rapid spread of pro-ANA sites, where patients come into contact with each other and bond around a glorification of the anorexic and bulimic identity, have rather, in fact, a role of political action in the active and militant propagandizing of the symptom and represent, in this area too, an internal trend in contemporary social discourse: the construction of social ties around identificatory signs, not correlated to one's own subjective history but to generic identities, often expressing themselves in a symptomatic condition denied as such and, rather, glorified as a way of life. A condition that can take the direction of solidarity against the disease or, on the contrary, support it. This fourth epidemiological phase characterizes the entry into the era of anorexia-bulimia as a virtual identity community, whose disturbing drift is realized when the destructive core of the anorexic symptom, that is to say the refusal of the Other, is elevated to the political dignity of a factor of aggregation and mission. In this perspective, the "identity communitarianism" (Laurent, *Ornicar? Digital*, 224) of pro-ANA sites manifests itself as a destructive self-segregationist agent, not intended, therefore, for a mutual and united struggle against the symptom (on the model of Alcoholics Anonymous) but, on the contrary, for a collective and exclusive reinforcement of the passion for the symptom as an alternative way to the social bond.

The enigma of anorexic jouissance

If we disregard a reading of anorexia that puts at the center the subject's way of enjoying in relation to the maternal Other, phenomenology could lead us to radically disconnect anorexia both from drug-addictive behaviors and, primarily, bulimia: positions in which, on a descriptive level, a drive to enjoyment, characterized by an unregulated dependence on a substance, is evident. In fact, the substance that makes the anorexic enjoy presents itself as invisible, as not objectifiable but no less irresistible for all that. It is around this knot, which cannot be traced back to the complexity of the practices of avoidance and control of the body, implemented by the subject, that the enigma of anorexic jouissance is constructed, which has challenged and continues to challenge the clinicians most involved in this field (Selvini Palazzoli, Cirillo, Selvini, Sorrentino, 1998, p. 2).

We can consider the enigma of anorexic jouissance as the common thread of this work. In this journey, Lacan's teaching will help us, in a particular way, to open up a passage for us, following the indication of one of his answers to the enigma that the anorexic embodies in their singular way of enjoying. This is an answer which is also, in certain aspects, enigmatic but nevertheless surprising in the way it sheds light on the question and which we will try to illustrate and make transmissible throughout these pages.

Lacan's counter-intuitive answer is that the anorexic is not, in reality, the one who refuses to eat; what happens, rather, in anorexia, is that the subject eats an unheard-of object: the nothing. This operation restores to the anorexic a full and limitless enjoyment, which they are not willing to give up for anything in the world. It will be a question, in the course of our investigation, of showing the clinical value of Lacan's answer to the enigma of anorexia, by the clear articulation of the logic that his formula condenses in an almost oracular way.

Two preliminary theses on les NFS: fetishistic forms of disenchantment, superegoic autotherapies

In this perspective, two definitions that we have formulated in recent years, in particular in the light of clinical experience in the field of anorexia-bulimia and obesity, around the status of NFS, to clarify the place of anorexia within these, can be useful to us beforehand. The first thesis determines as a unifying feature in the NFS a fetishistic disenchantment. This formula translates on the one hand the symbolic degradation of speech and the distrust of the Other that is amply identifiable in the clinic of the NFS. This is the side of "disenchantment" taken not in its critical-demystifying sense, but on the contrary in the sense of a degradation of the relationship with the Other which leads to a drift of denial of its function (Cosenza, 2005a, p. 60). On the other hand, it emphasizes the drive to blind enjoyment of the object (whether it be a substance as in the phenomenology of drug addiction or in bulimia or whether it is the body itself fetishized and invaded by differential modalities of jouissance as in anorexia, in depressive forms and in panic attacks), in the imaginary position of fetish condenser of jouissance. It is this "fetishist" side taken in its perverse sense, valued by the Kestembergs, where the fetish is not placed by the subject as a condition of desire but as an objectified condensation of jouissance.

The second thesis on NFS defines its status, in particular for the forms that can be traced back to the framework of pathological addictions, drug addiction and alcoholism, anorexia-bulimia, obesity, as forms of superegoic self-therapy (Cosenza, 2005b, pp. 67–72). By this definition, we wanted to indicate in a double movement a common thread that can be identified in particular in the clinic of NFS which takes the form of pathological addictions.

On the one hand, in fact, the subject finds through the onset of the symptom, for example the onset of anorexia, their own "autonomous" solution in response to an existential condition that they do not succeed in sustaining, in avoiding the passage through the Other of the word, and in this sense by treating themselves in an autotherapeutic way – in this clinic, the absence of a request for treatment and the extreme difficulty of activating a symbolic transfer, to which there corresponds a deadly narcissistic autonomism of the subject and an egosyntonia which accompanies it in particular at the beginnings of the drug addictive and anorexic symptom, are completely locatable traits. On the other hand, more radically, as the development of the NFS inexorably reveals, the supposed ego-narcissistic mastery over their symptom reveals itself to the subject as an illusion, because it is supported by an excessive superegoic push without limits to repetition and by a logic beyond the pleasure principle which does not take long to show its deadly and self-destructive economy. Any clinical history of a severe anorexic patient embodies in its pathological course, in a singular way, this double movement.

Anorexia as a "solution"

In any case, the different psychoanalytical approaches and psychodynamically oriented psychotherapies seem to converge around the thesis that anorexia and bulimia, even before being disorders or problems, are characterized by having been, for the subject, treatments, solutions. Of course, these are pathological solutions; solutions that lead to death (Kestemberg, 1981, p. 5), non-violent suicides (Lacan, 2001a, p. 35). More precisely, we are concerned with treatments produced by the subject, but not subjectivized, on which it is necessary to effect within the therapy a second-degree treatment which makes possible a subjectivation, a recognition and a symbolic elaboration of their unconscious causality in order to deactivate the self-destructive inclination that runs through them. This subjectivated treatment is oriented to produce an elaboration that has the strength and the efficiency to reduce, if not to eliminate, the symptom in the destructive effects that it entails for the life of the subject, by allowing him to construct his answer, at the same time more singular and more open to the encounter with the Other, compared to those constituted by anorexia and bulimia. These presented themselves to the subject as the only possible response, the best available solution in the face of something unbearable that the subject had to confront at a certain point in their experience (Recalcati, 1997, p. 29). It is obviously an unconscious solution that the subject has produced without knowing it to deal with an insurmountable difficulty that has arisen in his relationship to the Other. The conjunctures triggering this insurmountable difficulty are found in the clinical experience of the cure, and within the framework of a vast phenomenology; it is possible to reduce its structural invariants to a few essential nodes which refer to a difficulty for the subject in treating symbolically as much the traumatic experiences of loss as the no less traumatic experiences of the manifestation of desire as an excess thrust of the drive, as uncontrollable jouissance. In this regard, it is no coincidence that anorexia and bulimia are triggered above all in the puberty period, when the body of the adolescent is re-eroticized and installs the subject to occupy an adult position, although they do not yet fully have the symbolic apparatus which allows them to be able to do so. This disharmony that we can find in the relationship of the adolescent with his own body in transformation and with his own image, we find radically accentuated in the cases that will develop an anorexic-bulimic pathology. In these cases, in fact, the anorexic-bulimic solution presents itself precisely as the response to this unbearable disharmony and as the subject's attempt to anesthetize the encounter with the desire that runs through their body. In this sense, anorexia-bulimia presents itself phenomenologically as an anesthetic solution, which tends to disincorporate the sexual drive from its orientation toward the other, to divert it toward the autoerotic direction of an inanimate substance that can be located and controlled, food, or to orient it narcissistically toward the enjoyment of body image and the autarky of the anorexic lifestyle. The twisted ego-syntonia that anorexic anesthesia entails is evident in the effects also classified by the DSM-5 as disorders that make up the framework of the syndrome: "significantly low weight", "intense fear of gaining weight or of becoming fat", altered perception of body image (APA, 2022, p. 381). In the DSM-5, the reference to amenorrhea was eliminated, to include under the diagnosis of anorexia nervosa also males, and females in the infertile phase of life.

In the bulimic context, a destiny feared and very often realized in cases of anorexia, the subject finds a variant of the rigid drive autarky of anorexia: instead of freezing in the thrust of the drive at the origin, they realize it but only on condition of canceling its effects, of reducing its results to zero, of erasing its traces. The devouring of the object in bulimia – whether or not it is also, as in some cases, the sexual object – is functional and sustainable only on the condition that it is evacuated without residues by the subject. On this basis Bernard Brusset's thesis (1991, pp. 105–132) developed on anorexia and bulimia is supported, of the same anorexic-bulimic circuit held by the same logic of functioning where the anorexic ideal remains fixed on the horizon of the bulimia as a superegoic ideal lost but always to be recovered, whereas the bulimic collapse functions as a constant and terrorizing specter for the anorexic who, even if they do not consume food, always have it at the center of their thoughts.

Anorexia from the NFS to the real structure of the symptom

However, the anorexic solution appears to the clinician as a precarious and dangerous restorative operation for the subject and, at the same time, as a formation that reveals the structural status of the symptom in human experience. This is why defining it as a new form of the symptom, an effect of the paternal function crisis and the holding of the symbolic Other in the contemporary capitalist world, though it remains fair and productive, nevertheless involves a limitation to the context of the time and the historical-cultural perspective. To this is added the risk of misleading the more radical scope of its configuration and its consequences in the field of the clinic. As we will be able to show in the course of this work, what anorexia manifests, as being in action in the intransigent power of the subject's refusal to eat and to take care of themselves, is a tear between the self-destructive real where the patient finds themselves locked up and the word of the Other, the order of the symbolic. This heterogeneity between the real of the symptom and the field of the Other, which we find massively in the clinic of anorexia, from the first encounter with the patient, is, in the analytic clinic of neuroses, the residual product that we gradually succeed in isolating at the end of the treatment: the irreducibility of the partial object causing the subject's desire, in relation to the field of the signifier within which their story is constructed. This is what Freud indicated, in *Beyond the Pleasure Principle*, when he spoke of the object of repetition being impermeable to the work of symbolization operated by interpretation. And also what, *Analysis, Terminable and Interminable* at the end, therefore, of his parable of research in the clinical domain, he called when speaking of the "residual manifestations" of the repetition that one finds at the end of the analytic treatment.

The other radical difference consists, however, in the impossibility of recognizing, during much of the treatment, the macroscopic distance between the symptomatic jouissance taking hold of the anorexic and their speech, which remains empty and disconnected from the link to the Other. Exactly the opposite of what happens to the neurotic who, especially at the start of an analytic journey, shows himself to be hypersensitive to the discrepancies between what they say they want and what they want without being able to say it, between what they ask for and what they want.

In this sense, anorexia as a contemporary symptom reveals, by showing itself to the clinician and not to the subject who suffers from it, the radical structure of the symptom as such.

And in doing so, it shows all the limits of a purely metaphoric-semantic definition and of a purely semantic-hermeneutic symptom treatment practice, all centered on the production of meaning. In this sense, therefore, anorexia has a revealing scope since it revolutionizes the notion of the symptom by the revelation, at the heart of its fabric, of a jouissance irreducible to the signifier.

The restorative dimension internal to the anorexic solution, which allows the subject to elude the unbearable anxiety of a symbolically untreatable jouissance, such as imposes itself in the conjunctures of the onset of anorexia, is given by a narcissistic welding of the real drive, which materializes in the identification of the subject with the anorexic identity. This highlights, at the same time, the radically different treatment, which is at the base of the neurotic symptom, and the solution brought about by the construction of the anorexic symptom to the problem of the relationship of the subject with the real drive. The neurotic symptom, in fact, thanks to the action of repression and the return of the repressed, mediates between the subject and their relationship to the real, through a symbolic mechanism of signifying substitution. This allows it to function, for the subject, as a social link, as a point of connection between the real of the subject and the field of the Other. This is the meaning that can be given, in the language of Lacan, to the Freudian definition of the symptom as compromise formation.

The anorexic symptom, completely the opposite, treats the subject's relation to the real drive through the construction of a narcissistic hypostasis which provides them with an identity linked to the disease and detaches them from the link to the Other. For this reason, anorexics have a progressive tendency, in the evolution of the disease, to leave the social bond, to suspend all the activities and the associations previous to the manifestation of the symptom, until they abandon, sometimes, mealtimes and lock themselves in deadly isolation. As the contemporary trend toward the diffusion of virtual communities of anorexics on the Internet shows, the extra-familial relationships that they concede to each other are, at best, narcissistic-specular relationships that reinforce the identity of the jouissance linked to the symptom. On this axis are structured, moreover, many couple relationships when the anorexic has a companion during the illness: the partner is not configured as a partner of desire but as a narcissistic complement, an aid and a support for the sickness. In short, like a support partner who finds themselves in a position that is more anaclitic than erotic. While the neurotic symptom produces a divided, lacking, desiring, ego-dystonic subject, the anorexic symptom solidifies a narcissistic identity without apparent flaws, animated by an ideal of self-sufficiency, both euphoric and devastating, and by a state of fundamentally deadly ego-syntony.

The two paths of the anorexic symptom as real: nirvanic dimension and uncanny dimension (unheimlich)

We can introduce the encounter with the real of the symptom, with what is most irresistible and deaf that moves it, from two divergent paths that characterize it. We can already find both in Freud and see them massively at work in the clinic of food psychopathologies. The first path of the symptom as real leads us to the nirvanic dimension, eminently embodied in anorexia. On this path, we can identify clinical phenomena that are classically present in the work with our patients: disinvestment and withdrawal from social ties, the tendency to chronicity of the symptom, the push to death which takes the form of suicide deferred, non-violent and silent. Along this nirvanic path, the real of the symptom presents itself as something that puts to sleep, that extinguishes, like a deadly and lethal anesthetic. Death, in fact, does not function, here, as a symbolic limit but as a limitless horizon toward which the subject travels without brakes.

On the other hand, the second path of the symptom as real opens the doors to the uncanny (*das Unheimliche*) dimension of anorexia. If one follows this path, one experiences an effect radically different from anything encountered on the nirvanic path of the symptom. Indeed, if nirvana tendentially puts you to sleep until death, the uncanny wakes you up. The path of the uncanny is, indeed, a path that awakens, as Freud teaches us in his writing *Das Unheimliche*.

Certainly, the uncanny does not produce a happy awakening. On the contrary, it is an unpleasant awakening, the effect of the encounter with something foreign which, at the same time, embodies what exists most intimately for the subject but from which they keep a distance. The path of the disturbing induces the subject to a traumatic awakening. This traumatic awakening concerns a return and a reactivation of the real drive in the body of the subject, which the anorexic-bulimic subject, like the obese one, experiences with anxiety. However, what clinical experience teaches us is that, if they do not go through this passage, the subject will not be able to begin a real change in their condition, nor open up again to a relationship with the Other and reinvent their existence. They will remain chained in the deadly and autistic anesthesia of their symptom.

Note

1 See also in this regard, in the light of an ethnopsychiatric perspective, the classic study by R. Gordon (1990), *Anorexia and Bulimia. Anatomy of a Social Epidemic*. London: Basic Blackwell.

References

American Psychiatric Association (APA) (2022), *Diagnostic and Statistical Manual of Mental Disorders. Fifth Edition. Text Revision (DSM-5-TR)*. Washington, DC: American Psychiatric Association.

Ansermet, F. (1999), *Clinique de l'origine. L'enfant entre medicine et psychanalyse*. Paris: Payot.

Brousse, M.-H. (2006), L'amour du sinthome contre la haine de la difference. *La Cause freudienne*, no. 62, 2006, pp. 21–25.

Bruch, H. (1978), *The Golden Cage. The Enigma of the Anorexia Nervosa.* Cambridge, MA: Harvard University Press; (1979) *L'enigme de l'anorexie. La cage dorée,* tr. Fr. Paris: Presses Universitaires de France.

Brusset, B. (1991), Psychopathologie et métapsychologie de l'addiction boulimique. *La Boulimie. Monographie de a Revue Française de psychanalyse,* pp. 105–132.

Cliniques Mediterraneénnes (2005), *Cliniques Mediterraneénnes. Soigner, enseigner, evaluer?* no. 71, Marseille: Éres.

Cosenza, D. (2002), Lacan et l'héritage des Lumières. *Mental,* no. 11, pp. 39–43.

Cosenza, D. (2005a), La psychanalyse et les transformations contemporaines du Symptôme. *Mental,* no. 16, pp. 57–64.

Cosenza, D. (2005b), Angoscia e dipendenze nella clinica odierna. *Attualità Lacaniana,* vol. 2, pp. 67–72.

Freda, F. H. (1989), La toxicomanie: un symptôme moderne. *Analytica,* vol. 57, pp. 115–120.

Freda, F. H. (1992), Les nouvelles forms du symptôme. *Revue de l'ECF,* vol. 21, p. 85.

Freda, F. H., Lecoeur, B. (1997), Les nouvelles formes du symptôme. *Mental,* no. 4, pp. 139–148.

Freud, S. (1966), *L'inquiétant (1919), Oeuvres complètes,* vol. 15. Paris: PUF, pp. 151–188.

Guéguen, P.-G. (2005), À ceux qui pensent que nous pensons par nous-mêmes. *La Cause freudienne,* no. 61, pp. 15–17.

Kestemberg, E. (2001), *La psychose froide.* Paris: Presses Universitaires de France.

Kestemberg, E., Kestemberg, J., Decobert, S. (1981), *La faim et le corps: un étude psychanalytique de l'anorexie mentale (1972).* Paris: PUF.

Lacan, J., (2001a), *Les complexes familiaux dans la formation de l'individu (1938), Autres écrits.* Paris: Éditions du Seuil, pp. 23–84.

Lacan, J. (2001b), *Radiophonie* (1970). *Autres écrits.* cit., pp. 403–447.

Laurent, D. (2004), Inhibition, symptôme et angoisse aujourd'hui. *La Cause freudienne,* no. 58, pp. 56–60.

Laurent, É. (2005), Les deux plis du symptôme et de l'institution. *Ornicar? Digital,* no. 224.

Ménard, A. (1988), L'anorexie mentale, entre psychose et nevrose? Les anorexiques supposés sans demande. *Pas Tant,* no. 20, pp. 21–26.

Ménard, A. (1992), Structure signifiante de l'anorexie mentale. *Actes* ECF, no. 2, pp. 3–7.

Miller, J.-A. (2003), Intuitions milanaises (2). *Mental,* no. 12, pp. 9–26.

Miller, J.-A. (2005), Une fantasie. *Mental,* no. 15, pp. 9–17.

Miller, J.-A., Laurent, É. (2005), *El Otro que no existe y sus comités de ética (1996–1997).* Buenos Aires: Paidós.

Recalcati, M. (1997), *L'ultima cena. Anoressia e bulimia.* Milano: Bruno Mondadori.

Recalcati, M. (Dir.) (1998), *Il corpo ostaggio. Clinica psicoanalitica dell'anoressia-bulimia.* Roma: Borla.

Ruggiero, G. M. (Dir.) (2004), *Anoressia e bulimia nei Paesi dell'area mediterranea.* Milano: Deleyva.

Selvini Palazzoli, M., Cirillo, S., Selvini, M., Sorrentino, A. (1998), *Ragazze anoressiche e bulimiche.* Milano: Cortina.

Chapter 2

Anorexia as a frontier in the contemporary clinical debate

Anorexia between development and structure

While analytical approaches converge on highlighting the status of anorexia as a symptomatic solution and critically distance themselves from its reduction to a syndromic constellation of behavioral and cognitive disorders disregarding the singular subject who suffers and its history, their divergences however emerge with great clarity when the problem of the basis of the anorexic solution arises. If it is indeed essential, in a psychoanalytical approach to anorexia, to shift the accent, as Brusset underlines, from the syndromic dimension to the process dimension within which it occurred (Brusset, 1998, pp. 10–11), it is however on the nature of this process and on the clinical value of this solution that the different positions begin to emerge. Around this point, we are witnessing the complex deployment of readings of anorexia and its treatment, which reflect in this field the different orientations that make up the analytical field in the news. We do not intend here to make a historiographical catalogue of the different readings of anorexia produced in this field. We will limit ourselves to questioning a cardinal problem around which it is possible to order, by distinguishing them, the positions in play. This problem confronts the question in general terms because it questions anorexia in the light of the epistemological foundations of psychoanalysis that emerge from Freud's work. The terms of this questioning concern two perspectives that are found in Freud's work and which trace in post-Freudianism an essential dividing line between a psychoanalytic clinic based on a theory of development and a psychoanalytic clinic based on a structural logic.

Anorexia in the evolutionary-stadial paradigm of drive

Lacan made himself the author, in his return to Freud, of a clarification of the structural foundation of the Freudian unconscious, and first of all, he re-examined from the beginning of his teaching the epistemological foundations of the psychoanalytical clinic and traced a line of demarcation between the evolutionism of post-Freudians and the unprecedented structural logic that

DOI: 10.4324/9781003318439-3

can be identified in the Freudian text. The logic which contrasts with some scientifico-biological temptations internal to the work of Freud. By this operation, Lacan intended to question the developmental and teleological ideology of human psycho-sexual development which had taken root in post-Freudian psychoanalysis from an uninformed reading of some points of Freud's work, in particular *Three Essays on the Theory of Sexuality*. It is in particular in the work of systematization of the theory of the stages of psycho-sexual development carried out by Abraham that we can find, with the considerable clinical intuitions of one of Freud's best pupils of the first generation, the construction of a psychopathological installation codified as a tassonomy of the modes of arrest, fixation and regression of the subject at one of the evolutionary stages of the libido. Alongside this stadial determinism, we find a teleological inclination in the construction of Abraham which leads to the exaltation of the ideal of genital love as the concluding stage of completed human maturation, about which Lacan will not spare the irony of his criticism (Lacan, 2006, pp. 504–506). Within this complex doctrinaire construction, the place of anorexia nervosa is located by Abraham alongside the affections of nervous hunger, in an arrest of the development of the libido at the sadico-oral stage characterized by a cannibalesque relationship with the object, close to the melancholy position (Abraham, 1977).

This perspective only effectively develops one of the two fundamental indications proposed by Freud on the subject of the structure of anorexia nervosa: that which relates to its melancholic matrix, sketched out by the father of psychoanalysis in the *Manuscript G* of 1895 (Abraham, 1977) and taken up in 1915 in *Mourning and Melancholy* (Freud, 1957, pp. 91–97; Freud, 1968). What is highlighted there is precisely the non-separative side of anorexia as a melancholy expression of the fixation of the subject to the lost object. This melancholy version of anorexia is quite different in Freud from the declension of hysterical anorexia, where the refusal of food is based on the refusal/disgust circuit specific to the libidinal functioning of hysteria, where the refused object is, at the same time, object desired and refused as desired, and whose framework the father of psychoanalysis already indicates to us in his text of 1892, *A case of hypnotic healing*, which he will develop later in 1905 in the *Three Essays on the Theory of Sexuality* (Freud, 1987).

In the Abrahamian reworking of Freud's lesson, to this oral fixation is united the exercise of an anal mastery that we find in the symptomatic dimension of the omnipresent control in anorexia. Abraham will therefore become a promoter of a psychoanalytical reading of anorexia as a pathology of orality which highlights a central point of the anorexic question already sketched out by Freud, veiling however in a rigid determinism, codified and transmitted in the *Treatise* of Fenichel, the structural complexity involved in the anorexic question and in each case of anorexia. Lacan will assert from the beginning of his teaching of psychoanalysis, in total contradiction with this epistemological approach to the Freudian clinic – in particular in relation to the adaptive-psychologizing version of Ego-Psychology – a "structural perspective" which highlights in this context, as Ménard points out, the "signifying structure of anorexia nervosa" (Ménard, 1992, p. 3). This means that anorexia functions as a symptom, insofar as it is a signifier which represents the subject who suffers from it by another signifier whose precise symbolic value is found only within the signifying chain which composes the field of the historico-parental Other where he was constituted. Which is equivalent first, at least on one side, to considering anorexia, according to the classical definition of the symptom elaborated by Lacan, as a "metaphor" of the subject, as an unconscious message sent by the subject to the parental Other to questioning and summoning desire.

The psychogenetico-relational paradigm of anorexia: identity, narcissism and the family system

In his brief but illuminating considerations of the 1950s, Lacan made himself a precursor in his own way of a general displacement of the clinical problematic of anorexia which would impose itself in the mid-1960s, in the international symposium of Gottingen in 1965. In this symposium, in contrast to an organicist approach and above all thanks to the clinical work of Bruch and Palazzoli Selvini, we will see the affirmation of a psychogenetic etiology of anorexia centered on the problem of identity (Corcos, 2005, p. 14), narcissism, the relationship of the subject with the image of the own body and of its position inside the family system, in particular in relation to the mother.

In relation to this general shift in the issue, it seems appropriate to make some substantive clarifications. Above all, it seems that one can affirm that the contemporary psychopathological debate on anorexia remains still today anchored within the framework of this dominant general paradigm, which, as far as psychoanalysis is concerned, questions from different angles the anorexia in the context of a "clinic of primary narcissism" and the early mother/daughter relationship. Second, as we will specify later, the change of paradigmatic content in the reading of anorexia – passage from the centrality of the oral problem to the centrality of the narcissistic problematic – does not seem to agree with a change of general epistemological-methodological framework compared to the previous paradigm: it would seem that in the psychoanalytical field a deterministico-stadial evolutionism of drive development has been replaced by a narcissico-identity psychogenesis centered on the specular mother/daughter relationship with its psychopathological correlate of evolving breakdowns. These evolutionary stops manifest themselves within the framework of a narcissico-compulsive circuit, marked by Brusset with a drug-addictive quality, where the narcissistic fragility of the ego or of the "Self" corresponds to an excess in the search for immediate discharge through the action (acted, taking action) that compensates for it. This satisfaction assumes a negative autoerotic characterization (the reference is to an "autoeroticism of death") and is often realized through real practices of addiction to substances. Dependence in this field, often in conjunction with going through the conjuncture of adolescence, occurs as an alternative to an unsustainable relationship of symbolic exchange with another subject. It is within this perspective where the lines of psychoanalytic research are tied around an evolving epistemological paradigm that it is possible to situate, in the orientation of most post-Freudian approaches to anorexia, the beginning, course and result of the anorexic process and the unconscious value that it has for the subject.

Limits of a semantics of the unconscious: the criticisms of Bruch and Selvini Palazzoli on the analytic treatment of anorexia

In the clinical history of anorexia, a decisive point of no return has certainly been marked by the innovative, thorough and faithful to the purpose of research developed over more than half a century, by the two "true mothers" of the contemporary notion of anorexia nervosa: Hilde Bruch and Mara Selvini Palazzoli. Their long parallel work at a distance, characterized by a consistent reciprocal support, without however lacking differences in position, had two major objectives of common criticism which ended up being affirmed in the field of studies on anorexia nervosa. Above all, they have called into question the fundamentally organic nature of the pathology, affirmed by Simmonds, by providing clinical proof of the irreducibility of anorexia nervosa to a pathology of undernutrition of endocrine origin. The symptoms that invest the body in anorexia nervosa are necessary effects, in their perspective, of a syndrome of a psychogenetic nature.

On the other hand, the second critical objective concerns the analytical treatment of anorexia nervosa. Both, as psychiatrists and psychoanalysts, introduced themselves into the treatment of anorexia from the lines of orientation of the dominant psychoanalysis of the 1940s and 1950s which considered anorexia nervosa above all as a pathology of the orality and whose clinical practice placed at the center the knowledge of the psychoanalyst and the practice of interpreting the unconscious meaning of the symptom, referring to the oral sexual fantasy framework.

They both encounter on their way a fundamental obstacle linked to the clinic and a resource linked to a new general epistemology, to which they cling, but not with the same determination. The obstacle is constituted by the very clinic of anorexia nervosa, by the strong refractory nature of the anorexic to treatment, in particular to treatment by words, based on the interpretation of the unconscious meaning.

The resource, on the contrary, was constituted by the general theory of systems, conceived in California by Gregory Bateson in particular and developed in the clinical environment with studies on the family of the schizophrenic patient. The epistemological revolution of systems theory consists in shifting the axis of research from a linear causal paradigm to a cyclic paradigm, in which it is the complexity of the system which alone can enlighten us on the state of the elements who compose it. So, within the framework of a transformation that takes into account the system as a whole, the condition of the singular elements, which are inside, can also change. The application of this epistemological principle in the field of psychotherapy will find its greatest concrete realization in studies on organizations and in particular on the family, emerging from Selvini's research of the early 1970s, a translation in systemic therapy. family and a privileged object in the family of the anorexic (Selvini Palazzoli and others, 1978).

It is therefore against a precise theory and practice of psychoanalysis that the criticisms of Bruch and Selvini are directed; they can be summed up in three fundamental points: the first is the opposition to a psychoanalysis based on a linear idea of psychic causality, on an unconscious determinism which closely correlates in a biunivocal way points of libidinal fixation, fantasies linked to the erogenous zone and to the development of the personality and its symptomatic productions.

It is obvious that, in this doctrinal articulation of analytical knowledge where the theory of psychosexual development becomes an exhaustive and saturating reference code in the diagnostic classification of the case, Freud's discovery ends up losing its scope for innovation which was intrinsic to it in the time of its creation.

Second, on this basis, the practice of psychoanalysis ends up being reduced to a hermeneutics of unconscious fantasy meaning as predictable as it is ineffective, and which loses sight, in the centrality attributed to what the patient says, of the form that structures its discourse and the fundamental modality of interaction which characterizes its position, also in the treatment.

Thirdly, this translates, on the level of the technique of intervention, into a centrality of the semantic interpretation on the part of the analyst, which is produced from a position of knowing about the unconscious truth of the patient's suffering.

Well, faced with the anorexic patient, such an idea and such a practice of psychoanalysis are indeed ineffective and devoid of meaning. The frozen and monotonous chain of discourse, the evocative dimension of atrophied speech, the speech of the Other reduced to matter refused or swallowed and re-proposed in an adhesive and desubjectivated way, manifest themselves as impermeable barriers to Freudian practice reduced to a codified semantic machine.

But, at the same time, it is a question, in this version, of an idea and a practice of psychoanalysis which have lost the very heart of Freud's discovery: the real of unconscious desire as an irruption which presents itself structurally under the form of the unexpected and the surprise. In this sense, any semantic codification of the unconscious, posed as universal, inevitably betrays the real dimension of the unconscious as an unforeseen and singular production.

From meaning to structure: a new encounter between psychoanalysis and anorexia

In the post-war years, as the new epistemological perspective constituted by systems theory in its application to the clinical setting began to spread in the United States, and then spread in successive decades, an epistemological revolution was happening in Europe too. European California at that time was Paris; the new epistemology took the name of structuralism, as is well known.

Linguistics, anthropology, history, philosophy, literary criticism, in short, a complex field of knowledge, brought together in an academic way under the formulation of human sciences, had been crossed by this radical theoretical and practical restructuring induced by the concept of structure. On the basis of this concept, the reading of an event, a trace, a text, a said sentence, a symptom cannot take place without inscribing the message within the enunciative structure general from which it emerges. Indeed, it is this structure, and not, for example, the simple intention of the author, of the speaker or of the protagonist, of the patient, which determines its effective value and the effect of meaning that the utterance conveys. It is a revolution of method, scientific, which presents itself as an attack against any ideology of the humanist and teleological type. It advocates the primacy of the signifier and of the structure in relation to the semantic plane, the configuration of the signified as the structural effect of the signifying chain in a certain given point of the subject's discourse.

It is from this perspective that Lacan begins his teaching in the field of psychoanalysis and his "return to Freud". Lacan considers possible a return to the foundation of Freudian discovery, beyond ingenuous biologism and the sclerotized and predictable semantics of post-Freudism and the technicist reduction of its practice, through the encounter of Freud and Saussure. It connects the heart of psychoanalysis with the logic of the signifier and its primacy in the structural production of the effect of meaning, given that in an analysis it is essentially an exchange of words. The fruit of this meeting between Freud and de Saussure, acted out by Lacan from 1953, produced his most famous and classic statement: the unconscious is structured like a language.

Well, our opinion is that, in quite independent ways, starting from psychiatric traditions and analytical contexts autonomous from each other, and on the basis of totally different requirements, Lacan finds himself in agreement with most important researchers of anorexia nervosa on common ground: the critique, bordering on heresy[1], against the dominant analytic practice of the 1950s and 1960s. Bruch and Selvini arrive at this critique and develop it only in close connection to anorexia nervosa and the impossibility of treating this pathology using the parameters inspired by the practice in which they were formed, which prove to be ineffective. Lacan is rather driven by a much broader objective, which is to refound Freud's clinic, thus opposing its degradation into post-Freudiansm. However, anorexia nervosa presents itself punctually in his discourse as a clinical paradigm of an irreducibility which resists framing in the forms of dominant analytical knowledge, becoming in fact a syndrome "allied" to his attempt to criticize clinical orthodoxy, as hysteria had been for Freud with regard to the organicist psychiatry of his time.

The system as a resource and as a limit: the systemic-family pathway to anorexia by Selvini Palazzoli

The structural or systemic turn involves a change of position with respect to psychoanalysis which can take different paths. That of Selvini Palazzoli in the early 1970s manifests a radical position that leads her to a decision to break: the abandonment of psychoanalysis and the start of systemic-family therapy. The encounter with systemic logic cannot, according to the author, be integrated into psychoanalysis and reform its epistemological and technical status, with a view to a new commitment to the treatment of anorexia, the Selvini's fundamental object of research, who had nevertheless offered in 1963, through his *L'anoressia mentale*, a fundamental contribution for a psychoanalytical reading of the question, oriented on the Kleinian mode. A clear epistemological discontinuity characterizes her passage from the Freudian discipline to the systemic approach, throughout the common thread of her research, constituted by the enigma of anorexia nervosa.

However, a fundamental defect will be the basis of this turning point which will be recognized in a self-critical way at the end of her course. The optimistic emphasis placed on the system of family relations and on the therapeutic effectiveness of its treatment from the perspective of systemic purism, which puts the "black box" of the subject in brackets (as much in the anorexic patient as in her family), does not take into account the fact that the singular suffering of the patient cannot be entirely reduced to the structural effects internal to the order of the systemic transactions themselves. In the three logical times that punctuate the parable of the research of Selvini and her school on anorexia, the analytical time of the 1960s, the systemic purist time of the 1970s and 1980s and finally the reformed systemic time (systemic family therapy individual), we are witnessing the return to the heart of the family systemic device of the subjective variable that had been expelled from it (Selvini Palazzoli M. and others, 1998). Of course, this does not translate, in the renewed framework of Selvini's approach, into a return to psychoanalysis, but it nevertheless underlines the clinical evidence that Freud's work, in particular through the reading of Lacan, has rendered impossible to elude: the subject in his real singularity is irreducible to the determinism of the symbolic laws of the system, despite the fact that he constitutes himself within the system and in relation to its laws. When we take the subject out the door, the clinic teaches us that he can only come back through the window, generally more angry and in difficulty than before. This means, in terms that concern the clinic of anorexia nervosa, that the essential passage made by a clinical approach centered on the unconscious fantasy significance of the anorexic symptom to a systemic-structural logic which delimits its production as the result of internal interactions in the particular family system of the patient, does not say the last word or the decisive word on the question.

This passage reveals itself as a necessary condition to go beyond a psychoanalytical hermeneutics sclerotic of meaning, but it is not sufficient to isolate and untie the real knot that binds the anorexic to their symptom. Moreover, Selvini's latest book testifies to this, the high frequency of individual therapies in anorexic patients, following systemic-family psychotherapy interventions. In other words, this means that the anorexia nervosa of an adolescent girl is certainly also to be read as a metaphor for a dysfunction of the family system which finds in the symptom its pathogenic homeostatic solution, on condition of not reducing it entirely to this metaphorical status.

Moreover, the final turning point in Selvini's research, the abandonment of the reductionism of the position of the patient to the status of simple "designated victim" and "scapegoat" of the family system (Bruch, 1978, p. 95, 397), and the valorization of the position of subject of each member of the family in relation to their own family history, goes precisely in the direction of restoring to the anorexic subject his share of responsibility which cannot be evaded, even if it is unconscious, in relation to the choice of his own symptom and to the decision to keep it, transform it or abandon it.

The incongruous mother/daughter interaction and the learning deficit in anorexia nervosa: Hilde Bruch's way between psychoanalysis and learning therapy

Marked by a greater clinical realism and by a more accentuated epistemological prudence, Bruch's position criticizes the semantic-libidinal reductionism of the orthodox psychoanalytic doctrine, its linear mechanism and its therapeutic inefficiency in the field of anorexia nervosa, without however falling back in a systemic reductionism. In some ways, she is less radical than Selvini, she absorbs the new systemic wave in her thinking without however becoming a combative militant and she even realizes with a certain advance of some possible dubious consequences on the clinical level. At the same time and in the same way, she takes a critical distance from the practice of psychoanalysis, in which she was trained, to find herself, more happily, in an analytical version that shifts the axis of discourse beyond the psychosexual determinism of the phases of development of the libido. Bruch's perspective is more interested in deficits in personality development that occur within the framework of the subject's primary interactions by an internal insufficiency in the process of learning and transmission. Indeed, it is in this context that she situates the heart of the question of anorexia nervosa and at the same time that of obesity, considered as symptoms which are clarified, one in the light of the other. The logic of the system is thus integrated by Bruch into her theory of personality development within an analysis of the structure of mother/child interaction in the process of learning.

As she points out, from the particularized reconstruction of the history of their development, we have seen that they have certain misleading experiences in common, that is to say the absence or lack of appropriate responses and confirmation to the cues through which they indicated their demands and other forms of self-expression (Bruch, 1978, p. 73).

These incongruous messages, internal to the responses or to the maternal stimuli, addressed to the child, produce the corresponding mirror effect of a basic difficulty in the discrimination of stimuli and sensations on the cognitive and perceptual level on the part of the child.

Bruch traces these psychopathological frameworks, and among them anorexia nervosa, rather than to early traumas, to deviations that settle along the lines of orientation of personality development, from these dysfunctional interactions with the mother. The paradigmatic clinical example on this subject is that given by the incongruous response of the mother to the crying of the child.

Indeed, if in the experience of the infant, his cry is probably their most important instrument because it is with this means that he signals his discomforts, his desires and his necessities, on the side of maternal action the way in which one responds to the cry of the child, by satisfying it or by neglecting it, seems to be the determining factor in making him aware of his needs (Bruch, 1978, p. 73). Responding then to the cry with food, if it is a congruent response when his crying indicates the need for food, on the contrary becomes an incongruous and aberrant experience when this is not the case, just like not feeding him when her crying signals her hunger (Bruch, 1978, p. 76).

The reiteration over time of these incongruous experiences creates the bases for the construction of symptomatic nodes at the base of the onset of anorexia nervosa in adolescence, a syndrome which, in its typical form, for Bruch, revolves around three disturbed psychological functions: the pathognomonic disorder of the perception of the image and of the conception of one's own body, the lack of a precise perception and interpretation of the stimuli of the body, in particular those relating to the feeling of hunger and satiety, and finally, the crippling sense of inefficiency and helplessness underlying the indiscriminate negativism of overt anorexic conduct. In particular, the form of true anorexia, also called typical or primitive anorexia by the author to distinguish it from atypical anorexia, is characterized by the obsession with thinness which sustains the refusal of food on the part of the teenager.

In other words, anorexia develops as a desperate struggle out of a need for dominance to control their live (Bruch, 1978, p. 315). It is a struggle "to acquire mastery of themselves, their identity, to become competent and efficient" (Bruch, 1978, p. 295), pursued over time by a subject presenting a deficit of the

Ego, a fundamental narcissistic fragility which in its radical form refers, in many cases, to a real "schizophrenic foundation" (Bruch, 1978, p. 329). The translation of this approach in terms of treatment consists of "helping patients to break out of the locked circle of destructive thoughts, experiences and behaviors" (Bruch, 1990, p. 11), by supporting them "in their quest for autonomy and their own identity in the leading to awareness of the impulses, feelings and needs which have their origin in it" (Bruch, 1990, p. 12).

If the anorexia is the result of a fundamental deficit of self-experience, which arose in the patient's life from insane primary experiences of feedback from the mother, the therapy will mainly have a restorative function. If we leave aside the interpretation and the motivational and symbolic meaning of the symptom, which has turned out to be ineffective, even counter-productive, it is for Bruch to install the patient in the place of "active participant" Bruch, 1978, p. 386) of the treatment, to operate as an analyst a "constructive use of ignorance" (Bruch, 1978, p. 390), in order to establish the facts without interpreting them (Bruch, 1978, p. 388), and to emphasize listening to the structure of the discourse and the modes of interaction of the patient more than the content (Bruch, 1978, p. 411).

Bringing the anorexic patient, during the treatment, to a stronger adherence to the reality principle and to a correction of their own distorted cognitions and perceptions, is a permanent central objective in Bruch's therapeutic framework, even if it is anchored in a perspective of a work of transformation which concerns the personality as a whole, without ever being reduced to a simple orthopedics of perception and problematic conduct.

However, although the author emphasizes several times the irreducibility of his therapeutic position in relation to the frameworks of cognitive-behavioral therapies which focus on a practice of orthopedic re-education of the patient's cognitions and problematic behaviors, she does not foresee these therapies recognizing in the conception of the American psychiatrist, an essential point of reference from which they justify their therapeutic praxis. Indeed, Bruch's work is distinguished precisely by the emphasis placed at the same time on the deficit aspect as a whole of the Self of the young anorexic girl and on the cognitive-perceptual disorders at the base of anorexia nervosa, by the capacity to join with oneself in spite of oneself, as a central reference in the theory and in the treatment of anorexia nervosa, as much the cognitive-behavioral approaches focused on the orthopedics of the disorder as the psychodynamico-paychanalytic orientations inherited from the tradition of Ego-psychology, which point to a more general transformation of the personality.

A reversal of perspective: from the deficit of the self to the refusal of the Other

The path opened by Lacan to anorexia nervosa introduces, in our opinion, another way of reading the desubjectivized intractability that young anorexic girls present when the symptom takes hold in their lives. Intractability which is nothing other than the other side of the coin of their acquiescence, as much desubjectivated and impersonal at the request of the Other before the onset of anorexia. As we have seen, Bruch's thesis, which is the most shared in the clinical field, is that behind the negativism of the anorexic hides, in a defensive way, a deficit ego and that, therefore, the anorexic refusal is configured as a consequence, a spontaneous attempt at defensive self-repair of this fragility of the Ego. The logic of the treatment, in this perspective, goes in the strategic direction of a reinforcement of the Ego in the treatment which leads the patient to become autonomous and conscious, by gradually reducing the defensive negativism which characterizes her symptom. The perspective opened up by Lacan, and developed by his followers who are involved in the clinic of ano-rexia nervosa, goes in quite another direction.

For Lacan, the key problem of anorexia is not played out on the egoic narcissistic level and does not concern primarily the problem of the rela-tionship between the Ego of the anorexic and the level of reality. If the problem is framed in this way, as Bruch does, thus following the general lines of Ego-Psychology, even if this version is completely updated and enriched by the contributions of the Kohutian psychology of the Self and the clinical and epistemological instruments of the attachment theory, the treatment becomes a normalizing and restorative operation of a fragile ego and its deficits. And this is within a therapeutic relationship which is offered as an alternative to a maternal interactional modality which would have proved incongruous for the subject.

From the Lacanian perspective, if the anorexic has an altered perception of his relationship with the reality of their own body, with their external image as well as the proprioceptive sensations coming from the organism, it is because something has not intervened in the process of signifying constitution of the young girl's or boy's body. In other words, the degree of alteration of the Ego is the structured effect of a problematic signifying inscription of the body of the subject who will become anorexic. This means, in this logic, shifting the strategic axis of the question and the treatment of anorexia from the relationship between the Ego and reality to the relationship between the symbolic Other and the drive body of the subject. It is precisely the taking of the symbolic Other on the body of the subject, which encounters a special difficulty in the clinic of anorexia nervosa. It is the process that Lacan calls *signifying embodiment*, an operation through which the jouissance that invades the body of the child finds its regulation, which is lacking in the subject who, at the crossroads of puberty, will trigger the symptom of mental anorexia. as a spontaneous attempt to repair this lack of signifying inscrip-tion. This is clinical evidence that Bruch herself encounters when she speaks of a "schizophrenic core" of anorexia nervosa, while distinguishing it from schizophrenia in the proper sense. Selvini Palazzoli will in turn insist, at the level of the differential diagnosis, by emphasizing that it is a "psychosis in its own right" (Selvini Palazzoli, 2006, p. 162), distinct from both schizophrenia and melancholia.

For this reason, in our opinion, Lacan reverses Bruch's perspective. At the heart of the fragility of the Ego of the anorexic one must recognize, in the perspective opened up by the French psychoanalyst, a precariousness of the symbolic action of the Other.

In this sense, the formula "refusal of the Other", created by Jacques-Alain Miller to define the position of the subject in the new forms of the symptom and in particular of anorexia nervosa, reveals a structural dimension of the anorexic refusal which does not should not be confused with the denial negativism of the anorexic's behavior. The Lacanian subversion in the field of anorexia nervosa consists, therefore, over all, in the fact of situating, in the anorexic subject, the refusal of the Other in the core of the Ego.

Note

1   The use of the term "heresy" is not metaphorical here, but used by these same authors to define their clinical practice in relation to that which dominated in the 1950s and 1960s (Bruch, 1990, p. 14), or at least it is made manifest, in the case of Selvini Palazzoli, by the abandonment of psychoanalysis and the adherence to systemic-family therapy. In the case of Lacan, let us recall the "excommunication" that involved the expulsion from the IPA and the foundation of a new school of psychoanalysis.

References

Abraham, K. (1977), *Esquisse d'une histoire du développement de la libido fondé sur la psychanalyse des troubles mentaux (1916). Oeuvres completes.* Paris: Payot, II.

Bruch, H. (1978), *Les yeux et le ventre: l'obèse, l'anorexique.* Paris: Payot; *Eating Disorders: Obesity, Anorexia nervosa, and the Person Within* (1973). New York: Basic Books.

Bruch, H. (1979), *L'enigme d el'anorexie: la cage doré.* Paris: PUF; *The Golden Cage: the Enigma of the Anorexia Nervosa* (1978). Cambridge, Massachusetts: Harvard University Press.

Bruch, H. (1990), *Conversations avec des anorexiques.* Paris: Payot; *Conversations with Anorexics* (1988). New York: Basic Books.

Brusset, B. (1998), *Psychopathologie de l'anorexie mentale.* Paris: Dunod.

Corcos, M. (2005), *Le corps absent: approche psychosomatique des troubles des conduits alimentaires.* Paris: Dunod.

Freud, S. (1957), *Étude sur la melancolie dans le manuscrit G (1895). La naissance de la psychanalyse (1887–1902).* Paris: PUF, pp. 91–97.

Freud, S. (1987), *Trois essais sul la théorie sexuelle (1905).* Paris: Gallimard.

Freud, S. (1968), *Deuil et mélancolie (1915). Méthapsychologie.* Paris: Gallimard, pp. 65–121.

Lacan, J. (2006), *The Direction of the Treatment. Écrits: The First Complete Edition in English.* New York & London: Norton & Company, pp. 489–542; *La direction de la cure et les principes de son pouvoir (1958). Écrits* (1966). Paris: Éditions du Seuil.

Ménard, A. (1992), Structure signifiante de l'anorexie mentale. *Actes ECF*, no. 2, pp. 3–7.

Selvini Palazzoli, M. (2006), *L'anoressia mentale: dalla terapia individuale alla terapia familiare (1981)*. Milano: Cortina.

Selvini Palazzoli, M., and others (1978), *Paradoxe et contre-paradoxe (1970)*. Paris: ESF.

Selvini Palazzoli, M., and others (1998), *Ragazze anoressiche e bulimiche*. Milano: Cortina.

Chapter 3

The anorexic question in psychoanalysis between narcissism and dependence

Anorexia, primary narcissism and dependence: two current versions of the post-Freudian object-relationship paradigm

From the perspective of theoretical-clinical research on the psychoanalytical bases of anorexia, two lines of research within the framework of post-Freudiansm, currently in force, seem much more interesting to us. One goes back to the beginning of the 1970s in France and developed, within the framework of psychoanalytical child psychiatry, in public psychiatric institutions working in particular with adolescents, and its protagonists referred to the psychoanalytic schools of the International Psychoanalytical Association (IPA). The key authors were undoubtedly Evelyne and Jean Kestemberg, Bernard Brusset and Philippe Jeammet, the latter having headed the Department of Adolescent and Young Adult Psychiatry at the Institut Mutualiste Montsouris in Paris, where he carried out his clinical institutional practice with anorexic and bulimic patients. The psychoanalytical roots of the work of these authors can be found in the framework of a "French-style" reformulation of the Kleinian paradigm of object-relation theory, which includes within it the contributions of Winnicott, and which on certain points, particularly in Brusset, partially reflects the influence of Lacan's teaching. The second, on the other hand, was developed more recently. It is situated directly in the tradition of Anglo-Saxon psychoanalysis and in particular in the Kleinian-Bionian perspective. It also introduces a key clinical institution, the Tavistock Clinic in London, where in 1987 the psychoanalyst Gianna Polacco Williams founded, alongside the "Adolescent Department", the "Eating Disorders Workshop".

Narcissism and drug addiction: anorexia-bulimia in French psychoanalytical child psychiatry

The perspective of the Kestembergs: anorexia and the orgasm of hunger

This seam of psychoanalytical research on anorexia nervosa stems from the work of Evelyne and Jean Kestemberg and Simone Decobert on *La faim et le*

DOI: 10.4324/9781003318439-4

corps ("Hunger and the Body"). Published in 1972, and revised and updated in the following years, this work introduces important restructuring within the framework of an analytical-psychogenetic-evolutionary paradigm of anorexia. First of all, it shifts the fundamental peak of the anorexic question from the stadial-drive dimension to the narcissistic dimension. More than the anchorage to a fixation of the libido at the sadistic-oral stage of the drive, the strategic heart of the anorexic question can be seen rather in a "hypertrophic functioning of the Ego ideal" (Kestemberg and others, 1981, p. 144) which is realized in a megalomaniac ideal of control and mastery, exercised in particular by the anorexic on their own body. A megalomaniacal ideal counterbalanced by a real narcissistic deficiency of the Ego, a lacunary structuring of its organization (ibid., p. 177), the effect of a deficient narcissistic contribution on the part of the mother in the girl's childhood.

It is in the service of this megalomaniacal narcissistic ideal that the oral and anal libidinal satisfaction of the anorexic – linked to control and mastery – finds for these authors its *raison d'être*. Second, a fundamental autoerotism (ibid., p. 187), which passes not so much through masturbatory sexuality but rather through narcissistic gratification linked to hyper-invested activities like studies, motor skills and control of the hunger instinct, underlies their libidinal economy, where a narcissistic ideal of autonomy, often fascinating for the parents and transmitted by them, takes the place of an absence of sexual life and investments in the bonds of love.

Third, if the anorexic subject presents, alongside massive narcissistic investments, an extreme poverty and fragility of objectual relations (ibid., p. 201), for these authors, this is due to the fact of having been put by the parents, in particular by the mother, more in the place of an object of complete narcissism of his/her Self than in the place of a subject of desire other than Self (ibid., p. 130). In this sense, the clinic of anorexia nervosa presents itself for these authors as a clinic of primary narcissism and of the specular relationship which tends toward fusion and non-separation between the daughter and maternal desire. The mother tends to configure herself in the fantasy scenes of the daughter as an all-powerful and fundamentally asexual object, and the father presents himself as "maternized" (ibid., p. 124), more as completely narcissistic toward the mother than as a differentiated partner. The parental couple therefore often presents itself as a fusion: It is not internally differentiated and therefore incapable of representing for the girl the articulation of the difference between the sexes.

It is in the evolutionary passage through the period of adolescence that most often there emerges the anorexic response of the subject, which presents itself, for these authors, as a massive regression faced with an impossible access to genitality revealing a structural framework to be situated in a territory which cannot be traced back to neurosis and hysteria (ibid., p. 139). What is indeed present in anorexia, for these authors, is, in Kleinian terms, a refusal of the passage from the schizoparanoid position to the depressive position, a refusal of incorporation and introjection (ibid., p. 142) and an anchoring of the subject to a fundamentally projective functioning. For this reason, the division of the subject does not present itself neurotically as the product of repression which makes possible an interrogation on one's desire; rather, it takes the form of a splitting of the Self (ibid., p. 138) that brings to life the organization of a massive false Self. This split is situated in structural terms more on the slope of a psychotic organization of a non-delusional form – Evelyne Kestemberg would subsequently develop the clinic theory of cold psychoses, more precisely in a territory-bridge between non-delusional psychoses and a perverse structure. This is where another point of originality in the work developed in *La faim et le corps* lies: the valorization, alongside the narcissistic vector, of the perverse-fetishist dimension at play in anorexia (Bonifati, 2006, pp. 178–181).

It is no coincidence that for the Kestembergs, it is the Freud of narcissism and fetishism that is missing as a reference in the classic reading of anorexia developed in the evolutionary-drive paradigm. Indeed, the clinical originality of anorexia, which characterizes its specific functioning, is attributed precisely to the perverse solution that is found by the subject, in particular around the theme of the narcissistically invested body. It is this solution which basically marks for these authors the difference of anorexia compared to the psychotic framework of the melancholic type: the anorexic subject does not present themselves as melancholy, as petrified in the past; on the contrary, he exercises a negation of the past, and he is thrown forward in a megalomaniacal way (Kestemberg and others, 1981, p. 175). They do not see the seriousness of their bodily condition and project themselves egosyntonically into exhausting intellectual and physical performances from which they derive a narcissistic satisfaction. Anorexia presents itself, in other words, as a split not only of the ego, but also of the body. A split between an ideal body and a real body, the first narcissistically invested as a fetish; the second, the body proper, but above all the body inhabited by the drive pleasure, refused and subjected to a frenzied denial (ibid., pp. 189–190).

The perverse solution embodied by anorexia finds its most original point of expression for the authors in their reading of the theme of anorexic refusal of food. The authors do not make it a question strategically anchored in the drive field of orality. On the contrary, for them anorexia constitutes a libidinal regression which does not find its fundamental localization points in the coordinates of the erogenous zones (ibid., p. 149). Indeed, they read anorexic refusal as an experience that libidinally invests the body of the subject as a whole, to which they give the name of "orgasm" of hunger. In this cardinal experience of jouissance which is at the base of the refusal of food, the perverse solution at the base of anorexia reveals in its purest form its own radical imbrication with primary masochism and the death drive. The hunger orgasm is the effect of "a massive eroticization of the rejection" of food and "the pleasure of functioning from this rejection" (ibid., p. 200). This ultimately leads to a de-erotization of the oral zone as an erogenous zone in the strict sense, because there is no longer pleasure in food but the pleasure generated by the refusal of food. This special form of auto-eroticism, which is embodied in the pleasure of the sensation of hunger, is irreducible and calls into question for the authors "what could have been thought until today about the disgust aroused by food" (ibid., p. 187):

> This disgust, taken for a reactive formation, directly expresses the desire and the pleasure obtained, because in fact what the patients seek is hunger which leads to orgasm. We are also tempted to make this quest for hunger a specific sign of adolescent anorexia nervosa.
>
> (ibid., pp. 188–189)

The authors, therefore, make irreducible the anorexic refusal of food to hysterical disgust at food, metaphorically linked to the sexual desire of the subject and to his relationship with the desire of the Other who procures it. The "fascination for the state of emptiness" that we find strongly in anorexic patients is strictly correlated to the orgasm of hunger, whose research demonstrates the libidinal basis that supports the practices of emptying the body that we find in anorexia-bulimia such as vomiting and the use of laxatives (ibid., p. 188).

Anorexia as endogenous drug addiction by Bernard Brusset

Bernard Brusset's theoretical-clinical research on the foundations of anorexia nervosa, which developed from the second half of the 1970s, takes up the legacy of *La faim et le corps*, but at the same time it introduces innovations and important corrections compared to the theses which are already contained there. The fundamental thesis supported by Brusset as the guideline of his research is rendered by the conception "of anorexia nervosa as a process that must be situated in its relationship with bulimia, whether or not there is a passage to the bulimic act" (Brusset, 1998, p. 2). Brusset, therefore, presents himself as the theoretician of anorexia-bulimia, understood as a dynamic process supported by the same logic of functioning which oscillates between the two polarities of anorexia and bulimia. Beyond the phenomenological evidence which demonstrates how the majority of cases of anorexia fall into the bulimic transition, it is the logic of psychodynamic functioning which leads Brusset to support the relevance of thinking about the anorexic restriction in its structural relationship to the bulimic tipping and vice versa, in a closed circuit economic operation. The fear of bulimic tipping runs through the anorexic condition just as the megalomaniac ideal of control over the drive, typical of anorexia, is always on the horizon in a superegoic way, for the bulimic who is driven to find it again and again through bodily evacuation practices, vomiting, use of laxatives, frenzied motor skills (Brusset, 1991, pp. 105–132).

The thesis of anorexia-bulimia allows Brusset an important reformulation of the theoretical-clinical position of the Kestembergs which allows him to value what he defines as a drug-maniacal-addictive quality internal to the anorexico-bulimic circuit. If on the one hand, bulimia, according to Fénichel's definition of "drug-free addiction", "responds directly to the criteria for defining addiction with reference to constraint, repetition, slavery, excluding the effects particularities of the product", "the connection with anorexia nervosa of the restrictive type is obviously more debatable, but is not without justification, including from the point of view of risk behavior, defiance, denial or that of the quest for identity" (Brusset, 1998, p. 160). It is from this observation and from recent research on the neurophysiological foundations of anorexia which support this thesis, that Brusset welds the theme of anorexic refusal to the dimension of drug addictive enjoyment through the thesis of anorexia as endogenous drug addiction.

Indeed, while on the one hand, the anorexic position of refusal of satisfactions embodies a counter-drug addiction attitude that is realized in valiant defense of appetite perceived as "drug addiction"; on the other, it realizes, precisely in this operation of defense of satisfaction, a special and incessantly sought enjoyment whose effectiveness is confirmed by the data of biology – the increase in endorphins and the euphoric effect which is produced at following the practice of prolonged fasting – and which he defines as endogenous drug addiction (ibid.).

The dimension of jouissance functions for Brusset as a crucial point of articulation of the relationship with drug addiction. This is demonstrated by the disinvestment of other sources of satisfaction, primarily genital sexuality, and the overinvestment of satisfaction in action in the addictive process of drug consumption in the addict, refusal of food in its restrictive or bulimic form (devoring followed by evacuation). On this point, Brusset's analysis is in line with Abraham's classic indication, which united addiction to toxic substances and food pathologies in the common matrix of the refusal of genital sexuality, and of an autoerotic jouissance regression to the primary orality which takes its place. Moreover, the thesis of the addictive dimension at stake in anorexia, in the anorexic jouissance produced by the refusal, is identifiable in the process of anorexia, in particular in the phase of egosyntonic optimism – comparable to the honeymoon with the addict's drug according to Olivenstein's formula – where the anorexic experiences in the body the euphoric effects of his behavior of prolonged fasting. But also in the next phase where "objective self-destruction" and the risk of death reveal their common masochistic foundation (ibid., p. 161). In this respect Philippe Jeammet, who endorses and promotes the Brussettian thesis of the addictive dimension at stake in anorexia-bulimia (Jeammet, 1989, pp. 179–202), speaks of a "drug addict" type self-reinforcement mechanism pivoted on refusal and whose dual function is the control of fundamental affects and the "defense against the fear of not being able to do without the other, of being invaded by the latter" (Jeammet, 2006, p. 35).

Brusset, therefore, presents himself in a relationship of continuity, but also of rupture with respect to the work of the Kestembergs. The line of continuity appears, above all, in the perspective of epistemological-clinical background, where anorexia nervosa most often occurs as an arrest in psycho-sexual development at the crossroads of the passage from adolescence and as a regression to the pregenital and preoedipal dimension of the primary specular relation to the maternal object. This process is also characterized for Brusset by "a deadly narcissistic regression in which are manifested, to varying degrees, unbinding, negative narcissism and the auto-erotism of death" (Brusset, 1998, p. 222). He thus demonstrates that he assumes and develops the central theme for the Kestembergs of narcissism and auto-eroticism in their deadly version as supporting factors of anorexic functioning. The theme of anorexia as a pathology of "failures of narcissistic regulation" indeed constitutes the main axis of the continuity of clinical research on the anorexia of French psychoanalytical child psychiatry from Kestemberg to Brusset, up to the current work of Philippe Jeammet (1989, pp. 81–104) and Maurice Corcos (Corcos, 2010, p. 15).

Another point of continuity in Brusset's research with respect to the authors of *La faim et le corps* is that of conceiving of anorexia as a pathology which is situated on the structural level beyond neurosis, and which is characterized by a fundamentally anti-hysterical functioning (Brusset, 1998, p. 90). He does not share the importance that these authors attribute to perversion and tends rather to recover a centrality of the melancholic structure (ibid., p. 144) in continuity with Freud and Abraham, in many anorexias. That said, as far as the problem of structure is concerned, there remains with Brusset, as in all the evolutionary declensions of psychoanalysis and therefore also in the current versions of Kleinism, the possibility, as we observe in some clinical cases that he describes, that a subject with a psychotic organization can arrive at a neurotization of his position thanks to the analytic work. However, the points of discontinuity with respect to the Kestemberg approach turn out to be considerable. Above all, the importance attributed to the addictive-drug addiction dimension of anorexia-bulimia gives a new balance to the accentuation of the narcissistic side present in *La faim et le corps*, which however also maintains its centrality in Brusset. It is no coincidence for the author if the refusal produced by the drug-maniacal-addictive quality of anorexic jouissance is at the same time in anorexia the maneuver of the subject to seek to rediscover a feeling of identity and self-existence (ibid., p. 99). The paradox that anorexic refusal embodies here, already well circumscribed by the Kestembergs, is that the subject manages in anorexia to refuse desire in order to keep alive a narcissistic identity that is ideally autonomous, but in reality deeply rooted in a primary fusional relationship with the ideal mother. A relationship in which there is no place in maternal desire for the girl's subjectivity, but only the possibility for her to function as the double or narcissistic completion of the maternal imago.

It is thus within the framework of a narcissistic-addictive circuit that for Brusset the economy of autarkic enjoyment at stake in anorexia-bulimia is structured, the beginning of which sanctions the failure for the subject of the assumption of genital sexuality and the female position at the crossroads of puberty. In Kleinian terms, it reveals the infantile failure of introjection as a condition for passing from the schizoparanoid position to the depressive position which makes object loss and the work of symbolic repair possible. The shift in emphasis introduced by Brusset can be symbolized by the different rewriting of a famous phrase from Freud's *Mourning and Melancholy* to define the melancholic position – "the shadow of the object has fallen on the Ego" – used to signify in a formula his own reading of the key problem embodied by anorexia. In *La faim et le corps*, the sentence is "The shadow of the ego ideal invades the ego", where by the ego ideal we really mean the ideal ego of primary narcissism, the specular adhesion of the subject to the maternal image. On the other hand, the formula used by Brusset is the following: "The shadow of the object has fallen on the body" (ibid., p. 91), where the emphasis is placed on the primary object which parasitizes the body of the anorexic by rendering inoperative the process of separation-individuation.

Finally, we find in Brusset a partial consideration of the Lacanian approach in the reading of anorexia nervosa, within the framework of one of the four dimensions at stake in the perspective of development: the dimension centered on the "failures of paternal function". In this regard, Brusset highlights that for anorexia too, "as in drug addiction and in perversions, a partial foreclosure of the Name-of-the-Father is invoked" (ibid., p. 88), but he limits himself to sketching out this reference without making it his own and without deepening it.

The Kleinian-Bionian perspective in the field of anorexia and bulimia: the Tavistock experience of Gianna Polacco Williams

While, in the post-Kleinian reading produced by French psychoanalytical child psychiatry, the accent is placed on the double polarity of narcissistic deregulation and the drug-addictive libidinal circuit, the approach to anorexia formulated by G. Polacco-Williams and his collaborators at the Tavistock Clinic in London focuses on the theme of refusing dependency on others. It is in these terms that the author formulates the central axis on which their own theoretical-clinical research focuses: "The difficulty of 'taking from another', of internalizing a relationship of dependence", questioned here "in the context of the psychopathology of eating behavior" (Polacco Williams, 1999, p. 1). From this perspective, unlike the French authors who have most often questioned the clinic of anorexia and bulimia in the context of adolescence, the work of Polacco-Williams also extends, as directly testified by different clinical cases, to childhood to question the "relationship between the difficulties of internalization in the sphere of dependent relationships and the concrete nature of the problems related to the absorption of food" (ibid.). Indeed, a work coordinated by her is entirely devoted to this subject: *The Generosity of Acceptance. Exploring Feeding Difficulties in Children* (Williams and others, 2006).

Polacco Williams' approach is oriented by the reformulation of Kleinian theory translated into the thought of Bion, which mathematically formalizes the primary fantasy dynamics at play in the child-mother relationship, the mechanism of projective identification that characterizes it, as well as the passage from the schizoparanoid position to the depressive position. We know that Bion describes the unfolding of this passage by resorting to an analogy belonging to the field of food: it is a question of a veritable metabolism of thought, within which the mother plays the key role in that it has the function of welcoming, metabolizing and returning to the child in a pre-digested way these fragmented, chaotic and disorganized experiences that go through them and that they are not able, on their own, to metabolize. In the Bionian formalization, the beta elements are constituted by bizarre, chaotic, fragmentary and disintegrating contents which pass through the child and which they direct, through the mechanism of projective identification, toward the mother. The latter has the duty, first of all, to welcome these beta elements in themselves, and this is where her function as a psychic recipient of the child's anxieties of fragmentation lies. Moreover, through the exercise of the alpha function, which gives rise to the work of maternal reverie, the mother has the essential duty to transform these bizarre elements into metabolizable elements, and to return them to the child in a digestible form of their thought. It is within the framework of a failure of the maternal metabolization work of the child's projections, in a failure of the exercise of reception and the operation of symbolization exerted by the alpha function, that for Polacco Williams we must locate the origin of many cases of "Eating disorders", and in particular of anorexia and bulimia. It is effectively in response to this primary failure of the symbolic-metabolic function of the mother that the refusal to take from the other, to internalize a relationship of dependence, occurs.

This is indeed what the author maintains, giving as an example the commentary on a case of a child, Robert, who from birth had developed a refusal of food, in the first place, from the maternal breast, followed by a clear refusal of the feeding bottle and food. The mother, whose position has been reconstructed on the basis of experiences of "infant observation" by pupils of the Tavistock (observation of the mother/child interaction in the context of domestic life, according to the qualitative method developed by Ester Bick and Martha Harris (Francesconi, Scotto Di Fasano, 2009)), consistently experiences Robert's denial behavior as a challenge to her, and it prevents her from empathizing with her situation, from making sense of it. As Polacco Williams points out, we find here a failure of the container function. If the mother (the container) is not able to empathically accept the sensations and emotions which for the child are overwhelming and devoid of meaning, if she is unable to exercise the function of metabolizing the projections made significant in their head, these remain un-elaborated, indigestible for the child and they are returned to them as a "terror without a name" (Polacco Williams, 1999, p. 80).

This failure in the exercise of the alpha function is characterized first of all by a "reversal of the relationship between container and content" which emerges in the clinical experience of the mother/child relationship, where the mother, unable to function as a container of projections of the child, projects her own persecutory anxieties onto the child, putting it in the position of becoming the receptacle of maternal projections. This problem, verifiable "especially in cases where the parents of the patients are psychotic or borderline" (ibid., p. 89) finds a particular response in patients who develop food pathologies. They become not only the receptacle of external projections because of the failure of maternal reverie but of the contents coming from outside, in the first place; the maternal projections end up by assuming for the subject the status of "foreign bodies" whose subject feels overwhelmed. It seems clear that Polacco Williams moves in the field of a conceptualization of food pathologies beyond the hysterico-neurotic framework, where the proximity with psychosis appears clearly on the horizon, even if the instance of a difference which does not completely reabsorb the field of anorexia in the psychotic structure is maintained. For example, by comparing the case of a psychotic patient with eating problems to that of an anorexic adolescent, she introduces a clear distinction around the theme of the invasion of their body by foreign objects between the delusional creation of the first and the nightmare of the second.

In both cases, the fear, or even the terror, of something hostile that "enters" is experienced in a very concrete way. In the 17-year-old anorexic, it took the form of nightmares where every orifice of the body was invaded by tadpoles. In the psychotic little girl treated 20 years earlier, there was the concrete delusion of fleas which penetrated each orifice. Both patients suffered from severe eating disorders, and today I believe that in both cases one of the factors that contributed to the psychopathology was the early experience of being a receptacle for parental projections (ibid., p. 4).

To this fundamental organization of the relationship with the other, correspond specific responses that come into play in patients who develop anorexia and bulimia. In the first place, especially in cases of anorexia, Polacco Williams develops a conceptualization that offers us an interesting contribution in the direction of a reading of anorexic refusal as a defense in relation to another intrusive. Clinical experience with patients used as a receptacle for parental projections develops as a response what she calls an "access defense" syndrome (Polacco Williams, 1997, pp. 927–941), where in the absence of an internalized symbolic boundary the subject compensates by constructing a boundary that is exteriorized in a system of behaviors of refusal of the link, and in "symptoms of inaccessibility" (Polacco Williams, 1999, p. 106). Indeed, "the 'forbidden access' syndrome exercises the defensive function of blocking the entrance to each input felt potentially as intrusive and persecuting" (ibid.). An example that Polacco Williams presents and that we have personally noted in the discourse of many anorexic patients is the anxiety of the telephone ringing, which presents another invasion from which we must defend ourselves. They react, in general, by not answering the call, or by un-plugging the telephone.

The analogous operation is carried out by anorexic patients toward food, through refusal as a modality of defense against an object that contains all the basic difficulties that the subject has encountered with the maternal object, which could not have been internalized as a good object, but has maintained a persecutory connotation from which we must defend ourselves. What happens, on the other hand, in bulimia, according to the hypothesis of Polacco Williams, is that the body of the subject is invaded by projections (product of parents who "project anxiety instead of containing it" (ibid., p. 111)), now within it a par-asitic object which exercises a function antithetical to that of Bion's alpha function, and which is defined as an omega function (ibid., pp. 111–112). This is a disintegrating and disorganizing function, to which the bulimic patient tries to respond by refusing, through the evacuation behaviors typical of acting out (vomiting, use of laxatives, etc.), for the lack of a space that allows separation and takes the path of symbolization.

The "triangulation failure" (Williams and others, 2006, p. 8) in the child-hood experience of anorexia, the symptomatic effects of which manifest themselves in "continual attacks on paternal function" (ibid., p. 9) within the framework of the mother/daughter relationship, plays an important role in the work of Polacco Williams. The author establishes a clear distinction between the paternal function and the identification with the person of the father, defining the first as a third element that constitutes the existing space within the mother/daughter dyad. Indeed, she affirms:

> In a relationship between two people, a dyadic relationship, there is always a third element, namely the space existing between them, whereas in a mental state of fusion this space is absent. Thus, the dyadic relation is, in fact, always a triadic relation and the third element is constituted by the space existing between the subject and the object.
>
> (ibid., p. 23)

What happens in anorexia is that this "transitional" third space between mother and daughter is cramped and threatened by a thrust of fusion that the subject seeks and fears at the same time. This is achieved at the same time, by the anorexic, through a work of neutralization and weakening of the real bond internal to the couple of parents, aiming to keep the mother/daughter dyad compact in order to avoid the anxiety of separation that the recognition of the paternal function entails in the relationship of the subject with their mother. In this context, through a resumption of the terms of the second Freudian topic, we are witnessing a caricature of the paternal function operated by a cruel superego – in the formula of Bion, a "self-destroying superego" – embodied by absolutist morality and a disordered characteristic of the narcissistic mother/daughter dyad, whose destructive thrust mimics the elimination of the slightest third element which hinders the fusion (ibid., p. 15).

References

Bonifati, S. (2006), L'anoressia-bulimia nei modelli psicoanalitici contemporanei, Cosenza, Recalcati, Villa (dir.), *Civiltà e disagio. Forme contemporanee della psicopatologia.* Milano: Bruno Mondadori, pp. 164–194.

Brusset, B. (1991), Psychopathologie et métapsychologie de l'addition boulimique. *La boulimie, Revue Française de Psychoanalyse.* Paris: PUF, pp. 105–132.

Brusset, B. (1998), *Psychopatologie de l'anorexie mentale.* Paris: Dunot.

Corcos, M. (2010), *Le corps absent: approche psychosomatique des troubles des conduites alimentaires (2005).* Paris: Dunot.

Francesconi, M., Scotto Di Fasano, D. (Dir.) (2009), *Apprendere dal bambino: riflessioni a partire dall'Infant Observation.* Roma: Borla.

Jeammet, P. (1989), Psychopathologie des troubles des conduite alimentaires. Valeur heuristique du concept de dépendence. *Confrontations psychiatriques,* no. 31, pp. 179–202.

Jeammet, P. (2006), *Anoressia e bulimia.* Milano: Franco Angeli; *Anorexie et boulimie: les paradoxes de l'adolescence* (2004). Paris: Hachette.

Kestemberg, J., Kestemberg, E., Decobert, S. (1981), *La faim et le corps: une étude psychanalytique de l'anorexie mentale (1972).* Paris: PUF.

Polacco Williams, G. (1997), Reflections on some dynamics of eating disorders: "no entry" defences and foreign bodies. *International Journal of Psychoanalysis,* vol. 78, pp. 927–941.

Polacco Williams, G. (1999), *Paesaggi interni e corpi estranei: disordini alimentari e altre patologie.* Milano: Bruno Mondadori; *Internal Landscapes and Foreign Bodies* (1997). London: Karnac Books.

Williams, G. and others (2006), *La difficoltà di alimentazione nei bambini.* Milano: Bruno Mondadori; *The Generosity of Acceptance: exploring feeding difficulties in children* (2004). London: Karnak Books.

Chapter 4

Anorexia in Lacan's teaching

The revival of Freud's lesson: anorexia and structure

After this excursus around the most advanced perspectives internal to the neo-Kleinian evolutionary paradigm of anorexia nervosa, the transition to the approach of Lacan and his School is presented above all in the form of a transition to a structural paradigm of the psychoanalytic clinic. A passage that also represents a return to Freud, not only as the discoverer of the functioning of the unconscious as a signifying structure and the Oedipus complex as a structural crossroads in the process of constituting subjectivity. In particular, in the light of Lacan's teaching which developed from the beginning of the 1960s, the return to Freud is a return to the structure of the subject at the point inaccessible to the signifier which characterizes their mode of enjoyment (jouissance). This expression translates the functioning beyond the pleasure principle traversing the libidinal economy, isolated by Freud in his writing of 1920. The Lacanian clinic is, in this sense, a structural clinic, in the sense that it succeeds in isolating the position of the subject by reconstructing it in the light of its singular relation to the structure: to the Other, as a signifying system (historical-linguistic-familial) within which its existence is written, and to jouissance as an irreducible modality of satisfaction inhabited by a self-destructive entropic drive (what Freud eventually defines as *Todestrieb*). The Lacanian interrogation on anorexia thus revolves around this dimension that constitutes the structure of the subject, and its narcissistic-specular organization, as well as the system of practices and rituals which characterize anorexic behaviors are attached to this same structure of which they are constituted; and this, within the framework of the analytical work as well as in the clinical and theoretical construction.

This epistemological perspective has multiple consequences on the clinical level, and shows its incommensurability, despite the many interesting points of contact at the level of psychopathological and therapeutic phenomenology, compared to the analytical approaches of anorexia of an evolutionary matrix, linked to neo-Kleinian contributions, that we have already briefly quoted.

DOI: 10.4324/9781003318439-5

First, in the perspective of an evolutionary continuum, the structure presents itself in the genesis of each subject in terms of scansion in the arc of development, which progresses, going from its most primitive forms (the psychoses) to the most structured forms (neuroses), while having "psychic normality" as the ideal perspective. Lacan's perspective operates an "epistemological reversal" of this evolutionary scheme: it invites us, in other words, to think about the development of a subject from the effective possibilities internal to the structure that is specific to them. Rather than an evolution of the structure, Lacan invites us to think in terms of a "structural theory of the singular development of the subject". In this sense, the psychopathological exordium of anorexia, for example, is not conceived in terms of an evolutionary "breakdown" during development, but as a manifestation of the position of the subject, whose effective value must be identified at the level of the unconscious structure.

This has the consequence, second, that in the Lacanian perspective, anorexia constitutes a clinical phenomenon which can take on the character of a stable position, but is not in itself the index of a structure.

In this sense, Lacan's position on the question of structure in anorexia is a return to the position of Freud who, in his work, identified forms of anorexia of the hysterical type as well as psychotic anorexias of a melancholic matrix (Brusset, 1998, p. 1; Soria, 2000, pp. 28–29).

Although they do not fall into the temptation to attach anorexia to a single matrix, the continuing-evolutionary approaches of today, nevertheless feel the epistemological effects of their position, in the "substantial symptomatic disappearance of hysteria from their structural frames of reference for anorexia". Psychoses, perversions, "borderline" personalities, borderline states: here, as we have seen, is the structural frame of reference of the most advanced neo-Kleinian theories of anorexia, which – also because of the growing use of the "borderline" category of organization, underlined by Christopher Bollas (2001), which in the Lacanian perspective remains a phenomenological framework that confuses the structure more than it constitutes its own – erase the reference to hysterical anorexia, considering hysteria as a structure too evolved to be able to be represented by the anorexic symptom.

Third, if anorexia, in the continuing-evolutionary perspective, presents itself as a halt in the course of development, which manifests itself, for example, in adolescence by referring, in the neo-Kleinian perspective, to the absence of passage or an incomplete passage of the subject from the schizoparanoid position to the depressive position, the analytic treatment will function, through the analyst, as a stable and reliable container of the patient's projections; like the work of repairing the narcissistic deficiencies of the subject's ego, in the perspective of a completion of its passage – through the relation of transference with the analyst as a sufficiently good object in whom it is possible to entrust oneself – to the depressive position. In this sense, the treatment would effect a sort of evolutionary transformation of the structure, neuroticizing – in the passage to the depressive position – a subject who was not. In Lacan's structural perspective, it is impossible to change the structure, understood as the very stuff of which the subject is made. On the other hand, what is possible and what tends to be done in analytic treatment is to lead the subject to assume their own structure and to inhabit it in the most satisfactory way possible for them. This absolutely does not mean leading him to assume a depressive position of resignation to the determinism of the unconscious. The contrary is true, if we consider that the structure retains in itself a margin that cannot be fully structured by the signifying system, which precisely constitutes the space of the subject open to contingent and unpredictable encounters with something real that can change the course of its existence. It is in this sense that Lacan speaks, in his Seminar, Book XI, of the "unrealized" unconscious (Lacan, 1973, p. 31), as something that concerns above all the future of the subject, rather than his past.

Historical-critical preliminary to a Lacanian theory of anorexia

One Lacanian reading of anorexia nervosa that does not claim to be "innocent", in the sense attributed to this expression by Louis Althusser (Althusser, Balibar, 1968, p. 17) has its origins in the textual stratification previously carried out in this field with regard to anorexia. I would like to briefly address this question here, without aspiring to an ideal of exhaustiveness, and only in an attempt to trace the essential lines within the framework of which this reading – and in the very first place my reading – was produced.

In the first place, the "text of Lacan", in particular his writings and the published and unpublished transcriptions of his oral lessons, that is to say the text of his Seminars and his conferences. The Lacanian theory of anorexia is therefore above all the theory of anorexia, explicit or able to be deduced implicitly, and which can be identified directly from the text of Lacan.

We know that Lacan never entirely devoted writing or a lesson to this theme. Its references to the question of anorexia are rare and are found in a few specific textual articulations, where the reference to anorexia has no value as such, but serves, each time, to clarify a specific point of its current theoretical-clinical construction. In this sense, the elaboration of a theory of anorexia in Lacan is above all the realization of a linking, a tension, of the different affirmations concerning anorexia, always keeping in mind some epistemological conjunctures that occur in the different texts where these statements appear.

Lacan's four paradigms on anorexia

Lacan's main references to anorexia are found in four precise articulations of his production, in moments of his theoretical-clinical elaboration that are not homogeneous but rather epistemologically discontinuous between them, and which can be summarized as follows:

The *psychogenetic-regressive paradigm* in **Family Complexes**

Lacan's first original references to anorexia can be found in the 1938 text *Les complèxes familiaux dans la formation de l'individu*, written at the time at the request of Henry Wallon for the French Encyclopedia. The text, written by a Lacan who was a psychiatrist and still a young psychoanalyst, but already conquered by the teaching of Freud, is an attempt at psychogenetic reconstruction, strongly impregnated by the influence of the work of Mélanie Klein, by the passages of the complexes (complex weaning, intrusion and Oedipus) which establish the psychic constitution of the subject. It is within the problems of this Lacan, defined by Miller as "prestructuralist" (Miller, 2005, pp. 33–51), that the reference to anorexia is profiled around four fundamental nodes.

Weaning, psychic trauma, anorexia nervosa

Anorexia is presented here as one of the effects, alongside oral drug addiction and gastric neuroses, of weaning as "psychic trauma" (Lacan, 2001, p. 31). It is the "refusal of weaning" (ibid., p. 32) that reveals the stubborn fixation of the subject to the primary oral object, represented in this conceptual context by the primordial form of the "maternal imago" (ibid., p. 30). Anorexia manifests a failure in going through the Oedipus complex, a fixation with the original maternal imago and a nostalgic regression of the subject which is realized through anorexic pathology, toward fusion with the mythical object of primary jouissance.

Maternal imago, death appetite and anorexia

The maternal imago is therefore transformed, in this context, from "originally salutary" to "death factor" (ibid., p. 35) because it resists and works against the psychogenetic development of the subject. Anorexia is connoted here by a "fundamental appetite for death", which effectively brings it closer, as has been underlined, more to the framework of melancholy indicated by Freud, thus marking the non-dialectic-separative but rather "regressive-fusional" character of the pathological framework.

Anorexia, drug addiction, gastric neuroses: non-violent suicides

Anorexia, with its "hunger strike", presents itself, moreover, in continuity with the slow poisoning of oral drug addictions and the starvation diet of gastric neuroses, as a pathology of primary orality marked by an irresistible fusional push to the recovery of the experience of full enjoyment of the origin, and characterized by a self-destructive inclination which makes it one of the forms of non-violent suicide (ibid.). As Lacan writes, "the analysis of these cases shows that, in their abandonment to death, the subject seeks to rediscover the imago of the mother" (ibid.).

Lacan values here the intuition, already Freudian-Abrahamian, of an important clinical relationship that links anorexia and drug addiction, anorexia and psychosomatic disorder, an intuition later valued by Fenichel for bulimia and especially more recently by Brusset and Jeammet.

Anorexia and decline of the paternal imago

Anorexia finds its place in the historical-epochal context of contemporary civilization, characterized by a social decline of the "paternal" imago (ibid., p. 60) and in a family framework where the anorexic develops with the mother a relationship whose reference to the third function of the Oedipus complex does not intervene effectively, and is also characterized by a supremacy of the weaning complex which will condemn them "to repeat indefinitely the effort of detachment from the mother" (ibid., p. 82).

In other words, there seems to emerge from Lacan's text of 1938 the framework of a psychogenetic-regressive paradigm of anorexia which allows an articulation of the relationship of anorexia to the structural framework of melancholic psychoses.

The dialectical-hysterical paradigm in "The direction of the treatment"

We find the second scansion of Lacan's contributions on anorexia in the 1958 text, *The direction of the treatment and the principles of its power*, but there are also some other references in the seminars of this period, in particular in Books IV and V. We are here at the heart of the classic problem of the psychoanalyst and structuralist Lacan, built around the thesis of the "unconscious structured like a language", the primacy of the symbolic register and the field of the Other, and the pivotal function exercised within it by the signifier Name-of-the-Father. The text reflects this position at the level of the treatment, inviting the analyst to orient their position and their intervention in the treatment on the symbolic axis (on the signifying chain of the analysand's discourse) and not on the imaginary axis (on the meanings supported by the analysand's ego).

Within this theoretical framework, the reference to anorexia in the text revolves around a few important conceptual articulations, which can be summarized as follows:

• *Anorexia, need and desire*: anorexia is first understood by Lacan as the radical clinical embodiment of the structural irreducibility of desire to the register of need. The maneuver involved in the anorexic refusal of food carried to the extreme consequences of the risk of death is therefore read here by Lacan as the active operation of the subject to keep themselves alive alongside the Other as a desiring subject, even at the risk of their death as an organism affected by needs.

- *Anorexia and parental confusion of care with the gift of love*: the anorexia of the subject highlights a fundamental confusion in action with the parental Other, which the subject aims unconsciously to unmask and to highlight, to rectify: this subject, writes Lacan, "confuses the care it provides with the gift of his love" (Lacan, 2006, p. 524). In other words, the parents respond to the subject by scrupulously administering to them the care and the objects needed, remaining blind to the fundamental demand that animates his desire, which is fundamentally, like every demand, a demand for love. A request for a gift that is not an object of satisfaction, but a sign of the love of the Other for the subject. For this to happen, the Other must not fill the subject by administering to them the "asphyxiating porridge" of what they have, but rather they must offer them what they do not have, their lack, that is, their own love.

- *Anorexia, refusal and desire*: precisely in this perspective, the anorexic "employs his refusal as if it were a desire" (ibid.), or she/he makes the refusal function as an unconscious and mute request which challenges the Other to obtain the sign of love, the testimony of their desire for themselves.

- *Anorexia, thinness and phallus: the dream of the beautiful butcher* (ibid., pp. 518–524): this reference arises in the context of Lacan's commentary on Freud's dream of the beautiful butcher, in which the protagonist's renunciation of eating her favorite food is read as a modality, fundamentally hysterical, whose aim is to maintain unsatisfied desire by finding a libidinal compensation for this operation of renunciation which keeps the body lean. The thin body here embodies the body that is not satisfied with the object of need in order to remain alive for the Other as the object of desire. It is in this sense that the equivalence is asserted here: thin body = phallus, and thinness is phallicized as the object of the desire of the Other.

- *Anorexia and "feeding on nothing"*: Lacan's thesis, as it emerges from the Seminar, Book IV, is that the anorexic feeds on nothing (Lacan, 1994, p. 199), where the nothing assumes the value of signifier of the irreducibility of the desire of the subject to the seizure of the omnipotence of the Other, in particular of the maternal Other. In this sense, the nothing on which the anorexic feeds embodies the structural metonymy of human desire, the fact of being basically always the desire of the Other, its inexhaustibility.

- *"Mental" anorexia, knowing and eating nothing: the man with fresh brains*: in the initial part of *The direction of the treatment* (Lacan, 2006, pp. 499–503), Lacan also mentions, in a very subtle way, anorexia nervosa by commenting on the famous case of the man with fresh brains as formulated by Kriss. The key symptom carried by this patient was that of a great inhibition to have his own ideas, linked to the fixed idea of being a plagiarist. The intervention of Kriss in analysis restores to the patient that on the level of reality what he affirms does not correspond to truth, and that it is about his obsession.

To this, the patient responds to Lacan with acting: on leaving Kriss' office, he rushes to the restaurant to eat his favorite dish: fresh brains. This case highlights, as Laurent explains, the "mental" dimension of anorexia as a refusal to think with one's own head, to assume a thought on one's own account – it is moreover a trait that we constantly find in the clinic of anorexic patients – as an effect in this case of an attribution to the Other of the fact of being imaginarily the absolute holder of the thought which leaves no place for the subject. The attempt that this subject puts into action to preserve himself from the constant self-accusation of plagiarizing the Other is: "to think nothing". At the same time, his acting reveals an operation of reduction, underlined by Laurent, of the thought to the organ (the brain) which testifies to a reification of the symbolic phallus to the penis as an organ. The effect on the subject is an effect of alienation, and in this sense Laurent defines this form of anorexia as an "anorexia of alienation" (Laurent, 2000, pp. 131–137) which must be distinguished from the more classic form of hysterical anorexia as a separating maneuver (separation anorexia).

• *Bulimia and frustration of the demand for love*: in this same conceptual register, in *Le Séminaire, livre IV, La relation d'objet*, Lacan formulates a possible definition of bulimia (but also basically, or perhaps a better reality, neurotic obesity) as compensation, where he speaks of a satisfaction of fallback, obtained through food, of a frustration of the child's demand for love (Lacan, 1994, p. 188).

The horizon of this theoretical-clinical problematic of Lacan, based on the autonomy of the symbolic and on its primacy in relation to the imaginary register, clearly offers the framework of a dialectical-hysterical paradigm of anorexia (Recalcati, 1997, p. 196).

The causative-structural paradigm in the Seminar, Book XI

Finally, the third fundamental scansion in which Lacan advances theses on anorexia is located within the Seminar, Book XI, *The Four Fundamental Concepts of Psychoanalysis*, written in 1964. In this Seminar, which indicates a decisive theoretical turning point, Lacan is now far from his theses of the 1950s, which were based on the primacy of the symbolic, and he reforms the very notion of structure by inscribing it at the very heart of the notion of jouissance as real not reducible to the signifier, as "tuchè" which intervenes unexpectedly to break the regularity of the signifying "automaton". This jouissance is organized around the erogenous zones of the body thanks to the action of the partial objects (oral, anal, phallic, voice, gaze) which correspond to them and which function as objects causing desire for the subject. This acting of partial objects as objects that are the cause of desire, which Lacan formalizes with the notion of object *a*, means that the drive satisfaction that one obtains from any object whatsoever is produced by an indestructible push – the very core of our being as desire, according to Freud's definition – which finds its root not in the object of the drive as such, which can vary, but in the indelible trace of the lost mythical object of the first experience of satisfaction. The void left by this lost object thus becomes the cause of the subject's desire, the motor of drive functioning. Thus, the Seminar, Book XI embodies, in Lacan's teaching, the passage accomplished by the "classical" centrality of the concept of desire, to the new centrality assumed by the concept of drive (*Trieb*), from the centrality of the symbolic Other and of the Name-of-the-Father to the centrality of the real of jouissance and of its libidinal core constituted by the object *a*.

Lacan's reference to anorexia is located in this Seminar at the heart of this new problem, and maintains within it the central question of the hysterical-"classical" paradigm of anorexia as a maneuver that aims at the desire of the Other; but he complicates it by introducing the question of the real jouissance which comes into play in the anorexic subject through this operation. The epistemological passage in relation to the paradigm of *The direction of the treatment* is that of a dialectical reading of the anorexic refusal as a metaphor of the subject's desire, structured entirely on the signifying register to an inscription of the refusal within the dialectic of alienation and of separation which causes the constitution of the subject in its structural relation to the Other. An operation where, at the center, the object *a* is situated as cause of desire and key function of the separative operation of the subject. The anorexic maneuver is therefore questioned here, in its double status of maneuver on the desire of the Other and operation on jouissance. In this context, we are thus witnessing a resumption of the classic questions of Paradigm II (the anorexic refusal as a demand on the desire, "to eat nothing" of the anorexic), but in the new problem structured no longer around the centrality of the S-I (symbolic-imaginary) axis, but on the centrality of the R-S (real-symbolic) axis, and this displacement of the axis restructures the terms of the questions in subject. In addition, we are witnessing, or at least this is what emerges from the work of colleagues more engaged in a reading of Lacan's discourse on anorexia, a resumption of the key element of paradigm I (anorexia as a regressive response to the loss of the object of weaning, the appetite for death in anorexia, the non-violent suicidal dimension) within the framework of this third scansion of Lacan on anorexia (which we will now call paradigm III) to thematize the anorexic operation on real jouissance not identifiable at the level of paradigm II.

Lacan's fundamental references to anorexia in the Seminar, Book XI can be traced back to these essential nodes.

Anorexia and the nothing as an object a produced by weaning at the time of separation

This reference is at the heart of the dialectic of alienation/separation in which the subject is constituted, and it tries in particular to shed light on the decisive passage at stake in the time of separation. The constitution of the subject presupposes the separation of the object *a* as an organ which becomes a symbol of the phallus as lacking (-phi), that is to say of the castration of the subject itself. At the oral level, argues Lacan, the object *a* is the nothing, insofar as the subject weans himself from something which, from the start, is nothing for him. It is important to emphasize here that Lacan sees weaning as an active operation of the subject in the process of constitution, thus re-launching the idea of a "desire for weaning" in the child, formulated in *Le Séminaire, livre X, L'angoisse*. It is here, in fact, that Lacan clearly affirms that weaning is something that the child puts into action and not something that he undergoes (Lacan, 2004, p. 379).

The anorexic child eats nothing

It is at this point that Lacan introduces as an explanatory key the reference to anorexia, where he affirms that "in anorexia nervosa, what the child eats is nothing" (Lacan, 1973, p. 119). The reading of this sentence of Lacan is that it is in a relationship of discontinuity with the "nourishment of nothing" at the heart of the classic Lacanian paradigm of anorexia, and that it assumes, in the first place, for Lacan, the value of embodying an epistemological break at the heart of his teaching.

The "eating nothing" of the anorexic child shows here, first of all, the irreducibility of the object *a* to the field of the signifier, embodied by an invisible and contra-intuitive jouissance, nameable only through the para-doxical signifier "nothing". In other words, and this is one of the key theses of this work, the reminder of anorexia allows Lacan to embody paradigmati-cally the two fundamental epistemological cuts operated in the development of his teaching: the irreducibility of the symbolic function of desire on the level of need and demand in his classical doctrine, as can be seen in *The direction of the treatment*; the irreducibility of the function of jouissance as real and of the object (a) as cause of desire to the symbolic order of the significant Other in *Le Séminaire, livre XI*.

Anorexic "eating nothing" and the object of weaning functioning as deprivation at the level of castration

Lacan exposes the operation accomplished by the anorexic child in relation to nothing as object (a) in the logical time of separation. Faced with the loss of the oral object by the effect of weaning and the opening at the structural level of castration (-phi), the anorexic operation consists of an antiseparative maneuver – this is our own reading, which we also find in other authors like Soria – where, through the refusal to eat, the object nothing is retained in the empty mouth and positivized as real jouissance in action. It is therefore an object, the nothing, from which the anorexic subject does not completely separate, but which remains encysted in the mouth, and more generally in the body. In this operation, the anorexic cedes nothing to the Other; they retain primary jouissance in the mouth by disembodying it from the signifying structure in which it is constituted. By wanting to escape the effects of signifying alienation on the jouissance that inhabits the instinctual body in order to retain the full jouissance of the primary object of satisfaction, the anorexic thus loses the possibility of a recovery of jouissance at the level of the phallicization of the drive body as a body fully inscribed in the dialectic of desire and in phallic signification. Hence, the effects of a relapse into the real of one's body at the age of adolescence: amenorrhea in women, the reduction to a minimum of the sexual forms of the body, the prevalence of an entropic and inertial form of primary desire, which Lacan called in the *Family Complexes* "desire of the larva", situated between death and life. The fact that, precisely in *Le Séminaire*, Book XI, Lacan formalizes the ethical status of the Freudian unconscious, by freeing it from all forms of biological-evolutionary determinism, sheds light on this articulation of the anorexic question: it is ultimately the effect of a decision by the subject, their coming to be in the "zone of the larvae" (ibid., p. 31) from which they come, and the fact of not yielding to the desire of the larva which keeps them there. A mortiferous desire that Lacan in *Function and Field* called "desire for death", and which he defined in *Family Complexes* in the form of "appetite for death".

The anorexic, the fantasy of one's own disappearance and the question it embodies in the enigma of the desire of the parental Other: "Do you want to lose me?" (ibid., p. 240)

The other key step of the Seminar, Book XI, shows the operation activated by the child, in relation to the enigma of the desire of the parental Other and in relation to their own place in this desire, and which in anorexia shows itself in its radical status. The threat of disappearance, which the anorexic enacts with the body refusing food, is the fundamental maneuver that aims to put the love of the Other to the test until the risk of their own death. What the anorexic brings into play in this extreme position is the search for a lack in the Other that can become a sign of their desire for themselves. In doing so, they embody their own fundamental demand on the desire of the Other for them, in the radical form of a dramatic questioning: how much it matters whether they are alive or dead for the desire of the Other. The question "Do you want to lose me?" is indeed embodied in anorexia by a subject who addresses the Other in the condition of someone who is between life and death. The third Lacanian paradigm on anorexia, in the Seminar, Book XI, presents itself in the form of a causative-structural paradigm of anorexia, in which the anorexic position is found not only in its relation to the desire of the subject and to the dialectic with the desire of the Other, but also and above all in its structural relation to the real jouissance which sustains it and makes it possible: the object nothing as cause.

The Seminar paradigm of the refusal of knowledge, Book XXI

Lacan's passage on anorexia, the most radical and least valued to date, is found in a Seminar of his last teaching: to be precise, in the April 9 lesson of his Seminar, Book XXI, "Les non dupes errent", still unpublished (Lacan, 1973–1974, unpublished).

It is therefore a question of a reference situated after the turning point by Lacan in *Le Séminaire, livre XX, Encore* and which Miller, in *The six paradigms of the jouissance*, defines by an effective formula like the "Seminar of non-rapports" (Miller, 1999, p. 25). Lacan's formula "the sexual relation does not exist", already elaborated in previous Seminars and, in particular, in Book XVIII, *D'un discours qui ne serait pas du semblant*, here reaches an unprecedented degree of articulation, through the construction of a theory of femininity, based on a differentiated doctrine of jouissance and logically supported by what he defines as "the formulas of sexuation". In *Le Séminaire, livre XX*, Lacan defines the feminine position in relation to jouissance as a position taken between two possibilities of jouissance, between them irreducible, but which a woman experiences. The first is represented by phallic jouissance, structured from the laws of the signifier and symbolic castration; it finds in the phallic signification its point of coordination and, respectively, in the man and in the woman, two different positions from which it is possible to experience it: for the man, on the side of having and, for the woman, on the side of being for the man. In phallic jouissance, the position of the man vis-à-vis the woman is fetishistic: it is the search, in the female body, for this part of himself which he raises to the embodiment of his object, the cause of the desire. The position of the woman in relation to the man, in phallic jouissance, is erotomaniac: what makes her enjoy is being loved by the man. From the perspective of phallic jouissance, the sexual relation does not therefore take place, in the sense that the jouissances of man and woman do not converge in a unitary synthesis but they remain structurally unrelated to each other, although, in the sexual act, the meeting between the bodies occurs and the respective pleasures are realized in this union. Despite the phallic mediation and the search for what the subject lacks in the body and in the speech of the Other, the real experience of jouissance is essentially solitary.

The second possibility of jouissance, typical of the feminine position (which does not mean, in the absolute, that man cannot experience it) is represented by what Lacan calls the Other jouissance and which is characterized by a direct relationship with jouissance, without mediation operated by castration and by the phallic signifier. Its characteristic is to be a limitless enjoyment, neither measurable nor quantifiable, not localizable as it is, on the other hand, with masculine enjoyment, and which manifests itself in the form of a real dispossession, of a rapture, of a total loss of mastery which first affects the body as an enjoyable substance. It is not by chance that Lacan takes as an example of this enjoyment the experience of the mystics in their relationship to God.

This return by Lacan to the anorexic question therefore becomes essential, for us, immediately after *Le Séminaire, Encore*, which revolutionizes his theory of femininity and jouissance. And this by virtue of the fact that, first of all, anorexia is a condition experienced, in the majority of cases, by women: for several years, in international research, the epidemiological relationship between women and men has now been stable at a rate of one to ten. This is why, after *Encore*, it is more possible for us to ask ourselves in a more radical way why anorexia is a condition especially in women, beyond the rather weak explanations around the question, proposed today by sociology and mass-mediology, and can be traced back to the centrality, in contemporary social discourse, of the image of the thin female body.

A hypothesis that we will try to put forward and to verify clinically, in our work, is that according to anorexia nervosa it would be possible to find the trace of a defect of symbolic inscription of the female subject which would harm the enjoyment in the phallic register and would leave the girl, as the only tolerable experience, the limitless Other jouissance, degraded in the form of a contemporary pathology of feminine excess (Francesconi, 2007; Eldar, 2009), as with other pathologies, anorexia nervosa.

The context of the Seminar, Book XXI, where Lacan takes up the reference to anorexia, concerns a question that has always been at the heart of Lacan's questioning on anorexia: the status of knowledge in the anorexic subject. However, in this context, the notion of knowledge (*savoir*) is radically rethought by Lacan, compared to its classical conceptualization where it is reduced to the completely symbolic structure of the signifying chain. According to the progressive advance in Lacan's teaching, thought is jouissance (Lacan, 1975, p. 91), the exercise of knowledge represents jouissance (ibid., p. 173) and, for psychoanalysis, the very essence of knowledge is to be "check in knowledge" [*savoir en échec*] (Lacan, 2008, p. 116). These are definitions that bring us back to the non-signifying and non-signifiable real core, to the very heart of knowledge. In this radical re-conceptualization, which is essentially a reformulation of the status of the unconscious since, for Lacan, knowledge is essentially unconscious knowledge, we are witnessing a progressive displacement of the unconscious, conceived as a signifying machine, toward the real unconscious. To use a conceptual couple, highlighted in recent years by Jacques-Alain Miller, it is a passage from the transferential unconscious, a signifying structure that produces meaning, to the real unconscious, a repository of letters and waste of lalangue hors-sense.

It is therefore important for us to verify how Lacan changes the way he conceptualizes the relationship of the anorexic to knowledge in the light of this unprecedented status of unconscious knowledge as real outside of meaning.

Let us therefore, in this lesson of the Seminar, Book XXI, note the following key passages:

- *"Very little for me"*: the anorexic, like some children who represent the exception compared to most children, does not harass adults with questions to find out more about several aspects of reality, by attributing to them a knowledge about the things of the world. They maintain a relationship with knowledge similar to that which they have with food and which can be expressed with the phrase: "Very little for me".
- *Anorexia as an action that says: "I eat nothing"*. "Anorexia is an active position whose implicit sentence, in the silent action of the anorexic, is "I eat nothing".
- *The worry about whether they are going to eat or not is such that they do not even notice that they are starving to death.* Asked by Lacan why they did not eat, the anorexics replied that they were so preoccupied with knowing whether they were going to eat or not, that they did not even notice that they were starving to death.
- *It is not desire that governs knowledge but horror.* This thesis according to which, at the heart of the subject's relationship with unconscious knowledge, there is not desire but the horror of knowledge, is for Lacan a structural thesis which is valid for the subject in themselves. But the clinical example of anorexia nervosa makes it possible to highlight it in a striking way. Anorexic rumination around knowing whether they are going to eat or not is a practice of limitless enjoyment that completely absorbs the patient while eclipsing their subjectivity. This limitless enjoyment, which keeps them immobile around the knowledge of whether they are going to eat or not, causes their body and the vital necessities that must be satisfied in order to survive to fall into oblivion.

Concluding considerations on anorexia in the last teaching of Lacan

The theses of the Seminar, Book XXI introduce, in our opinion, an epistemological break, in Lacan, compared to his previous formulations on anorexia nervosa. An obvious tension appears very particularly between the theses on anorexia, contained in *Le Séminaire*, Book XXI, and those which are found not only in "La direction de la cure" of 1958 but also in *Le Séminaire*, Book XI, in particular concerning the function of anorexia in relation to the field of the Other. Whereas in 1958 and 1964, the thesis of a sort of dialectical matrix of anorexia remained present, despite the passage, in *Le Séminaire, livre XI*, to a paradigm of the unconscious including the real and jouissance, as maneuver of the subject aiming to open a lack in the Other, in the Seminar, Book XXI, the anorexic action "I eat nothing" does not operate at all to open a lack in the Other.

On the contrary, here *Le Séminaire* rather accentuates the refusal of the Other as such, the refusal of unconscious knowledge as something that causes horror to the point that the subject lets themselves die rather than encounter it.

The knowledge by which the anorexic allows himself to be absorbed is, rather, a desubjectivized knowledge: a knowledge-jouissance-without-limit, strictly anchored to eating behavior and which nourishes its pathological solution by leaving the patient immobile and undivided. Moreover, the avoidance of the encounter with castration, that is, with the lack of the Other and with one's own subjective division, constitutes the basis of this anorexic position. The obsessive demand on food and on the fact of eating or not eating, which occupies them entirely in their rumination, serves here to cover for themselves the encounter with the horror of knowledge which concerns the structure of the unconscious as only a hole in the real, without security.

This position therefore aligns well this reflection of Lacan's last teaching on anorexia with the first Lacanian paradigm contained in *The Family Complexes*, particularly in the non-separative and non-castrating thrust, internal to anorexia, and in the sharing of the same instinctual destiny with drug addiction pathologies. Indeed, already in the 1938 text, the refusal of marriage with the phallus and an economy of enjoyment, structured on direct access to an inanimate object, caused food pathologies and drug addiction to intersect.

For this reason, this fourth paradigm on anorexia could be well defined as the Lacanian paradigm of the "refusal of the Other", to use the formula created by Miller, as we will see later, that is to say, the essential characteristic anorexia nervosa.

References

Althusser, L., Balibar, É. (1968), *Leggere Il Capitale*. Milano: Feltrinelli; Althusser, L., and others (1965), *Lire Le Capitale*. Paris: Maspero.

Bollas, C. (2001), *Isteria*. Milano: Cortina; *Hysteria* (2000). London/New York: Routledge.

Brusset, B. (1998), *Psychopatologie de l'anorexie mentale*. Paris: Dunot.

Eldar, S. (Dir.) (2009), *Mujeres, una por una*. Madrid: Gredos.

Francesconi, P. (Dir.) (2007), *Una per una. Psicoanalisi e femminilità*. Roma: Borla.

Jacan, J. (2008). *Le Séminaire. Livre XVIII. D'un discours qui ne serait du semblant, 1970-1971*. Paris: Le Seuil, p. 116.

Lacan, J. (2001), *Les complexes familiaux dans la formation de l'individu (1938). Autres écrits*. Paris: Seuil.

Lacan, J. (2006), *The Direction of the Treatment and the Principles of Its Power (1958). Écrits. The First Complete Edition in English*. New York/London: Norton & Company, pp. 489–542; *La direction de la cure et les pricipes de son pouvoir. Écrits* (1966). Paris: Seuil.

Lacan, J. (1994), *Le Séminaire. Livre IV. La relation d'objet, 1956–1957*. Paris: Seuil.

Lacan, J. (2004), *Le Séminaire. Livre X. L'angoisse, 1962–1963*. Paris: Seuil.

Lacan, J. (1973), *Le Séminaire. Livre XI. Les quatre concepts fondamentaux de la psychanalyse*. Paris: Seuil.

Lacan, J. (1975), *Le Séminaire. Livre XX. Encore, 1972–1973*. Paris: Seuil.

Lacan, J., *Séminaire XXI. Les non dupes errent, 1973–1974*, inédit.

Laurent, É. (2000), *Improvisación: anorexias, Gorali, V. (Dir.), Estudios sobre Anorexia y Bulimia*. Buenos Aires: Atuel Cap., pp. 131–138.

Miller, J.-A. (2005), *Lecture critique des "Complexes familiaux" de Jacques Lacan, La Cause freudienne*, no. 60, pp. 33–51.

Miller, J.-A. (1999), Les six paradigmes de la jouissance. *La Cause freudienne*, no. 43, pp. 7–29.

Recalcati, M. (1997), *L'ultima cena. Anoressia e bulimia*. Milano: Bruno Mondadori.

Soria, N. (2000), *Psicoánalisis de la anorexia y bulimia*. Buenos Aires: Tres Haces.

Chapter 5

Lacanian readings of anorexia

From Lacan to the Lacanian orientation

For those who have ventured to investigate the clinical question of anorexia from the teaching of Lacan, the indications of the latter have functioned as enigmatic clues used as vectors of orientation in the reading of the discourse of anorexic patients.

In the light of a first reading, Lacan's statements on anorexia seem to function as an "other discourse", in comparison with that formulated by post-Freudian analysts, including in the most advanced neo-Kleinian versions that we have attempted to summarize in the third chapter.

First of all, it is clear that *Lacan does not approach anorexia starting from narcissism*. Moreover, he says nothing about the issues relating to the narcissistic hold on the body and its particular effects – narcissistic-identity fragility, altered perception of body image – which, however, are at the heart of the debate on anorexia nervosa, at least since the early sixties. As the theoretician of the mirror stage, he could easily have chosen this path and located the heart of the problem of anorexia at the level of a defective passage through the structuring intersection of subjective identity. But Lacan chooses another path, which consists in situating the heart of the problem of anorexia beyond the imaginary, in the dialectic of desire between the subject and the Other, and in the action which causes jouissance in the articulation of the anorexic position. This absence of reference to narcissism, on the part of Lacan, therefore reveals, in our opinion, a certain rigor which is coherent with the fundamental orientation of his lessons: it is only in the light of his relationship to the Other and to jouissance that the narcissico-imaginary structuring of the subject can effectively be highlighted in its effective status. To be able to orient oneself in the imaginary field without being trapped there, it is necessary to find a point of support beyond this field, in the domain of the symbolic: this is the methodological indication that Lacan makes his own, in reference to Spinoza and Freud, and which is lacking, at varying levels, in post-Freudian orientations, by conditioning at the root of the reading of clinical experience.

DOI: 10.4324/9781003318439-6

Second, Lacan places, in his own way, at the center of the anorexic question the problem of the family bond, without however articulating it in terms of the early specular relationship of the child to the mother and the insufficiency of the care of the mother (as it is in the context of post-Freudian approaches), nor in terms, specific to systemic theory, of a lack of communication within the family system which traps the patient, confining them to the role of scapegoat and designated victim. Lacan places at the heart of the question of anorexia the relationship of the subject to the Other, of which the parents, and in particular the mother, constitute the first concrete embodiment. Indeed, it is to the desire of the parental Other that the subject addresses themselves through the anorexic refusal, to challenge the enigma and ask for the gift of love.

Third, in *Le Séminaire*, livre XI, Lacan (1973) once again addresses anorexia as a drive question, updating, however, the classic clinical theme that revolves around orality. Indeed, by a counter-intuitive operation impracticable within the framework of a phenomenological-egoic perspective, he isolates the object which causes the oral satisfaction, by detaching it from the series of oral objects, breast included, and calls this object, the object nothing. In Lacan, the drive enigma of anorexia thus becomes the singular relationship of the anorexic subject with the nothing as the object that causes it.

It is from these points of reference proposed by Lacan, that it was possible to develop over the decades following his death, thanks to the clinical-theoretical work of several Lacanian psychoanalysts particularly involved in this field, an original, and fruitful clinically, theory of anorexia nervosa. A field that has become very important because of the epidemic spread of anorexia and bulimia (but also obesity) over the past fifty years.

In this work, we will try in particular to indicate the key elements of the development and the progress made in this field by the colleagues who study the clinic of anorexia from the Lacanian orientation transmitted by Miller, in his multi-decade works of writing and reading Lacan's texts. It is indeed to the latter that we owe the most significant contributions and it is also from these same readings that we orient ourselves.

They are characterized by the dialectical tension of Lacan's teaching and clinical experience in the field with anorexic patients, on the part of psychoanalysts who, in more than one case, have been working for a long time, not only in private practice but also within therapeutic structures. As we will see, the data that emerge from intensive clinical practice with anorexic patients will have a decisive weight in the development of the Lacanian theory of anorexia nervosa. We will limit ourselves here to succinctly pointing out, among the Lacanian readings of anorexia after Lacan, those which, from an organic point of view, because of the continuity of research and originality, have, in our opinion, distinguished themselves in particular, by contributing in an important way to the construction of a Lacanian theory of anorexia nervosa. We will examine these contributions in more depth, as well as those of other authors who have written on this theme, when we discuss the reconstruction of the main points of advance reached in the clinical theorization of anorexia.

A structural theory of the anorexic process: Augustin Ménard and logical time elided in anorexia

It is to the work of Augustin Ménard that we owe the first attempt at an overall reading of anorexia nervosa, carried out in the light of an intense clinical experience as a psychoanalyst alongside these patients, within private practice as psychiatric institutes. In a series of articles written between the mid-1980s and the 1990s, Ménard values, in particular, the innovative discontinuity of the reading of Lacan, in relation to the evolutionary approach in psychoanalysis, placing at the center of his research the "signifying structure of anorexia" and the problem of anorexic jouissance, as a crucial question of theory and treatment. Ménard therefore clearly places the problem of anorexia in the tension between the signifying logic of desire and the economy of enjoyment.

Second, Ménard shows how, in Lacan's "structural perspective", anorexia is not the product of an evolutionary stage which has not been passed, but rather that of "an elided logical time" (Ménard, 1992, p. 3). From this thesis, he develops a short but essential and convincing theorization of the three logical times at play in the process of subjective constitution, in an attempt to show where the elision of logical time that anorexia embodies lies, and the passage that must be produced in the treatment.

This theorization, as we can see in its articulation, summarizes them in itself, by integrating them, in a movement of *Aufhebung*, all the main references of Lacan on anorexia, and in this sense it presents itself as a true reading in the strong sense of the Lacanian text. Indeed, the three logical times indicated, which are articulated through the resumption of the frustration-deprivation-castration triad of the Seminar, book IV can be synthesized in this way.

Frustration and the dialectic of exchange and gift

In this first stage, Ménard valorizes the indications given by Lacan in *The direction of the treatment* (Lacan, 2006, pp. 525–526) and the conceptual triad of need/demand/desire to show the basis of the anorexic refusal of food. This operation in anorexia aims to divide the object of need from the sign of love in order to verify in the desire of the Other who offers it, in particular in the desire of the mother, the presence of a lack which denotes love for the subject, not just administration of the object of need. The essential problem in the time of frustration, which Ménard also questions about its "bulimic side", consists in the fact that, in the relationship of the anorexic subject with the parental Other "it is the lack itself which has failed" (ibid., p. 5). In other words, the anorexic subject in the time of frustration seeks, through the refusal of food, to provoke in the desire of the Other what he does not succeed in finding there: the gift of a sign of love for them.

The appetite for death and the time of deprivation

The time of deprivation is the time which presents to the anorexic subject the real loss of the object realized in the weaning. This is the crucial time of anorexia, because faced with the real loss of the object, the subject finds themselves having to make a choice: accept it or refuse it. For this reason, Ménard situates in this second phase Lacan's reference to the anorexic's appetite for death as a response to the weaning indicated in the *Family Complexes* (Lacan, 2001, p. 35). It is in this time that the anorexic refusal of the loss of the object is situated and its operation to eat the object nothing as a means to avoid "eating the signifier, or assuming the loss of the object as structural effect of the law of castration". It is in this sense that Ménard seems to read Lacan when he asserts in *Le Séminaire*, livre XI that "the object of weaning can come to function at the level of castration, as deprivation" (Lacan, 1973, p. 119).

Castration and access to desire and the law

This is indeed the logical time elided by the subject in anorexia: the condition of full access to the dialectic of desire in fact implies that the subject, by assuming the law of symbolic castration, accepts a structural loss of enjoyment. The elision of this passage to the logical time of castration in the experience of the anorexic subject, and its anchoring in the time of deprivation through refusal is, in our opinion, well exemplified in the clinic of the anorexic exordium in adolescence. The elision of this passage is revealed in the inability of the young anorexic to settle into the sexual position of woman or man in the dialectic of desire between the sexes, and in their autistic entrenchment in the asexual jouissance that the symptom offers them. The decisive clinical question at stake in the treatment of anorexia for Ménard is that of how to allow the subject to accomplish the passage from logical time II of deprivation to time III of castration: a passage that he elided by the construction of the symptom.

Alongside this general formalization which finds its cardinal point in the thesis of elided logical time in anorexia, and which the author supports by resorting to various references from clinical cases which he himself has treated, Ménard anticipates in his articles almost all the key elements of development of the Lacanian theory of anorexia after Lacan. I limit myself here simply to naming them: the questioning of the reduction of anorexia to the structural framework of hysteria and the openness to psychotic frameworks and in particular to melancholic ones, more obvious, according to him, for psychoanalysts who are confronted with serious cases in the context of psychiatric institutions; the determination of two levels of functioning of the object nothing in anorexia, one on the side of desire and the other on the side of jouissance; highlighting the clinic of anorexia as a clinic oriented by a "latent demand", and not by an absence of demand as might appear phenomenologically. Finally, some fundamental indications to guide the treatment, for instance, shifting the axis of the discourse from food to something else, do not answer the patient's question on the level of the need, temptations to which the anorexic pushes the treater, so as not to drag the axis of the treatment to the time I of the frustration and to its imaginary dialectic by taking the place of the nursing mother; do not miss the intervention when the anorexic brings into play the threat of disappearance, which is often a prelude, if it is not symbolized under transference, to the interruption of the cure; do not resort in extreme situations to hospitalization, taking care to pass it off as the subject at the level of the logical time of castration (Time III), an encounter with a limit that dams up deadly jouissance, and do not, as often happens, re-propose the logical time of deprivation (Time II).

The anorexic aporia in the reading by Jacques-Alain Miller: "structure of all desire" and "refusal of the Other"

In the construction of the anorexic problematic in the Lacanian orientation, it is essential in our opinion to relate to anorexia in the reading of Miller. As with Lacan, with Miller also the references to anorexia are episodic and developed in the general context of his work of reading the foundations of the psychoanalytic clinic. And yet the weight of his statements on this subject is just as important for the orienting effects that he produced on the theoretical-clinical research in depth around the anorexic question in the Lacanian field. In particular, we seem to be able to grasp an antinomic tension in action in his discourse on anorexia, in particular in the course in collaboration with Éric Laurent from 1996–1997 "The Other who does not exist and its ethics committees" (Miller, Laurent, 2005), between the classic reading in the Lacanism of anorexia as a radical form of hysteria and a reading that introduces on the other hand a beyond of hysteria at the heart of the anorexic question. The first aspect, the one which can be traced back to the paradigm of hysterical anorexia, is taken up several times by Miller, and is expressed in the thesis of anorexic refusal as a radicalized version of the hysterical "no". In this context indeed, as he affirms in "Silet", the refusal of food is presented as a maneuver "essential to the subject to show that he exists outside the omnipotence of the Other" (Miller, 1998, p. 222). From this perspective, anorexia is on the side of the barred subject; it is more "on the side of separation" than alienation in relation to bulimia; and one can even wish to say, according to Miller, that anorexia is "the structure of every desire" (Miller, Laurent, 2005, p. 378). This thesis, which proposes anorexia as a radicalized clinical embodiment of desire, we could say as "pure desire" but also – in a definition that shows its deadly effect at work – as a "terrorist" which goes toward death in the name of the ideal of an angelic body (Miller, 2001, pp. 162–163), a contemporary figure of Antigone, seems to us to enter into tension with the definition of anorexia proposed by Miller himself as "refusal of the Other":

> What is in the foreground in anorexia is the rejection of the Other, and in particular of the nurturing mother, and more broadly the rejection of the great Other.
>
> (Miller, Laurent, 2005, pp. 378–379)

Indeed, the notion of "refusal of the Other" introduces a more radical form of negation of the hysterical-neurotic "Verneinung" which is formulated dialectically from a fundamental "yes" to the big Other, by a "Bejahung" inscribed in the structure of the subject. Miller moreover clearly underlines, in his 1991 Spanish lecture, *Modalidades del rechazo*, this logical division between the two fundamental forms of refusal in the psychoanalytic clinic, by taking up the theme of the Freudian text *Die Verneinung*, already commented on by Lacan (Miller, 2006, pp. 271–282). Here, he clearly distinguishes the hysterical refusal as negation starting from an affirmation, from the structural refusal which is a "no" to the Other as such, and therefore takes more the preclusive-psychotic form of the rejection of the "*Bejahung*" in a more primary form. The formula, refusal of the Other, seems in other words to open the clinical field of anorexia to something beyond hysteria. This passage allows the space for a thematization of the psychotic forms of anorexia, and offered the decisive impetus to the direction of the research on the new forms of the symptom. And in fact, beyond Miller's intentions, this is the fate that this formula has met with those who have deepened the anorexic question in the light of its statement.

A new scansion in the Lacanian clinical orientation and its effects on the reading of anorexia: the transition to the Borromean clinic and the theory of ordinary psychoses

Another fundamental passage which, in my opinion, has had a considerable impact in the most innovative readings of anorexia, is located in the general reorientation of the Lacanian clinical problematic, fixed above all by the reading of its foundations that Miller developed in the light of Lacan's last teaching. This reading, which shifts the axis of the primacy of the symbolic and of the Name-of-the-Father to the centrality of the real and of the notion of jouissance, leads to rethinking the foundation of the clinic of the dysfunctions of the symbolic in action in the symptom at the libidinal holding of functioning which makes it exist as a way of singular jouissance of the subject. This displacement marks the passage in the Lacanian problem from the centrality of the classical structural clinic to the formulation of a Borromean clinic in which the symptom is placed at the center as a singular knotting of the three registers (real, symbolic and imaginary) around the object *a* cause of desire. If in the clinic of neuroses the knotting is made possible by a fourth ring which binds the others together and which is given by the signifier of the Name-of-the-Father, in the clinic of psychoses this signifier is lacking, and in its place a more solid stabilization of the psychotic symptom implies that another signifier comes to function for the subject as a knot. In this passage, an epistemological rupture is accomplished, because the clinic is founded around this real point of the structure, jouissance, which is outside the logic of the signifier. In this sense, Miller reads this passage from Lacan as an invitation to think about neurosis starting from psychosis, as a subset, anchored in the Name-of-the-Father, of a larger whole which has jouissance as a common denominator, in the specific- ities of its articulation. This passage found its consecration in the clinical conversations on the psychoses carried out by the ECF in France at the end of the 20th century, where there arose, in the light of the new epistemological framework indicated, a new conceptualization of the psychoses, no longer reducible to the framework of language disorders (hallucinations, delusions) evident in the more classic psychotic forms and which can be obviously traced back to a foreclosure of the Name-of-the-Father. The introduction of the notion of ordinary psychosis (IRMA, 1999; Miller, 2009) extends the field of psychoses to psychotic frames not characterized by the classic forms of lan- guage disorder, but more generally by those subjective frames whose structural functioning shows an enjoyment that is not fundamentally anchored by the operation of the paternal metaphor.

This passage turns out to be essential to our discourse, because in my opinion it makes it possible to radicalize in the Lacanian clinical reading of anorexia the thematization of the psychotic forms which present themselves in our experi- ence, and which most often assume the traits, as Evelyne Kestemberg also noticed, of "non-delusion", "cold" psychoses, anchored in a psychotic treat- ment of the body and jouissance. In fact, the most significant and in-depth Lacanian readings of anorexia in the last decades are characterized, as we will see, by the progressive clinical accentuation of this psychotic dimension. This dimension is already clearly present in the precursive reading of Ménard, who anticipated this passage in the clinic of anorexia, in his writings straddling the 1980s and 1990s, like almost all the fundamental themes that would be devel- oped later, even if there is almost no explicit trace of his work in the following more innovative contributions, which we will now try to describe succinctly.

Anorexia/bulimia in the new forms of the symptom: the reading of Massimo Recalcati

While Ménard's work comes in the form of solitary research brought to the attention of the ECF, the most important contributions we will now analyze, those offered by Massimo Recalcati in Italy and by Nieves Soria in Argentina, are characterized by the fact of having developed in the context of psycho-analytic research groups which they themselves guided. Recalcati has produced his most important contributions to this field to date, based on his clinical experience within a therapeutic institution for the treatment of anorexia and bulimia, the ABA, of which he was for a long time the scientific director; Soria develops her research within the framework of a working group on anorexia and bulimia of the "Instituto Clinico" of Buenos Aires (ICBA) of the Freudian Field, and within the Faculty of Psychology of the University of Buenos Aires.

Recalcati's research, begun in the early 1990s and whose most important works date back to the period between the end of the 1990s and the beginning of the 21st century, can in my opinion be summarized in two fundamental phases. The first is constituted by the elaboration of a theory of anorexia and bulimia based on the teaching of Lacan, able to guide clinical work with anorexic and bulimic patients. The second phase, begun in the year 2000, is characterized in the current context by the development of the research paradigm on new forms of the symptom (Recalcati, 2010), including ano-rexia, following Miller's indication.

Recalcati's essential theses on anorexia can be summarized schematically in a few essential points. In the first place, it takes up Brusset's theory of anorexia-bulimia as a unitary circuit animated by the same logic of func-tioning (Brusset, 1991; Recalcati, 1997, p. 25), where the anorexic position cannot be thought of except in dialectical relation with bulimia and vice versa, and which engages it – it is in this that lies the originality of the operation – within the framework of the Lacanian differential structural clinic. It is an attempt, one might say, to bring the phenomenology of ano-rexic and bulimic malaise back to a unitary logic (anorexia-bulimia) and to circumscribe its specific value for the subject through its inclusion in the structural framework which is specific to them (psychosis/neurosis). Second, Recalcati isolates in Lacan what he defines as a fruitful aporia around the status of anorexia: the tension, already present in Freud, between a hysterical-dialectical side and an autistic-melancholic side, which at first complicates a Lacanian reading of anorexia reduced to the sole framework of hysteria. Third, this analysis leads the author to situate beyond the problem of the differentiality of structures an antinomic tension in the anorexic-bulimic position, between a version of anorexic refusal as an unconscious call ad-dressed dialectically to the desire of the Other and a version of refusal which, on the other hand, shows autistically, according to Miller's definition, a fundamental "refusal of the Other", an enjoyment of one's own symptom detached from the Other, without Other. It is this second side of the refusal, which pushes the author to speak of a "psychotic quality" of anorexia-bulimia, verifiable in the clinic beyond the reference to a psychotic structure of the subject. The "holophrastic inclination" that characterizes the stereo-typed and anonymous discourse of the anorexic-bulimic subject around weight, food and the body would be a clinical manifestation that testifies to a "weak desire" and little subjectivized even in its neurotic forms, the structural effect of a "weak paternal metaphor" (ibid., p. 77). This "weakness" is translated by Recalcati through an effective formula relating to the anorexic position in Lacan's dialectic of alienation and separation. A formula according to which the anorexic refusal would bring into play a maneuver of separation, as Miller indicates, which however does not occur from an assumption of the constitutive alienation of the subject in the field of the Other, but presents itself rather as a maneuver against this alienation, as a refusal of alienation: "Separation counter-alienation".

Recalcati's attempt to frame the anorexic phenomenon of the dysmorphoperception of the body image, in the light of Lacan's theory of the mirror stage, is just as original: in the relationship of the anorexic with the image of one's own body the encounter repeats with what the author calls "the grimace of the Other" in the mirror, which occurs at the time of the constitution of the unitary image of one's own body. By this formula, Recalcati accounts for the effect of mortification which is imbued with the encounter of the anorexic with the image of his body, as a repeated manifestation of a superegoic judgment of inadequacy on his body originally received from the other.

To the duplicity of the anorexic refusal corresponds, in the reading of Recalcati, the thesis of a "double status of nothing" in anorexia, where Ménard's analysis of the double "function" of the object nothing, one anchored on the symbolic plane of desire and the other on the real plane of jouissance, is taken up and radicalized. The two nothings of anorexia, which Recalcati articulates based on a distinction by Serge Cottet between the clinic of lack and the clinic of emptiness, refer on the one hand to the nothing as the signifier of desire, underlying a clinic of nothing as lack – a dialectical-neurotic declension of nothing; and on the other, to nothing as emptiness, pure jouissance that cannot be subjected to the hold of symbolization, the foundation of the psychotic side of the anorexic position (Recalcati, 2002, pp. 17–25). It is precisely on the basis of this second definition of the status of the anorexic nothing that Recalcati directs his current research path – the second phase of his research – which he defines as "clinic of the empty". Through this, he proposes to probe the new forms of the symptom – anorexia/bulimia, drug addiction, alcoholism, panic attacks, depression – understood as monosymptomatic variations of the fundamental refusal of the Other which characterizes the contemporary era. Based on Miller's reading of the contemporary Other, the author determines in the decline of the symbolic dimension and in the unprecedented apogee of jouissance which characterizes it, which pushes the subject to have to enjoy without limit, the horizon unprecedented in today's clinic. This horizon is no longer based on the centrality of the process of repression and the return of the repressed, as it returns in the classic psychoanalytic clinic of neuroses, but on a "generalized foreclosure" of the symbolic law which places the contemporary subject before an imperative to enjoy limitless as the superego imperative of contemporaneity.

Failure of the equation body = phallus, refusal of the semblance and imaginary nomination: anorexia in the reading of Nieves Soria

Nieves Soria's research, which developed in Argentina in the early 1990s, is less ambitious in its theoretical-programmatic horizons, but no less radical in its conclusions. Instead of following the same research direction of Recalcati on the new forms of the symptom, her work presents itself rather as a probe focused on the clinic of anorexia and bulimia which uses the internal potential of Lacan's last teaching. Compared to the reading of Ménard, who systematizes Lacan's remarks on anorexia in the light of clinical experience, Recalcati and Soria question anorexia in relation to Lacan's theory as a whole and in particular – especially the Argentinian psychoanalyst – based on the more advanced developments of Lacan in the 1960s and 1970s. Soria's research is based on her private practice as a psychoanalyst who receives anorexic and bulimic patients. Her working method does not take the form of a general theorization, but consists in bringing out from the clinical case the theoretical question around an essential point of the clinic of anorexia. This does not prevent, especially in the more recent developments of her production, her situating the status of anorexia and bulimia as radicalized expressions of a tendency internal to the contemporary horizon, characterized by a "difficulty embodying the father" into his symbolic function; this therefore produces a return effect of "generalized melancholy" (Soria, 2006).

Her more original contributions gradually converge, parallel to the trajectory of Recalcati and the work of Manuel Férnandez Blanco (2000, pp. 51–62), toward a questioning of the reduction of anorexia within the hysterical framework, and therefore toward a problematization of the classical Lacanian doctrine of anorexia. This "parallel convergence" signals, in our opinion, the effect of change in the general problem internal to the Lacanian clinic to which we alluded a little earlier, and the orientative indication put forward by Miller to think neurosis from psychosis, and no longer vice versa. This indication was also, in a way, assumed in the field of anorexia nervosa and produced effects of transformation of the acquired coordinates of reference.

This manifests itself in the course of Soria not only in a clear demarcation between the melancholic forms and the hysterical forms of anorexia (Soria, 2000, pp. 26–32) which are based on a return to Freud. This is expressed above all through a tight clinical interrogation of the anorexic position in the light of the subject's relationship with the object a, with the phallus and the body as phallicized, and with the structure of the subjective fantasy. It is around these structural knots of the constitution of the subjective position that Soria's work produces a clinical deconstruction of the classic identification anorexia = hysteria. The author highlights a fundamental failure in anorexia of the equation body = phallus, which does not account for the drive to be the phallus for the Other at the heart of hysterical identification. Whereas in hysteria the subject knows how to make use of the phallic semblance, and their body is presented as phallicized in the seductive dynamics of the feminine masquerade, in anorexia we are witnessing a fundamental "refusal of the semblance" (ibid., p. 52), which calls into question the equation: thinness = phallus at the heart of hysterical anorexia. This failure reveals a difficulty for the subject to embody the father as a signifier and manifests itself from troubles in the functioning of the paternal metaphor, of which Soria extracts two variants from Lacan. The first concerns the Gide case, and manifests itself in the form of a failed knot in the mother between desire and love: the mother who is all love and who desires nothing transmits the phallic signifier to the child in a deadly version, without desire, which pushes him to identify with this dead phallus, at the origin of the successive anorexia and homosexuality of the writer.

The second comes from Lacan's reference to the anorexic child in *The Seminar*, Book XI, and takes the form of the reduction of desire to the level of need in the maternal position.

In her more recent contributions, Soria manages to question the fact that one can speak, in the case of anorexia, of a real structuring of subjective fantasy, since the object around which anorexic jouissance revolves, the object nothing, does not detach itself from the body, but continues to remain encysted inside without being able to effectively assume the logical consistency of object *a*. This parasitization of the object nothing in the body of the anorexic, the effect of the refusal of the symbolic embodiment of the father, leaves the anorexic outside the very framework of phallic jouissance, which supposes the passage of the subject through castration and loss of enjoyment as a condition of its exercise. In this sense, Soria, following an indication of Javier Aramburu, manages to support the thesis that with the refusal of the Other, in anorexia, we are witnessing a "refusal of the enjoying substance" (ibid., p. 120; Lacan, 1975, p. 33) which is manifested phenomenologically by the deadly dephallicization of the anorexic body, in the refusal of the feminine position (Eidelberg and others, 2003) and in the autistic closure of the subject in a enjoyment without Other.

From this framework, the reading that Soria develops, around the theme of the image of the body in anorexia and its dramatically alienating effect for the subject, is quite original. It can be read as a structural effect of the return to the real of what has been rejected: the deadly appearance of the gaze object as a point of real around which the frame of the specular image of the anorexic body pivots. In this sense, Soria can affirm that "anorexia is the body in anamorphosis", the skeletal caricature imbued with jouissance which breaks the perfection of semblances as in Holbein's painting "The Ambassadors" commented on by Lacan (Soria, 2000, p. 96). However, the author also engages in the attempt to analyze, with reference to the later teaching of Lacan, the dimension of functioning in action in the anorexic position, characterized by a fragility of the process of symbolic embodiment. In this respect, the symptomatic behavior of the anorexic is situated, in the context of the Borromean logic and following Lacan's *The Seminar*, Book XXI, in a form of knotting that passes through an imaginary nomination, which finds its own root in the body and in its image (ibid., p. 74). The special consistency that the ideal image of the body ends up by assuming in anorexia leads Soria to situate it as a knotting point of the three registers (real, symbolic and imaginary), which supplements, in a rather inefficient way, the absence or the precarious inscription of the phallic signifier.

A reading of anorexia from anxiety: true anorexia by Carole Dewambrechies La Sagna

An unprecedented Lacanian perspective on the reading of anorexia nervosa emerged from a recent contribution by Carole Dewambrechies La Sagna, a Lacanian psychiatrist and psychoanalyst from Bordeaux, who introduces, on several points, important innovative aspects compared to Ménard's thesis, Recalcati and Soria. In this new approach, the effects of a radical rereading of the clinic of anorexia, carried out by the author in the light of Lacan's *Seminar L'angoisse*, intertwine with certain fundamental theses, matured during her psychoanalytic practice and, above all, of her practice as head of department within the psychiatric Institution, in the light of the experience of hospitalization of anorexic patients.

The first key thesis, which introduces a discontinuity in the framework of Lacanian readings, consists in positioning anorexia nervosa beyond the classic dichotomy between neurosis and psychosis. What the author defines as "true anorexia", and which corresponds strictly speaking, in her opinion, to what Lacan defined as anorexia nervosa, cannot be traced back either to the framework of hysterical anorexia or to the anorexic symptoms inherent in psychotic framework (Dewambrechies La Sagna, 2006, pp. 58–59). For this reason it is essential, in the treatment, to be able to arrive at a diagnosis of structure which makes it possible to distinguish true anorexia from hysterical and psychotic frames, in order to orient the treatment according to the requirements that the structural specificity entails. This is a new thesis which, as such, opens up, in Lacanian territory, a classic question: should anorexia, therefore, be conceived as a structure in its own right? Or, should we read its specificity rather within the framework of the Lacanian clinic of knots, as a particular form of knotting of the three registers: imaginary, symbolic and real?

On the side of the relationship with the hysterical anorexic, true anorexia is radically different both structurally and in terms of treatment. The clinic of hysterical anorexia presents itself as a "clinic of the phallus" where the refusal of food functions for the subject as a modality of self-phallicization making his body desirable in the eyes of the Other. In this sense, the clinic of hysterical anorexia is structured around desire in its relation to the phallus, as a structurally missing object, which the hysterical subject plays at incarnating through the thinness of the body in order to capture the desire of a man or partner, as happens in the Freudian dream of the beautiful butcher. In this context, hysterical anorexia presents itself, at the treatment level, as a condition in which, for most cases, hospitalization is not necessary (ibid., p. 63). The analysis is often effective on its own in the treatment of hysterical anorexia. When, on the other hand, we are concerned with true anorexia, we find ourselves, as for the psychoses, within the framework of a "clinic of the object" where the pivot is constituted by the relation of the subject to the partial object which reactivates the relation of the little girl with the partial object in the body of the mother. It is in relation to true anorexia that Lacan, in *Le Séminaire*, Book XI, introduces the affirmative declination of "eating nothing" which we must clearly distinguish from the desire for nothing of which Lacan speaks in *The direction of the treatment* in relation to hysterical anorexia where nothing is synonymous with lack. Lacan "elevates the nothing to the dignity of an object", exactly "to answer the question posed by anorexia" (ibid., p. 65), and situates its most probable collocation, according to the author, at the level of the oral object (ibid.). The framework of true anorexia presents itself with its own characteristics: it expresses, in a paradigmatic way, in the clinic, "the attachment of a subject to his own symptom" (ibid., p. 57); it manifests, in an extreme way, the "power of refusal" of food as well as of any cure; in true anorexia the subject asks for nothing; the symbolic power of speech is canceled.

In other words, and in most cases, when the symptom has set in, the conditions for a talking cure and for starting an analysis cannot exist. According to Dewambrechies, the therapeutic response to true anorexia, once it has set in, is primarily hospitalization (ibid., p. 67).

As we said above, it is necessary to distinguish at the same time true anorexia from psychoses presenting anorexic symptoms. This is a distinction whose meaning is reinforced by the fact that true anorexia does not respond effectively to pharmacological treatment, while psychoses also benefit from it in terms of food symptoms. The essential distinction that the author proposes is between being "outside the discourse of structure", as is the case with the psychoses, and being "outside the discourse of fact", as is the case with the anorexia nervosa where the subject's speech is absent or has no value and runs completely empty. Under these conditions, this position outside of discourse, when it is established, constitutes an impossibility for the realization of psychoanalysis understood as an ambulatory analytical cure. It is necessary, on the other hand, to give hospitalization as an indication (ibid.).

Hospitalization as a first step in the treatment of anorexia nervosa makes it possible to introduce the second key thesis, articulated by Dewambrechies: the clinic of anorexia nervosa is a "clinic of anxiety" (ibid., p. 70). The value of this thesis lies at the strategic heart of the treatment question. Indeed, the starting point of anorexia nervosa is represented, on the one hand, by a state of indifference of the patient vis-à-vis their condition and, on the other hand, by a devastating anguish of the people around them, first of all the members of his family. As the author points out, the patient, immersed in their own symptom, does not present any state of anxiety and yet anxiety is always present in the clinical setting in a special form, that of the anxiety of the other (ibid., p. 66).

Anxiety to the Other is a typical action of the anorexic position: the anorexic anguishes insofar as they make themselves for the Other, first of all, an "object impossible to nourish" (ibid.). But if on the one hand this constitutes a impasse to the treatment, from another point of view it is also a question of the perspective from which a therapeutic intervention becomes possible (ibid.).

In this perspective, well-managed hospitalization already presents itself as a first decisive therapeutic operation. Indeed, it allows us, following the lesson of Charcot, to separate, through the isolation of the anorexic subject from his family, "the subject of the anguish of the parental Other" (ibid., p. 70). This operation creates the conditions for a decisive passage to occur in the anorexic subject. A passage that can happen provided you do not let yourself be made anxious by them and do not ask them for anything.

This passage consists in the encounter of the anorexic subject with his own anxiety, an essential condition for them to be able to get out of the indifference in which they have positioned themselves, to resume feeding themselves and to manage to re-subjectivate their own position while modifying. When this happens, it is often the subject's unconscious that is the first to respond through a resumption of dream production.

It is important to emphasize one last point according to which the reading proposed by Dewambrechies differs from the other main Lacanian contributions that we have analyzed: the denial of the existence of an essential relationship between anorexia and bulimia (ibid.), highlighted, on the other hand, with different degrees of connection, by the other analyzed Lacanian authors.

Second, the author calls into question the thesis, which was once that of Freud, of melancholic centrality in psychotic frames characterized by anorexic symptomatology. In his view, indeed, in contemporary developments in psychiatric intervention, melancholia is now diagnosed and treated before it assumes the possible form of the anorexic symptom. It is rather the paranoid forms that dominate in the psychotic frameworks of anorexia and no longer in the classic version of the poisoning delirium but in the more contemporary form of an anxiety of contamination linked to the object of food.

Open questions on anorexia in Lacanian orientation

This concise review of the main readings of anorexia within the framework of the Lacanian orientation leads us, first of all, to notice a fundamental result that is obvious: there is no Lacanian reading of anorexia that is single and homogeneous. On the contrary, we are faced with paradigms of reading, inspired by Lacan, which present themselves as openly heterogeneous and, in certain aspects, conflicting with each other. In our opinion, this represents more of an asset than a limit insofar as it allows the clinical problems of anorexia nervosa to remain open, and encourages greater demonstrative rigor for those who espouse the different theses. This makes it possible to keep alive, in this field, the style of clinical research of Lacan, research aimed at a rigor which does not close the questions but which allows them to be framed with greater precision and to be relaunched.

In this regard, a further merit of the reading proposed by Dewambrechies La Sagna resides precisely in the fact of having rendered problematic the Lacanian question on anorexia nervosa, by the opening, in fact, of a conflict of reading around important critical nodes. I limit myself here to pointing out two that are absolutely central.

The first is an obvious conflict between the paradigm of true anorexia, proposed by Dewambrechies, and the paradigm of anorexia/bulimia, present in the authors analyzed and, in particular, in the reading of Recalcati. Deciding whether anorexia nervosa has a structural relationship with bulimia or whether it presents itself as an autonomous and independent framework of the latter is not a simple question of nosography and classification, since this has important repercussions at the level of the logic of the treatment and its technique. If a value is attributed, in the logic of the anorexia/bulimia paradigm, to the fact of treating anorexic and bulimic patients together, for example within the group system or within a therapeutic community, this value, in the event that we assume the paradigm of true anorexia, is decidedly lacking and could result, in certain aspects, completely contradictory.

The second point concerns the problem of the structural framing of anorexia nervosa, problematized by Dewambrechies through the indication of the irreducibility of anorexia both to hysterical-neurotic frames and to psychoses. The conflict of readings therefore presents itself in these terms: is anorexia nervosa irreducible to the structural binomial psychosis/neurosis (Dewambrechies' thesis) or is it a question of a subjective position conceivable only within of the binomial psychosis/neurosis, as one of its possible variations? On this point, the thesis of the autonomy of the framework of anorexia nervosa ultimately problematizes Lacan's classical structural clinic as a whole, although the author cites Lacan to affirm it. Should we recognize on this point also, as we have shown in this work, a typical function of anorexia nervosa in the work of Lacan: that of situating oneself on a fault line, of epistemological passage, of turning within the framework of a structural clinic toward the framework of a clinic of knots, such that it imposes itself in the most advanced teaching of Lacan?

References

Brusset, B. (1991), Psychopatologie et métapsychologie de l'addition boulimique. *La Boulimie. Revue Française de Psychanalyse*, Paris: PUF, pp. 105–132.

Dewambrechies La Sagna, C. (2006), L'anorexie vraie de la jeune fille. *La Cause freudienne*, no. 63, pp. 57–70.

Eidelberg, A. and others (2003), *Síntomas actuales de lo femenino*. Buenos Aires: Del Bucle.

Férnandez Blanco, M. (2000), La posición anorexica, Gorali, V. (Dir.). *Estudios sobre anorexia y bulimia*. Buenos Aires: ATUEL CAP, pp. 51–62.

IRMA (1999), *La psychose ordinaire: la Convention d'Antibes*. Paris: Agalma/Le Seuil.

Lacan, J. (1973), *Le Séminaire. Livre XI. Les quatre concepts fondamentaux de la psychanalyse, 1964*. Paris: Le Seuil.

Lacan, J. (2001), *Les complexes familiaux dans la formation de l'individu (1938). Autres érits*. Paris: Seuil.

Lacan, J. (2006), *The Direction of the Treatment and the Principles of Its Power (1958). Ecrits*. The First Complete Edition in English. New York/London: Norton & Company; *La direction de la cure et les principes de son pouvoir. Ecris* (1966). Paris: Seuil.

Ménard, A. (1992), Structure signifiante de l'anorexie mentale. *Actes ECF*, vol. 2, pp. 3–7.

Miller, J.-A. (1998), *Silet (1995), La Psicoanalisi*, no. 24, pp. 215–235.

Miller, J.-A. (2001), *Lettres à l'opinion éclairée*. Paris: Seuil.

Miller, J.-A., Laurent, É. (2005), *El Otro que no existe y sus comités de ética, 1996–1997*. Buenos Aires: Paidós.

Miller, J.-A. (2006), Modalidades de rechazo (1991). *Introducción a la clínica lacaniana: conferencias en España*. Madrid: Gredos.

Miller, J.-A. (2009), Effet retour sur la psychose ordinaire. *Quarto*, no. 94–95, pp. 40–51, janvier.

Recalcati, M. (1997), *L'ultima cena: anoressia e bulimia*. Milano: Bruno Mondadori.

Recalcati, M. (2002), *Clinica del vuoto. Anoressia, dipendenze, psicosi*. Milano: Franco Angeli.

Recalcati, M. (2010), *L'uomo senza inconscio: figure della nuova clinica psicoanalitica*. Milano: Cortina.

Soria, N. (2000), *Psicoanalisis de la anorexia y bulimia*. Buenos Aires: Tres Haces.

Soria, N. (2006), Anoressia-bulimia. *Scilicet del Nome-del-Padre*. AMP (CD Room).

Chapter 6

The four functions of refusal in anorexia nervosa

Refusal as a key to anorexia

Following the methodological indication proposed by Lacan in *The Seminar*, Book X, *Anxiety*, we have sought a key that could open the door to the field that intrigues us: anorexia in its strategic core, in its logic of functioning, beyond the nosographic and comparative references that abound in the tradition of psychiatric and psychoanalytic psychopathology. References which we have, in any case, taken into account during this work. The key that we have found, and which will be the main thread of this chapter, is that of refusal as a strategic node in the clinic of anorexia nervosa. We found this key as much in Lacan's affirmations as in the reworking of them by Lacanian authors deeply involved in the clinic and in the theory of anorexia nervosa. Now it is a matter of defining in a specific way the status of refusal in the clinic of anorexia nervosa.

The reasons that led us to this choice are different and can be summarized in four fundamental points.

First of all, the "phenomenological evidence" that the clinical experience shows us and that institutes refusal as a paradigmatic factor unifying the various "negative" behaviors put into action by the anorexic: the refusal of food, of the female body, of sexuality, of the social link.

It is this evidence that situates anorexia as the radicalized incarnation of refusal in the clinic. This evidence is presented in all its destructive force in the refusal of the treatment. As Dewambrechies La Sagna recently affirmed, as a clinician, what we are confronted with when we meet the anorexic is indeed the power of this refusal (Dewambrechies La Sagna, 2006, p. 66).

This phenomenology of the anorexic refusal allows us, second, beyond the references to the narcissistic fragility of the Ego and to the cognitive-behavioral deficit aspect that would be correlated to it – central factors not only in psychiatry and psychology, but also in the evolutionary approaches of post-Freudian psychoanalysis – to question its function in its affirmative or "positive" status of solution, even if it is a pathological solution, in relation to a constitutive difficulty of the subject's relationship to the Other. In this sense, the

DOI: 10.4324/9781003318439-7

anorexic refusal is presented more as a position taken with the Other than as a deficit or negative behavior. It is therefore better to avoid the normalizing reconduction to a supposed developmental normality and to insist on the unveiling of what supports it symbolically and libidinally.

Third, questioning the function of refusal in the field of anorexia nervosa, allows us to raise anorexic refusal from the purely mute status of behavior to the structural dimension, from the plane of phenomenology to the plane of logic. This leads us to situate the core of the anorexic position beyond the narcissistic-specular dimension, as a mode of articulation of the subject's relation to the Other and to jouissance.

Finally, exploring the function of refusal in the clinic of anorexia nervosa allows us to reveal, beyond the phenomenological monotony of refusal behaviors, the differential polyphony not only of the subjective structures of anorexic patients, but ultimately their singular and irreducible modes of jouissance.

In this chapter of our work, we will try to take advantage of the indications of Lacan and his students to deepen, with the help of clinical situations, the status of anorexic refusal. As we have seen, it is presented as a function with a double status: on the one hand, in the clinic of neurosis, it is a function of desire; at the same time, refusal in anorexia is characterized as a function of jouissance that assumes functional structures that are differentiated in psychoses and neuroses:

$$\text{refusal} = f\,(d) \qquad \text{refusal} = f\,(j)$$

This bifrontal status of the function of refusal we find on the other hand in the structural duplicity of the object cause in anorexia, that is to say the object nothing, which functions on one side as a signifier of desire as structurally desire for something else; and at the same time as the object cause of desire which gives rise to a jouissance structured around dissatisfaction and deprivation (this is the case in particular in hysteria), when it is not a psychotic jouissance structure declined in a melancholic-toxicomaniac way, if not more clearly schizophrenic or paranoid:

$$\text{object nothing} = f\,(d) \qquad \text{object nothing} = f\,(j)$$

What we are trying to propose in this part of the research is the determination of a quadruple root of refusal in anorexia nervosa: a dialectical-hysterical matrix that structures refusal as an unconscious demand addressed to the Other; a matrix of refusal as a defence of the real; a matrix of refusal, also identifiable in the clinic of psychoses, as an attempt to separate (in psychosis this often takes the form of disconnection) the subject from the Other and the social bond; and finally, the matrix of refusal as jouissance, which constitutes the fundamental enigma of the clinic of anorexia nervosa, and the object around which this work in particular revolves.

Refusal as a metaphor for desire: the conjunction between anorexia and hysteria

Hysterical anorexia: between forgetting and discovery

A first root of the phenomenon of refusal in anorexia nervosa finds its clinical and conceptual frame of reference in hysteria. It is indeed from the solid psychopathological research axis developed by Lasègue – who formalized the syndrome in 1873 in the medico-psychiatric nosography by the definition of hysterical anorexia – which then passes through Freud to finally arrive at Lacan, that we can determine a definition in neurotic terms, more precisely in hysterical terms, of anorexia nervosa.

This definition is not exhaustive and does not intend to reduce the anorexic phenomenon entirely to the framework of the hysterical structure, but it nevertheless determines in hysteria the structural terrain of a specific version of anorexia. The highlighting of hysterical anorexia and its functioning, and the special function of the refusal that is exercised there, assumes a specific topical value, especially today, when the reference to hysteria is veiled not only by the descriptive-classificatory nosography of the DSM – which has erased the very notion of hysteria from its lexicon – but also by the dominant tendency among authors of psychoanalytical matrix engaged in research on anorexia, who favor the exclusive reference to the borderline organization or to psychosis (Appeau, 1992, p. 172; Brusset, 1998, p. 221). This is a counter-tendency to the dominant inclination which sidelines the reference to hysteria, reducing it to a syndrome which had its moment of glory in the psycho-pathological context of bourgeois societies with classical capitalism – the Victorian era would be the paradigm – and which would be in the process of extinction today, (let us stress that some important authors belonging to the IPA such as Cristopher Bollas totally disagree with this point of view), that the position of the School of Lacan and of the Lacanian orientation is affirmed. There is indeed in Lacan's perspective something imperishable in hysteria, especially because we can recognize in it the functioning of a discursive structure (what Lacan will rightly call the discourse of the hysterical), and because hysteria marks the very feature of human desire as a desire structurally for something else in relation to what we say we want, a desire for something else in relation to the object of demand. No object of demand can indeed totally satisfy the subject's desire, and it is in this margin of structural dissatisfaction that the unconscious motor of the subject itself is situated, its structural division, raised to the mathema of the hysterical position.

It is because of this structural dissatisfaction of human desire, which in hysteria is thus highlighted, that the hysteric functions in the environment and in the bonds of belonging (family, work, love, society) as a factor of tension and of questioning the status quo and as an opening to change (Brousse, 2002, pp. 66–71; Naveau, 2001, pp. 72–92).

For this reason, there is a very heated clinical and psychopathological debate around the reading of hysteria as a syndrome in the process of disappearing, supplanted by the mass diffusion of new forms of the symptom, or, on the contrary, as a syndrome that would be hidden under the forms of NFS (in particular in anorexia and bulimia) through an operation of historical-social metamorphosis of the clinical figures of hysterical desire, as Bollas (2000) argues. In this perspective, anorexia as well as bulimia, as pathologies that predominantly affect women and their bodies, would fully result, in different cases, from contemporary, postmodern versions of hysteria.

From the perspective of the Lacanian orientation, anorexia and bulimia are phenomena that, even if persistent, are not reducible to a structure per se; nor can they be reduced entirely to a Freudian clinical structure. On the contrary, as we will see in this work, there are singular variations of anorexia and bulimia in the different clinical structures (psychosis, neurosis and perversion), where the anorexic-bulimic phenomenon exercises differentiated functions for the subject in relation to the specific requirements that the structure entails for him.

In this sense, hysterical anorexia undoubtedly constitutes, for the Lacanian orientation, one of the essential structural frames of reference that allows us to read, in many neurotic anorexic-bulimics, the function and the field of refusal in their pathological experience.

Functions of refusal in hysterical anorexia

Refusal as a condition of desire

Lacan, a reader of Freud, highlights that the hysteric, through the practice of refusal, deals with something that concerns the very structure of human desire. This means, first of all, that if the subject does not have the possibility of saying "no" to what happens to him or her from the Other, the space for a possible and sustainable desire cannot be created. Only if the subject succeeds in withdrawing, at whatever level, from the necessity of consenting to the demand of the Other, does he or she become able to articulate a difference, however slight, between him or herself and the Other, which manages to distinguish him or her from the Other, allowing him or her to assume his or her own position. In this sense, the subject's refusal of the Other's demand becomes the very condition of his desire. Based on this argumentation of Lacan, Jacques-Alain Miller, more recently, has radicalized the Lacanian indication, by assuming, in *The Other Who Does Not Exist*, anorexia as a structural paradigm of human desire as a desire for nothing, as a refusal that creates this void of being indispensable to the articulation of desire (Miller, Laurent, 2005, p. 378; Ansermet, 1999, p. 162). It is basically this fundamental anorexic operation that the child puts into action in early childhood to introduce a hiatus that separates his position, what he wants, from the parents' demand to take care of him and feed him: he refuses food when he wants to transmit to them that what he lacks, at that moment, is something else. A child who cannot refuse, who can never say "no" is a child who cannot desire, who is completely prey to the demand of the Other. He is the exclusive object of this demand, he is One with the Other.

Refusal as a metaphor for the demand for love: unconscious demand for
rectification of the subjective position of the Other in relation
to the subject

The dynamic of refusal in hysterical anorexia presents a double side. On the one hand, it is the essential maneuver that allows the constitution of the subject as differentiated from the Other and not totally reducible to the grasp of the Other. On the other hand, through refusal, the subject exercises on the Other, in particular on his parents, a maneuver unconsciously oriented to rectify the unbearable position they occupy in relation to the subject. Lacan clearly expresses this point in *The Direction of the Treatment*, when he shows the state of fundamental confusion in which the parents of the anorexic find themselves. The girl's anorexia is at the same time the result and the denunciation of this confusion. Lacan says that the parents do not distinguish, in their relationship with their daughter, the care of the gift of love, they do not distinguish the satisfaction of needs from the gift of the sign of love that comes into play on the symbolic level in relation to the desire of the girl as subject.

Indeed, responding to the demand for love with the object that satisfies the need produces an effect of structural dissatisfaction in the one who asks. As Lacan teaches, one can only respond to the demand for love on the level of love, by giving the other, through the sign of love, one's own lack, what one does not have and not what one has. There is thus a symbolic side to the refusal at work in hysterical anorexia, which challenges the Other so that it can respond to the subject at this radical level of demand, that is, at the level of the demand for love. The refusal in hysterical anorexia presents itself precisely, in the Lacanian reading, as a radical operation that tends to show to the Other, in particular the parents, the irreducible difference that structurally separates the symbolic level of desire from the level of need and satisfaction.

The ample phenomenology of refusal that constellates the clinic of hysterical anorexia, from the refusal of food to the refusal of bonding, is crossed like a thread by this function of silent and acted message in the body that asks the Other for the sign of love that it cannot give. In this logic, then:

Refusal = unconscious demand (versus desire).

This is what Lacan's teaching consists of, in his text *The Direction of the Treatment*, when he says that the anorexic plays her refusal as a desire, thus teaching us that refusing is the anorexic-bulimic mode of asking. We find this form of demand in its paradigmatic and radical version in hysterical anorexia.

In Claudia's case, the father's departure for a job abroad and the fact of staying at home with a mother totally absorbed in caring for her daughter produced the conjuncture for the triggering of the anorexic symptom at the age of 14. Faced with the overflow of maternal anguish and the absence of the father, the anorexic response was the only solution available to the subject to face this new situation. The father's concern about the girl's condition and his decision to return to Italy permanently (giving up the prospect of a career abroad to look after her), resulted in the girl's recovery in the following months and the end of a physical condition in which Claudia's life was seriously at stake. In this case, the daughter's anorexia takes on the double function of a demand for love addressed to the father to return, and of a barrier to the excess of maternal anguish poured out on the daughter.

Metonymic dimension of desire in anorexic-hysterical refusal: refusal as desire for another

However, in hysterical anorexia, the function of refusal is not reduced to radicalizing the difference between desire and need and the irreducibility of the former to the latter. The refusal reveals, at the same time, the irreducibility of desire to the field of the demand. As Lacan says, desire is beyond and below demand (Lacan, 2006, p. 530). Indeed, whatever the object of the demand, the subject will always remain partly unsatisfied, i.e. with an unfulfilled desire, but at the same time and more radically, desire presents itself as structurally irreducible to the demand. In this sense, we find in hysterical anorexia the metonymic structure of desire understood by Lacan, in *The Direction of the Treatment*, where he affirms that "desire is the metonymy of the want to be" (ibid., p. 520).

In the case of Clementina, a 20-year-old patient, whom I followed in individual consultation in an institution for almost a year, and who subsequently continued her analytical work in my private practice, the metonymic trait of desire emerged in an obvious way after an initial period of treatment for a "restrictive" anorexia that had abruptly interrupted her affective life at the age of 16, pushing her toward a progressive isolation. During the first year of consultation, the stagnation of her discourse around the food symptom functioned as the main theme, the young girl strongly insisted on her autonomy in relation to affective relationships and social ties and on being self-sufficient. Only one vital passion animated her in the dark period of anorexia: the passion for theatre, which led her, a year ago, to pass the entrance exam to the most prestigious Italian theatre school (this important institution of Milanese cultural life trains new generations of actors).

For Clementina, the satisfaction of entering the school was immediately followed by anxiety: the demanding activity of the school's theatre training exposed her to continuous contact with other students and teachers, to a social life from which she could not escape. She was particularly uncomfortable during the festive and social moments typical of the theatre world, such as late-night dinners after rehearsals. Moreover, her anorexia was put to the test because of the requirement of a physical muscle tone indispensable to support the obligatory physical exercises in certain subjects of the school's didactic program. Thus, in this context, the spectre of the subjective division that distressed Clementina was introduced: to keep the anorexia or lose the theatre? The introduction of the anxiety, as Dewambrechies La Sagna has pointed out (Dewambrechies La Sagna, 2006, p. 67), breaks the presumed ego-syntonic plenitude of being that anorexia guarantees to the subject and opens the door to the malaise of the subjective division, making the subject responsible for her unconscious decision. Anorexia becomes symptomatic and the space for a subjective rectification of the subject's relationship with the real can open up. It is at this point that the metonymy of desire, frozen for a few years, begins to manifest itself again as an effect of this shift in position. It was in the relationship with men that Clementina experienced the effects. She began to dream again, to dream about herself with boys, in particular, with colleagues from the theatre school. Only that every time she dreams of a boy, and there is a chance of meeting him in reality, or even of starting an affair, the patient feels and carries over into analysis the immediate affective chill that leads her to drop the relationship. Each time, she repeats, "I thought it was him, but in reality it wasn't".

In the treatment of hysterical anorexia, the shaping of the hysterical dialectic of desire and its laws in the subject, as well as the manifestation of anxiety and subjective division, are a sign of effectiveness of the work in act.

The "fantasy of one's own disappearance" in hysterical anorexia and the unconscious demand that expresses: "does he want to lose me?"

The metaphorical aspect of refusal in hysterical anorexia finds its most radical manifestation at the moment when the anorexic restriction, the refusal to eat, exceeds the critical threshold for the survival of the organism, and the state of the body that risks death becomes for the subject itself the mute embodiment of a radical demand for love that questions the Other on the place it reserves in its desire for the anorexic subject and for the fact that he or she is alive or dead. Lacan clearly expresses this point in a passage of *The Seminar*, Book XI, where he speaks of the anorexic child as the embodiment of a desperate and silent demand addressed by the subject to his parents in order to verify the love they have for him. This is why the anguished response of the parents to the worsening of the anorexia only consolidates the strength of the symptom and the pathological power of the anorexia because the subject expects from the parental Other a response that functions as a sign of love, as a word that gives an irreplaceable place to the subject in the desire of the Other, and not as a manifestation of the Other's anguish. The anguish of the Other has the effect of consolidating the anorexic solution, by feeding the subject with the trait of perversion that anorexia presents in its functioning: to anguish the Other by reducing it to impotence. This is what we see in many cases, where the parents, in the grip of anguish, collude with the girl's symptom, supporting and feeding it concretely. This is most evident in purging anorexia, where the parents very often become slaves to the girl's symptom, buying food to order for the subject to binge on. In "restricting" anorexia, we also find, in various cases, a support of the symptom by the parents which serves to relieve their own anguish. This is the case, for example, of a mother who, in front of her hospitalized daughter who is risking her life, prevents the doctor from applying a nasogastric tube for parenteral nutrition because she cannot stand her daughter's crying. It is only the non-anxious response from the Other that allows a limit to be set to the narcissistic-imaginary omnipotence of the anorexic symptom, thus opening up a possible space for the patient's subjective speech.

The threat of disappearance in the analytic transference: the push to interrupt the treatment and its symbolic side

Something similar occurs in the transference toward the analyst or the nursing staff on the part of the anorexic patient: the refusal of the treatment, the threat of interruption, the symptomatic aggravation, can only be read if we take into consideration the metaphorical aspect of the message, of the testing of the analyst's position of desire. One must, in fact, suppose a structural ambivalence in the demand of the anorexic-bulimic subject (Cosenza, 2001, p. 233), and try as an analyst to occupy in the transference the place of another Other than the one the subject has already met in his history. An Other capable of recognizing, in the neurotic refusal that the subject addresses to us, the symbolic thickness of an unconscious demand. This is the precious indication that Lacan suggested to us for the treatment of anorexia when he tells us that the anorexic "… emplys his refusal as if it were a desire" (Lacan, 2006, p. 524). This is why we pay particular attention to the moments and modalities of emergence in the treatment of the dynamics of refusal, to the negative transference, to the absences and the "acting out" of the patients. In these situations, in fact, what manifests itself revolves around an unconscious demand that is addressed to us as analysts. In some ways, it is precisely through this testing of the holding of the Other, which we embody for them as analysts, that these patients provide us with the opportunity to bring out, through our intervention, the presence of an unconscious demand. This demand alludes to what we might call their preliminary questioning of the treatment, through the threat of interruption. Through this maneuver, the anorexic subject reactivates the fantasy of disappearance by which the girl, in childhood, questions, often through the refusal of food, but also through the refusal of speech, the parents' desire for her, her place in the parental desire, in the form of a fundamental questioning: "Does they want to lose me?"

(Lacan, 1973, p. 240). This maneuver by the patient produces an effect of intensification of the transferential dynamic, which removes the subject from the empty stereotypy, typical in these patients, of an anonymous discourse. This brings into play the object of a phantasmatic repetition that challenges the analyst by putting his position to the test. It is up to him, in fact, to show the subject that what happens in analysis is not reduced to mere empty words. And that, on the contrary, the call contained in the refusal, in the threat of interruption of the treatment, arrives at the destination of the one who knows how to restore it to the subject in its form of enigma inherent in his desire. This fundamental maneuver is often carried out, in the contingency of a treatment, by the analyst's interventions which contain the subject's exit from the treatment, by sheltering him from the autistic-autodestructive push internal to the anorexic refusal. In some cases, the treatments held together at this difficult moment, thanks to the subtle thread of one or more telephone interventions by the analyst, to letters or messages written or sent to the patient during periods of temporary interruption or hospitalization. These means gave the subject back the minimum of confidence in the Other that was indispensable for continuing the work. In each case, the structuring of a symbolic transference was only possible through the encounter with an analyst who did not respond either with anguish or with indifference to the patient's threat of disappearance. Rather, the analyst found himself occupying the place of the object that is the cause of the subject's desire, of the vital thrust that orients the subject to say what he wants, to produce his desire in the analytic work.

Clelia, one of my patients who suffers from "purging" anorexia, has a love life closely linked to the manifestation of the symptom. When she meets a man and begins a relationship, the symptom disappears. However, her problem reappears from time to time during the building and consolidation of the relationship. Each time, the partner becomes anxious about her infinite demand for love and escapes. This results in a devastating reactivation of her symptom. In these circumstances, she comes to analysis with the idea of interrupting the treatment and displaying an overwhelming aggressiveness toward the analyst. One of my interventions had the effect of placating her anger and producing the attenuation of the symptom; indeed, I said to her: "It certainly won't be your vomiting that frightens me and makes me run away!" Her attempt to reproduce in the relationship with the analyst the dynamic put into act with her partners had found a stop in an interpretative act that had emptied its imaginary consistency.

Refusal as an unconscious demand for interpretation

It is only at this level of the analyst's position that we can read in the treatment the emergence of refusal in hysterical anorexia as a demand for interpretation addressed to the analyst herself. It is precisely from the installation of this basic position of the analyst in the transference relation during the course of the analysis that a practice such as that of interpretation becomes possible and effective, which, on the contrary, in the early stages of the work with anorexics, often proves ineffective. This is because of the nominalistic reduction of speech to the simple flatus vocis that characterizes the anaesthesia of anorexic discourse in the preliminary phase of treatment. Indeed, the encounter with an Other who is reliable for the patient and embodied by the analyst, the fact that he functions as subject-supposed-knowledge, makes the reopening of the subject's unconscious possible. The production of a dream or a missed act no longer appear to the subject as meaningless phenomena, but as events that have a relationship with his or her existence and that can be deciphered. This passage, which can be defined in terms of the hysterization of the subject's unconscious productions (dreams, slips of the tongue, symptoms ...), makes the effectiveness of the analyst's interpretations possible for the subject. The reopening of the unconscious allows the subject to symbolize his history, to determine the place he has occupied in the family discourse, the network of identifications around which his phantasmatic identity has been structured.

In neurotic anorexia, we can thus observe that the refusal of treatment conveys, above all, to a certain extent, the value of an unconscious demand addressed to the Other, embodied by the analyst in the treatment, which tends to verify the desire that the latter introduces in the work with the patient.

Refusal as a defence

The anti-metaphorical side of anorexic-bulimic refusal

If it is true that the clinic of anorexia finds its fundamental knotting point by presenting itself as a clinic of refusal, the status of anorexic refusal cannot be reduced to its symbolic-metaphoric declination of unconscious demand toward the Other. On the contrary, this dimension, even if it is essential in the reading of the functioning of neurotic anorexia, does not exhaust the value and the function that the dynamics of refusal also embodies in the framework of neuroses. Indeed, we always find, along with the metaphorical-dialectical side of the refusal, in hysterical anorexia, an anti-metaphorical and anti-dialectical side of the refusal itself, which does not imply and does not allow the interpretation of the refusal as a metaphor of an unconscious demand. The first level of reading of this anti-metaphorical dimension of anorexic refusal is found in the definition of refusal as defence. To move from the definition of anorexic refusal as an unconscious demand to the definition of refusal as a defence means, above all, to change the sign of the subject's orientation toward the Other: to move from a search – even if paradoxical – on the part of the subject – for desire in the Other, to a protection of what happens to the subject on the part of the Other. Thinking of anorexic refusal as a defence leads us, beyond the dialectic of recognition, to isolate the relation of the anorexic subject in relation to the real that he defends them-selves from and that the encounter with the Other presents for them.

The definition of anorexic refusal as a defence of the drive real is clinically more generalizable than the definition of refusal as a metaphor of an unconscious demand, since, unlike the latter which concerns above all the field of neuroses, it has a universal value in anorexia, even if in a different way, as much for neuroses as for psychoses.

The refusal of food as a defence

This function of refusal as a defence is found in action at all levels of the anorexic experience and also involves the dimension of eating disorder. Indeed, in the discourse of anorexic and bulimic patients, the refusal of food – whether in the anorexic form of abstinence from food consumption, or in the bulimic form of evacuation – cannot be reduced to an absence of appetite. On the contrary, the food that is refused and that the subject has stopped eating at the beginning of the illness is often the most coveted food. In its place, the subject chooses a food characterized by the value "light", very low in calories and which induces at the lowest its evocative function of appetite.

In this sense, the anorexic refusal of food is presented as a defence of appetite rather than as an absence of appetite. In this respect, in their famous book, *La faim et le corps*, Kestemberg and Decobert underline the counter-intuitive paradox embodied in the anorexic relationship with food: at the basis of this refusal, there would be something other than an absence of hunger, but rather an "orgasm of hunger", where "pleasure is concentrated in the silent intoxication of hunger, sought, chased and found" (Kestemberg and others, 1981, p. 231). In this sense, the refusal of food divides the anorexic subject, by defending him from something he covets. However, when the treatment is already well advanced, the anorexic-bulimic subject begins to find the way back to the food-appetite, and he/she can rediscover the ex-perience of feeding himself/herself by experiencing the oral pleasure that this entails. For example, an anorexic patient in a therapeutic community was able to resume eating ice cream, her favorite food, after ten years of absolute prohibition of eating this food. She recalled the repressed memory of her childhood discovery of ice cream, when she had her tonsils removed and, immediately after the operation, the medical staff offered her an ice cream. This particular pleasure of tasting ice cream, which for her was originally linked to an experience of loss that affected the body, was no longer acces-sible to her at the onset of anorexia in adolescence. The attenuation of the anorexic symptom, the partial loss of the enjoyment that the illness entails, was necessary for her to recover this experience of pleasure.

The institutional experience in a therapeutic structure allows us to ex-amine in more detail the issue of food refusal on the part of anorexic and bulimic patients. With our colleagues from the therapeutic community

"La Vela", we made another clinical "discovery" in this respect, by observing what was happening at the time of meals shared by anorexic and bulimic patients and noticing a singular operation in which the patients with hysterical dynamics were involved. The first time I became aware of this phenomenon, 25 years ago, was when I observed Agnese, an anorexic patient with a hysterical structure, who, during the meal, tended not to eat, but on the other hand, pushed a bulimic friend to eat, trying to sneak her food into the latter's plate. When she managed to get her classmates to eat her food, or when a community educator sat at her table and she served him, her face clearly expressed a satisfaction that I would describe as "starving". Similarly, her anger was clearly visible when someone refused the food she offered. Agnese's example led us to examine food refusal from another angle, in the light of this dynamic consisting of the patients' passionate haste to make others eat. A dynamic, moreover, that underlies a rather well-known phenomenon, namely the inclination for cooking of anorexic patients, who often prepare dishes for their families and, in general, for others: a phenomenon that associates with a refusal a disproportionate interest in it. The theoretical hypothesis that I was able to formulate in this respect is the following: the anorexic patient eats what she wants by identification, identifying herself with the Other that they push to eat. The anorexic eats by proxy, by pushing the Other to eat in their place and by deriving satisfaction from this in terms of identification.

Refusal to eat   "Vicarious" eating

(−)   (+)

In our opinion, this applies absolutely to hysterical anorexia, in which case the anorexic does with food what, as Freud teaches us, the hysteric does with sex: she can consume it by proxy, by identifying herself in the sexual relationship with a man (or a partner) with whom she is in contact, as in the case of Dora, where the relationship is with another woman. Feeding by proxy through identification with another person compensates, in an imaginary way, for the refusal of food that the anorexic puts into action in reality. This said, there is a third essential level of the anorexic subject's relationship with food involved in the refusal, a level that no longer touches the imaginary dimension, nor the symbolic one linked to the refusal of food, but the register of the real, to which we will return when we address the definition of refusal as a mode of jouissance, where an enigmatic libidinal positivity emerges in the refusal. This is what Lacan expresses when he affirms, in *The Seminar*, Book XI, that it is not true that the anorexic does not eat: on the contrary, she eats, but what she eats is "nothing", and the refusal of food is the element that allows the anorexic to consume this nothing to which she is libidinally attached.

Food refusal   Eating "nothing"
(−)   (+)

In psychotic anorexia, the refusal of food functions as a defence which is not, however, directed against the subject's appetite: in this case, unlike hysterical anorexia, it is not the subject who defends themselves against something they desire, even if it disgusts them. In psychosis, the refusal of food protects the subject against something threatening, which for them is epitomized by food. In cases of paranoia, e.g. delusions of poisoning, the refusal of food obviously becomes the immediate consequence of the paranoid certainty by which the subject maintains that someone, a persecutor, wants to poison him. But also in some less obvious forms of psychotic anorexia, food appears as a contaminated and threatening "object" from which the subject must preserve themselves at all costs. The anxiety of contamination and contaminated food is a rather frequent phenomenon in restrictive anorexias, especially in psychotic forms, and effectively testifies to the function of anorexic refusal as a defence against a real that threatens the subject in an invasive way.

Refusal of the body image in the mirror: partial failure of the mirror stage and defence against the return of the real in anamorphosis

Besides the refusal of food, the central disorder of the dysmorphoperception of the body image is also characterized – this is one of our theses – by a declension of the anorexic refusal in the framework of the scopic experience. Indeed, we can read the radical disorder that runs through the experience of the anorexic subject in his or her relationship to his or her body image as a phenomenon that does not find a cause in the obsession with fatness and thinness, but rather a secondary and failed attempt to repair a constitutive alteration, which concerns the primary narcissistic constitution of the subject itself. In this respect, the Lacanian contributions of the last three decades offer the most solid conceptual bases for illuminating this singular clinical phenomenon.

The first important thesis is the one put forward by Recalcati, who identifies the matrix of the anorexic-bulimic dysmorphoperception of the body image in a failed passage of the subject through the structural crossroads of the mirror stage. The author reconstructs this passage, formulating the thesis according to which the little girl perceives in this critical situation the "grimace of the Other" as a surmised judgment of contempt or devaluation in relation to her body image. This would have the consequence that, beside psychoses characterized by a structural fragmentation of the image of one's own body that leaves the subject in a state of perplexity or in the grip of persecution, in neurotic anorexias and also bulimias the subject's relationship to the image of the body takes on an exorbitant and derealizing traumatic character, which goes beyond the normal structural alienation linked to the "primordial discord" that accompanies the unifying effect of the encounter with the "Gestalt" of one's own body. Beyond the somewhat imaginary reference to the Other's grimace, there is no doubt that in the history of anorexic patients, we can identify an early encounter with traumatic signifiers – judgments, sentences – uttered by important figures in their lives, which have had a lethal impact on the subjects' relationship with their bodies. These are formulations that have reached the subject as superegoic judgments, which have functioned in the course of his or her life as true master signifiers (S1), to which the anorexia was an unconscious attempt to respond on the part of the subject. For us, it is therefore from the identification of these S1s by the subject in analysis that it is possible for him/her to come to terms with what is happening to him/her in the anorexic relationship to his/her body.

However, it is to a clinical intuition of Soria's that we must recognize, in our opinion, the determining factor at the level of the libidinal real that is at the basis of the dis-perceptive phenomenon typical of anorexia. Indeed, by taking up in an original way the theses expressed by Lacan in *The Seminar*, Book XI, on the functioning of the scopic drive, and by applying them to the clinical field of anorexia, Soria manages to identify, as we have seen, the drive foundation of the anorexic altered perception of the body image in a return of the drive real rejected at the level of the anorexic image of the body in anamorphosis. This is translated in the experience and in the language of anorexia in terms of too much fat in the body image, which is its mode of saying a *plus-de-jouir*, both unbearable and irresistible (Soria, 2000, p. 37). It is in relation to this excess of enjoyment, in defence of this surplus of enjoyment that the return of the scopic drive into the real intervenes, that the anorexic is pushed toward the mirror while refusing to recognize their own image in the mirror.

Refusal as a defence against the drive: the refusal of enjoyment (jouissance)

Alongside the refusal of food and the altered relationship to one's own body image, the third crucial point that comes into play in the symptomatic dimension of anorexia is the relationship to sexuality. It is not by chance that amenorrhea, generally accompanied by an absence of sexual life and, in any case, by substantial anorgasmia, characterizes the condition of most anorexic female subjects for several years. Seen from this perspective, the anorexic refusal is presented as a stubborn defence of the anorexic subject against the fact of occupying a feminine position and the implications that this position entails. The fact that most of the onset of anorexia occurs in young girls during the pubertal or prepubertal period confirms the classical reading of anorexia as a refusal to move into the female position at the crossroads of adolescence. In this respect, anorexia presents itself as a position that defies the laws of biological development in an anti-naturalistic way, by demonstrating in the real that the problem of the passage to the sexual position of man or woman cannot be resolved within the framework of the evolutionary determinism of the organism.

However, on this point too, it is necessary to differentiate hysterical-neurotic anorexias from psychotic forms of anorexia. In the former, the refusal of the sexual drive is structured as a desire, it makes dissatisfaction a mode of enjoyment and is thus inherent to the symbolic logic of the signifier that pivots around the phallic signifier. In this sense, the clinic of hysterical anorexia is a "phallus clinic". On the other hand, the non-neurotic forms of anorexia fall within the framework of a "clinic of the object" (Dewambrechies La Sagna, 2006, p. 62), where the exclusion of the Name-of-the-Father blocks the subject's access to the phallicization of the body and to sexuation, producing the effect of a radical refusal of the semblant linked to sex (Soria, 2000, pp. 51–52).

In fact, in the case of psychoses, we are faced with a function of refusal, also embodied by the food symptom, which responds to a different logic. Indeed, in psychoses, refusal, embodied, for example, in the anxiety of contamination, in the practices of introduction and forced evacuation of substances through the body, but also in the refusal or the abrupt rejection of the bond, functions as a way of containing the invasion of an Other without limits who wants to enjoy the subject. We could write this logic using the following formula:

$$\text{Refusal} = \text{limit (to the invasion of the Other)}.$$

In working with psychosis, the subject's trust can be gained if he or she is helped to deal with the all-powerful and sadistic Other, which he or she defends as best he or she can by trying to distance himself or herself from it through food refusal, vomiting and evacuation. If the omnipotence of the Other is reduced, then the eating symptom of the psychotic subject can also be tempered and function as a stabilizing compensatory self-therapy, which does not expose him to the risk of death or triggering, opening the way to the delicate and difficult work of constructing other points of stabilization that can function for the subject, in parallel to a smaller eating symptom, as points of support.

Anorexic refusal as a mode of separation from the Other

"Refusal of the Other", new forms of the symptom and anorexia

There is a third dimension at play in the dynamics of anorexic refusal, in which refusal is presented as the way in which the anorexic subject seeks to find autonomy from the Other. From this point of view, refusal functions for the anorexic as a key to operate a modality of separation from the Other on which they depend. It is, however, a modality of separation that presents itself in a functioning detached from the dialectic with the Other, as a push to rupture with the Other and as a progressive passage at the imaginary level from dependence to autonomy. This is what constantly emerges from the very discourse of anorexic-bulimic patients. It is frequently found in the treatment in the moments of rupture when the anorexic patient operates the rupture that leads them to interrupt the treatment in the name of an imaginary self-sufficiency, which, instead of emancipating them, alienates them in a kind of autonomist "delusion" of which they remain a prisoner without knowing it.

This passage in the treatment also takes the form of a refusal of the unconscious, an erasure of one's own history, an absence of the past. The anorexic subject presents themselves in most cases without history and without memory. Our problem will therefore also be that of bringing out from their discourse whether their rejection of the unconscious is structural or whether it is a closure of the unconscious, a condition that assumes a preliminary opening and the possibility of a re-opening (Schejtman, 2004, p. 184).

In the course *The Other that does not exist* and its ethical committees Miller introduced the formula "refusal of the Other" to define the status of the relation to the Other in the new forms of the symptom. Here, the refusal of the symbolic dimension corresponds to the autistic closure of the subject around the substance of jouissance (drugs, food, psycholeptics, etc.). The refusal of the Other as a diffuse subjective position is an effect of the epochal crisis of the Other in the contemporary era, which had already been announced by Lacan through the figure of the decline of the paternal imago in the *Family Complexes*. In the age of the non-existent Other and the decline of symbolic authority that it entails, the refusal of the Other as a subjective position expands. The general formula that Miller provided to define the new forms of the symptom is "jouissances without an Other". This indicates the operation of the subject in these new symptomatic forms: the push to preserve the impossible integrity of a full mythical jouissance that would not be undermined by the alienating action of the Other, by the lethal effect of the signifier that involves a structural loss of jouissance. From this point of view, the refusal of the Other that can be spotted in anorexia loses the imaginary-emancipatory framing on which it is often built, to show its true aspect of irresistible nostalgia toward the One jouissance of the "Thing", jouissance without limit.

A pathology of the link to the Other

On the reverse side, in fact, anorexia-bulimia is configured as a pathology of the link to the Other. This is clearly shown in the first place by phenomenology, when it illustrates to us the tendency to isolation, the desertion of meal times, the inclination to the refusal or devouring of the Other which is the characteristic of the relational experiences of the anorexic-bulimic subject. In this sense, if we can give value to the thesis that humans do with food what they do with the Other, the metaphorical significance that the eating disorder includes in anorexia-bulimia becomes clear (Cosenza, 1998, pp. 129–159). The dietary "disorder" refers to a relational "disorder" of the subject, and the clinic of anorexia-bulimia, taken on the side of the relational life of the subject, teaches us this. Second, anorexia-bulimia is already configured as an attempt to respond to an unbearable relationship with the Other, which sinks its roots into the most intimate substance of the subject. At the level of this dimension, the clinic of anorexia-bulimia presents itself as a clinic in deficit of separation in relation to the Other, above all in relation to the maternal Other. In this perspective, the all/nothing logic is established that animates the devouring/refusing dynamic through which the anorexic sketches out their unbearable links. It is as a response to this aporia that anorexia-bulimia emerges as an imaginary attempt at separation from an invasive or abandoning Other, through the dynamics of refusal (of food, of the relationship, of the body ...). However, this pseudo-separation does not allow the anorexic-bulimic subject to obtain real autonomy, but alienates him or her in a kind of autarchic delusion, in a pathological autonomy that is supposed to be the fruit of the overcoming of all dependences. In reality, this supposed autonomy is only the reversal of a cannibalistic dependence on the Other, which in the critical conjunctures of the life of the anorexic-bulimic subject, is represented as inevitable. Each treatment of anorexia-bulimia is then confronted with the problem of how to allow the subject to go beyond this split between dependence and autonomy that they put into action cyclothymically, by supporting them in the invention of a particular, less destructive mode of articulating to one another. There can be no desiring autonomy of the subject without it assuming the dependence on the Law of the Other, without it inscribing its own position in the history that has constituted it.

The all-powerful Other of the anorexic

The anorexic refusal of the Other does not function as a maneuver of symbolic separation but only as an imaginary distance from the Other. This malfunctioning is linked to the fact that it preserves the integrity of the omnipotence of the maternal Other. If the mother maintains herself for the subject in a status of omnipotence, giving no sign of her structural castration and lack in being, then it will not be possible for the daughter to experience her own lack as irreducible to the field of maternal desire, and thus to transform such a lack into a desire that seeks its object beyond the structural dependence of the maternal Other. It is only on this condition that, as Freud taught us, the girl can in the course of her psycho-sexual development change her object, passing from the link to the phallic mythical mother to the orientation of love toward the father, as happens in the development of infantile hysteria. In relation to this itinerary of the psychosexual development of the neurotic girl, anorexia seems to manifest itself – when it is not a question of a real underlying psychosis where the function of the Name-of-the-Father has not been instituted to separate the child from the maternal desire – an impasse in this passage, a massive libidinal anchoring to the pervasive demand of the maternal Other. An unchastened Other, which lacks the lack, and from which it is not possible to disengage. In this conjuncture, the development of anorexia in the pubertal phase often becomes the construction of a compromise formation, which for a long time does not make enigma for the anorexic, between the link of exclusivity of the maternal demand and the subject's requirement of separation. Consequently, the cardinal point in the analytical treatment of neurotic anorexics revolves around the knot of the castration of the maternal Other and the loss of jouissance that it entails in the psychic economy of the anorexic subject. This loss, however, if it is assumed by the subject, opens the doors to a recovery of jouissance that occurs in the process of symbolic separation from the Other, and whose effects in the treatment of anorexia are clearly represented, even at the level of the body that re-pulses.

The anorexic pseudo-separation

Miller, in *L'Autre qui n'existe pas*, indicates in anorexia a declination of the new forms of the symptom which is situated, as in heroin addiction, on the side of separation, contrary to bulimia which seems to be declined, like cocaine addiction, rather on the side of alienation. The anorexic is in fact phenomenologically situated, like the heroin addict, in a position of waste and scandal in relation to the functioning of the Other, on the margins of family and social functioning. As we indicated earlier, we know that this operation of separation from the Other is paradoxically put into action by the anorexic who aims to preserve the imaginary integrity of the object from which they are trying to separate themselves. Here lies the fundamental separation defect that is at the heart of the clinic of anorexia. The anorexic dreams of a separation without loss, thus an imaginary separation, which does not question the real economy of jouissance where the subject is caught in the meshes of the Other. For this reason, the denial of loss is omnipresent in the clinic of anorexia, and the absence of the other is treated by the anorexic by means of its reduction to non-existence: the other who is missing becomes a non-existent other, upon whom the subject brings down the freeze of indifference.

This emerges in an impressive way in the group treatment of anorexic-bulimic patients, where the absence or abandonment of the group by one of the participants tends not to arouse comment, and where the analyst has the duty to lead the group back to symbolize this absence, to elaborate the loss.

In this sense, Recalcati has effectively used the formula "separation versus alienation", in an attempt to define the anorexic maneuver within the framework of the dialectic of separation and alienation formulated by Lacan in *The Seminar*, Book XI. The topological error at stake in the anorexic refusal as a maneuver of separation from the Other is given precisely by the attempt to operate a separation without there being a preliminary assumption of the loss of jouissance produced in the subject by the effect of the alienating action of the signifier. This modality of separation from the Other, which does not involve the assumption of the law of symbolic castration, allows us to understand the imaginary and fundamentalist autonomism that is often present in the discourse of the anorexic subject.

In the clinic of psychoses, the anorexic pseudo-separation from the Other takes, through refusal, more precisely the form of a disconnection from the Other, of a drifting away, of an identification with the waste, of an exit from the social link which often becomes the only way for the subject to stem the persecution, the only alternative to the suicidal act. In the case of Luana, a patient in a community setting, the anorexic refusal to eat became the only alternative to what happened to her periodically, each time she regained weight and returned to social life: she gave herself over to an unrestrained sexual pleasure, where anyone, man or woman, alone or in a group, could enjoy her without restraint. Anorexia curbed, each time, this devastating urge to become the object of the Other's jouissance, at the cost of substantial social isolation within the framework of the institution.

Refusal as jouissance

From the refusal of jouissance to the jouissance of refusal

The most enigmatic dimension that anorexia embodies, however, manifests itself in the construction of a particular modality of jouissance, which occurs precisely from the refusal of jouissance that characterizes its position. It is at this level that we can isolate the fourth root of anorexic refusal, in which the refusal itself presents itself as a modality of jouissance of the subject, or as the jouissance of the refusal as such. It is precisely this side at stake in anorexic refusal that challenges clinicians more, because it shows a satisfaction in self-destruction – embodied in the anorexic's complacency in "restricting" conditions, at the risk of their life – a manifestation of the death drive in the body, which cannot be read exhaustively within the sole defining framework of refusal as a defence of the Other and of the jouissance. There is, in fact, an erogenous dimension of anorexic refusal, a particular libidinal thickness that comes into play from the moment when the anorexic traps themselves in the jouissance of their disorder (Ansermet, 1999, p. 64). If, on the one hand, the anorexic refusal as a defence of the Other and as a rejection of the "jouissante substance" is presented as the negative operation that underlines anorexia nervosa, on the other hand, the specificity of the anorexic operation emerges from the singular libidinal positivization that leads the subject to install themselves in a special modality of jouissance, which is self-referential, outside the dialectic with the Other, which raises the refusal itself to the level of jouissance. It is in this perspective that we put forward the thesis that refusal is the specific mode of jouissance of anorexia nervosa.

In this logic, the pseudo-separative and negative operation that is contained in the anorexic "no" to the jouissance linked to the presence of the Other (refusal of jouissance) finds a form of libidinal recovery in a non-dialectical "yes" that the anorexic formulates in relation to the jouissance of her symptom (jouissance of refusal):

Refusal of jouissance   Jouissance of refusal
(−)   (+)

The jouissance of refusal between hysteria and anorexia

The hypothesis that there is an affirmative jouissance of refusal in anorexia explains the radical attachment, the true love that the anorexic bears to her symptom. It is important, however, to try to isolate its specificity, by differentiating it from other clinical manifestations of jouissance in the form of renunciation. The clinic of hysteria is par excellence a clinic of refusal and jouissance in refusal. However, in hysteria it clearly emerges that the function of refusal is configured as a way of preserving the desire and as a metaphorization of jouissance that passes through the way of compromise of the symptom. The hysterical jouissance of renunciation aims to keep the subject's desire alive by making dissatisfaction a special modality of satisfaction, a circuit of jouissance that metonymically keeps itself in circulation without being exhausted. The jouissance of refusal, in the clinic of hysteria, is hooked to the function of refusal as desire that Lacan talks about in *The Direction of the Treatment*, but also in *The Seminar*, Book XI about anorexia as a – hysterical – maneuver of opening up a lack in the parental Other (Soria, 2000, p. 28). For example, in conversion and in hysterical somatizations we always find a trace of a message that the subject unconsciously sends to the Other in encrypted form.

Thus, in hysterical anorexia we encounter the knotting of a double function of refusal: as desire linked to the field of the Other, and as jouissance of the own symptom.

Refusal   Refusal
----------   ----------
Desire   Enjoyment (Jouissance)

We also encounter in hysterical anorexia, in the clinic, in particular in the periods of major consolidation of anorexia, a prevalence of the autistic jouissance of refusal over the metaphorical function of refusal as desire. The mode of jouissance that the symptom embodies, prevails, at different moments of the anorexic hysteric's course, over the exercise of its symbolic-metaphorical function. It is the effect of the analytic work that makes it possible for the hysterical subject to articulate more affirmatively the function of her anorexia as a refusal that metaphorises a desire addressed to the Other, that questions her place in the desire of the Other. This should, in my opinion, warn us against the risk of undervaluing the jouissance of the anorexic symptom in hysteria, which does not allow itself to be reabsorbed in its entirety within the framework of the dialectic of desire between the subject and the Other, but maintains its own residue of autistic and non-dialectic functioning.

The anorexic jouissance atrophies in fact the metaphorizing function of the symptom that the hysterical structure predisposes, hypostatizing anorexia as a position of the subject itself. It takes the whole time of treatment to allow the hysterical subject to recognize in their own anorexia an enigmatic symptom. When this passage occurs, the jouissance of the anorexic refusal has already lost part of its libidinal consistency, and for the subject a door beyond the autarchy of his own symptom has opened.

Eating "nothing", libidinal positivization of anorexic refusal

The reading of anorexic refusal not only as a privative-negative key but also as an affirmative-positive key is the fruit of one of Lacan's most acute clinical intuitions in the clinic of anorexia nervosa. It is realized around the interpretation of the eating act in anorexia and produces a paradoxical effect of surprise, indicating at the heart of anorexic behavior, in the core of the anorexic refusal of food, the reverse side of an abstinence or a loss of jouissance. On the contrary, the refusal of food becomes in anorexia an affirmative practice of jouissance that revolves around a special object, inaccessible to the gaze, which Lacan calls the object "nothing". The affirmative translation of the anorexic refusal of food in Lacan's famous passage from *The Seminar*, Book XI, is "eating the nothing", eating the object nothing. The nothing is here conceived by Lacan as the object *a* that comes into play at the level of the oral drive in the process of subjective constitution. We know that in order to constitute itself, the subject is called upon to separate itself from the object *a* as organ. And that an object can function as (a) if it has two structural characteristics: (a) to be an object and as such separable from the subject's body; (b) it has a relation to lack, which allows it to function as a symbol of the phallus insofar as it produces a lack (-φ). To illustrate clinically this logical structure of the object *a* as a constitutive function by which the subject is called upon to separate itself in order to constitute itself as such, Lacan uses the example of anorexia:

I will immediately embody for you what I mean. At the oral level, it is the nothing, insofar as what the subject has weaned himself from is no longer anything for him. In anorexia nervosa, what the child eats is nothing. In this way, you understand how the object of weaning can come to function at the level of castration, as a privation (Lacan, 1973, p. 119).

In this passage, Lacan reinterprets the anorexic question from the centrality of the function of jouissance as the real organized in the drive body, in particular around the erogenous zones. This allows him to highlight the affirmative-positive dimension at stake in the anorexic position at the level of the constitutive dialectic of separation and alienation, and to frame anorexia as a solution in impasse at the level of separation with a grater precision. First, he highlights that the drive object of weaning at the oral level is not the mother's breast, but it is the nothing because "what the subject has weaned himself from is no longer anything for him". This differentiates the nothingness as a real object, for example, from the faeces as an object of the anal-excremental drive which for the subject operates as an object of symbolic exchange in the dialectic with the demand of the Other. But the aspect that is more important for us here is given by the highlighting of anorexia as a particular operation that the child puts into act in relation to the object of weaning, that is to say, to the object nothing. This operation is formulated here by Lacan first as a logical forcing, indicative of a difficulty of the anorexic subject to situate the object of weaning, the nothing, at the level of symbolic castration (-φ) as an object structurally lost because existing only at the mythical level. Consequently, Lacan describes the operation of the anorexic child on the object of weaning as an attempt to make it function at the level of castration as privation. In this operation the nothing as object of weaning is not negativized as in the process of separation that weaning involves for the neurotic subject. On the contrary, it is positivized as a real object retained in the subject's mouth, an empty object not lost, the heart of the anorexic's oral jouissance. Lacan thus illustrates the effect of this operation of the anorexic child on the object of weaning by the paradoxical and counter-intuitive act that is its consequence on the clinical level: the anorexic child who eats nothing. This thesis of Lacan's leads us to identify in anorexia an affirmative and anti-separative drive response to the loss of jouissance implied, in the subject's experience, by the passage through weaning. In this sense, if weaning structurally implies a loss of jouissance, the anorexic response goes in the direction of a closure of this loss and a positivization of the object nothing as a non-lost object, an object of jouissance that remains in the mouth, non-metaphorizable.

Weaning	Anorexia
(−)	(+)

Soria effectively expresses this passage, where she points out that here "Lacan signals a common position in anorexia: by making castration a privation, it positivizes the jouissance lost in weaning, recovering a plus-de-jouir in eating nothing" (Soria, 2000, p. 27).

In this perspective, in accordance with the general framework of *The Seminar*, Book XI, which substitutes the primacy of desire for that of jouissance, Lacan reduces the value of the anorexic refusal as a metaphor of desire, central in *The Direction of the Treatment*, to highlight in the anorexic refusal an operation of jouissance and on jouissance. In this respect, Soria interestingly indicates in the anorexic refusal of food a "transformation of jouissance" which, we would say, gives life to the construction of a sui generis modality of jouissance, refractory to entering the dialectic of desire (ibid., p. 34).

In the anorexic refusal, therefore, the negativization of the object-food, a phenomenologically evident dimension, is the condition of the positivization of the object-nothing as the invisible heart of the oral jouissance of the anorexic subject:

Object-food   Object nothing
   (−)   (+)

Cannibalistic jouissance of refusal: anorexia versus melancholy

In this logic, the pseudo-separative foundation at stake in the anorexic refusal of food becomes more evident, as does the cannibalistic matrix – a cannibalism of the object nothing – that supports it at the libidinal level of the oral drive. The more the anorexic refuses food, the more they enjoy without limit devouring their object nothing, as an object that they do not to evacuate from her mouth, that does not come out, that does not detach itself from their body. The jouissance of refusal is thus a cannibalism of nothing. The anorexic subject takes the bread out of their mouth to continue devouring their nothing. This push of the anorexic subject to become One with the object-nothing becomes evident in the clinic at the moments of radicalization of the anorexic symptom, when the conditions of the body go beyond the minimal parameters necessary for survival. In this critical conjuncture, we often observe, beyond the subjective structure, a double effect: (a) a substantial eclipse of the subject who withdraws into a total and a-dialectic refusal toward the Other; (b) an attitude to present oneself in the position of an object full of jouissance, which is one with the object-nothing. This critical conjuncture, frequent in the clinic of anorexia, embodies in a paradigmatic way the formula elaborated by Miller for the new forms of the symptom: jouissances without Other. She radically shows how in anorexia the refusal of the Other and of the jouissance substance that animates the body through the effect of signifying alienation (the refusal of the phallicization of the body and of the structuring of phallic jouissance), finds as a positivo-affirmative libidinal correlate in anorexia the production of a mode of jouissance in which the drive object – the nothing – does not detach itself from the subject's body, but remains trapped inside. In this sense, Soria has recently argued that in anorexia "the object *a* has not acquired its logical consistency" (Soria, 2006), precisely because jouissance has not been extracted from the body and continues to fill it inside. In this sense, we share Dominique Laurent's thesis that "far from being a clinic of emptiness, the clinic of nothing is a clinic where lack is missing. It is therefore rather a clinic of the full, centred on the subject's relationship to the object nothing, which more specifically affects the oral sphere" (Laurent, 2004, p. 56).

If we can locate trans-structurally traces of this phenomenon of missed separation from the object during the phases of symptomatic aggravation also in severe hysterical patients, we find it constantly in the forms of anorexia where a "drug-addicted" functioning, and a psychotic structure of melancholic type, prevails. In these cases, it is not an enjoyment of deprivation that sustains the libidinal economy of the anorexic subject but rather an autistic, nirvanic enjoyment, where the death drive finds its own clinical embodiment in refusal.

My experience with the therapeutic community "La Vela" has allowed me to witness several situations where the aggravation of the symptom of one of the anorexic patients led them to risk death because of the weight loss caused by the abstinence from food. In hysterical patients, too, this condition did not allow them to deal symbolically with the moment of crisis; in these cases, the introduction of a separating act, such as hospitalization, proved much more effective for them than an interpretation in confronting the emergence occurring.

The case of Marta is a paradigmatic example of this kind of situation. Marta is a young girl who arrived in the community at the age of 18, after having interrupted psychotherapy, suspended school attendance and spent most of her time locked in her room. The problem she had at school was that she could not pass the tests, even though she had studied the subject in question. In the mornings, her father would drive her to school, but when Marta arrived at the entrance, she would start to have panic attacks, and her father would get anxious and drive her home. After an infinite number of absences, Marta did not dare to go to school again and had to repeat the year. All of this took place in an atmosphere of great disappointment and bitterness on the part of the parents, who had assigned to Marta the task of redeeming them by obtaining the diplomas they had failed to obtain. At home, Marta tyrannized and distressed her family, who, under the threat of the girl's anorexia, obeyed her every demand. The decision to stay in the community was taken by the parents in agreement with Marta, but not without strong resistance from both sides. In the community Marta acted in two ways: with the staff and the companions she had a compliant and complacent position, while with her parents she spoke negatively about what was happening in the community, telling them that she felt bad there and thus made them anxious. Marta's anorexia was a response to very specific oedipal coordinates that emerged during the community treatment. The first one was linked to the absence of the father from the house, who had to help the anorexic sister (who died in a wheelchair in an institution). Marta's entire childhood was built around this scene: the absent father, she and her mother alone at home, the anorexic aunt who took away her father and husband through illness. Marta's identification with the anorexic aunt is thus central to the construction of her anorexia. On the maternal side, Marta was supported in her anorexia by her mother's over-judgment of her body and of sexual behavior, which was connoted as something dirty. In the prepubertal period, the anorexic symptom bursts out, based on a double function: to call the father back to her in the way that proved effective, even if lethal, for the aunt; to satisfy the mother's superegoic ideal by becoming a skinny, asexual and studious girl. For this reason, the school failure, more than the anorexia, was a symptom for the parents.

Marta's anorexia did not stop when she entered the community; however, she was satisfied with the relationship with the companions and with life in the institution. We had to apply the nasogastric tube to her to get her to eat, but this was not enough. We then called the girl, together with her parents, and told her that we could not help her if she did not accept hospitalization in a clinical nutrition ward. Only after hospitalization, when her body's survival conditions had been restored, would we welcome her back into the community. The girl's reaction was heartbreaking: desperate cries because what she wanted was to continue losing weight while remaining in the community. Only afterwards did the identification with the anorexic aunt who had died in the institution, the one who had taken the father away from her through illness, become clear to her. This case is a good example because it shows how, at the moment of the aggravation of the illness, a subjective functioning of the symptom as a metaphor that appeals to the father is outclassed by an adialectic thrust toward the realization in extremis of a mortifying jouissance without limit. "In community we don't want her dead, but alive" was the interpretation that came to her from the treating team. This sentence, in this circumstance, was going to detach the subject from her adhesive identification with the anorexic aunt who had died in the institution. Identification therefore on the melancholic side with the anorexic who dies devouring her own object-nothing and realizing her "appetite for death". The firm position of the team, supported by that of the parents, succeeded in convincing the girl to be hospitalised, which allowed her to return to the community in a different position.

The case of Alessia, a patient I treated in a monosymptomatic analytical group with the ABA, shows more clearly the melancholic trait that runs through her anorexia, structuring it. This patient remained stuck to a traumatic scene from her childhood life, which she worked on in the advanced phase of her treatment: she saw in the car's rear-view mirror the desperate and tearful look of her father who said to her: "Now you have to take Mummy's place!" Alessia's mother had died of cancer when she was eight and her brother was only three. Alessia, a slightly chubby child, began to lose weight, slowly at first and then rapidly during her pre-adolescence. Her response to her father's desperate call for her to take the place of her dead mother set her on a mortifying identification, of which anorexia became the answer. She entered the group at eighteen in the midst of "restricting" anorexia, saying she was only doing it because her maternal grandfather and her boyfriend had asked her to, but that she hads no intention of getting better. Alessia attended all the sessions, because it was impossible for her to break her word. After two years in the group, she would miss a session in a critical situation that would highlight the structure of the subject. That afternoon, some boys had stopped to look at her while she was kneeling down to arrange clothes in the window of the shop where she worked. Alessia was certain that they were looking at her backside. She sent a message to the ABA in the afternoon for my attention, saying that she could not come because of the eyes. In the message she had drawn several menacing eyes looking.

The return of the gaze object as a non-symbolizable object to the real had the effect of cracking the compensatory hold of her anorexia. For about a month, she could not leave her house because she could not bear to be looked at. I gave her daily telephone appointments, which she answered punctually, until she was able to return to the group and thus continue and complete her work. The persecutory effect of the gaze object weakened and then disappeared within a month. She finished her law studies with a master's degree in children's law, her goal being to work as a lawyer for the defence of abandoned children. Her mother's death was for her, as she said, an unbearable abandonment, she had felt unavoidably let down, stuck in a dead end. This would put her in a position to speak in a group about her infinite anger against the dead mother, who had abandoned her to her fate.

Alessia's case clearly shows the anti-metaphorical functioning of anorexia as a position of the subject that does not structure itself to achieve a separation from the lost object, but which, on the contrary, becomes a modality for retaining it and eternalizing it in the body, working in the opposite direction to the elaboration of mourning. The early death of the mother and the father's desperate appeal to his daughter to take her place reached the subject as unsymbolizable events to which she responds, structuring anorexia as the return into the real of a loss that cannot be symbolized by the subject, as the melancholic nostalgia for the Thing that is realized through the rejection of symbolic castration. The narcissistic identification with the lost object found in Alessia's case an imaginary emphasis because of her striking physical resemblance to her mother, which we were able to observe on the day she brought photos of her to the group. Alessia reached the end of her anorexia only after a long work of differentiation of her own position from that of the dead mother, during which the supplementation that made the project of becoming an advocate of abandoned childhood emerge in her played a considerable role. This operation enabled her to find a solution beyond anorexia, to distance herself from the maternal object, and to find in the law a mooring capable of covering the imaginary inoperative function of the father.

Soria underlined how at the heart of anorexia we must locate on the paternal side a missed embodiment of the father in the girl's experience, radical in the case of melancholic anorexics. It is precisely through this symbolic incorporation that the Name-of-the-Father becomes operative, and that the paternal function can exist in the subject's experience, allowing the loss of the object as an experience that can be treated by the work of mourning. A return in the real of this failed incorporation can be seen for Soria at the level of the anorexic refusal of food, which testifies to the failure of the function, formulated by Lacan, of the father as an aperitif (*a-père-itif*) which detaches the child's mouth from the mortifying jouissance of the object-nothing in order to stimulate its appetite.

Enjoyment of the gaze in the mirror in anorexia

A homologous effect can be found in the functioning of the scopic drive in anorexia, as the case of Alessia shows. Here, the anorexic passion for the mirror is given by the failed separation of the gaze object from the subject's body. The gaze object does not present itself for Alessia as symbolically treated by the signifier, as a metaphor for the desire of the Other, but presents itself in the real, without veils, as an object that invades the subject by looking at it from all sides. Thus Alessia finds herself disarmed, without the help of the phallic signifier, when she encounters the boys' unveiled gaze on her body. It was in an identical situation where she was completely disarmed that she had encountered the desperate gaze of the father who had nailed her to the place of the dead mother: Alessia's response produced, instead of the impossible phallicization of her own body as desirable, the sick body of anorexia. Anorexia had thus functioned for her as a knot that was able to sustain her for ten years, until the moment when the conjuncture of the unleashing produced the return of the gaze-object into the real, with the effect of a real hole in the fabric of the body image. Indeed, the plus-de-grease that the mirror gives back to the anorexic in her own body image, producing the effect of altered perception, is only the topological reverse of the structurally invisible gaze object, the authentic source of anguish of the anorexic.

Indeed, in the clinic of anorexia, the father's function of aperitif fails not only in the regulation of the oral drive but also in the inscription of the scopic drive in the regime of symbolic castration. The father does not effectively introduce in the daughter the function of the veil, the phallicization of the body and the inscription in the dialectic of the semblance; hence, the extreme difficulty for the girl to function in the dialectic of the feminine masquerade in relation to the other sex. If, structurally, the subject cannot see herself as a result of the structural schism between eye and gaze, in the clinic of anorexia the gaze as a drive object is not fully detached from the subject's body, which is, so to speak, hunted down, prey to the subject's own gaze. The less the anorexic's body is phallicized, the less it is a catalyst of the Other's desire, the more the anorexic experiences the excess of the gaze on her body in ana-morphosis.

Anorexia as addiction to "nothing" (Dewambrechies La Sagna, 1996, pp. 149–157)

A different declination of the jouissance of anorexic refusal, which tends to be situated beyond the dialectic with the Other, to burn the bridges with the Other, presents itself alongside and sometimes with melancholic cannibalism, in the addictive version of anorexia. Fenichel, who reworked some of Freud's and Abraham's clinical indications on the oral drive and the pathologies of addiction, was the first to intuit its importance in the definition of bulimia as "drug addiction without drugs". Indeed, the bulimic condition lends itself, in a phenomenologically more obvious way than in anorexia, to a knotting with the field of addictions. The irresistible link to a substance, food, the impossibility of controlling the impulsive thrust that surges in the eating crises and in the successive compensatory behaviors of evacuation, the coactivity and the constancy of the symptomatic repetition: all this highlights an operation of intersection, if not properly of inclusion, of bulimia in the field of pathological addictions. It is clear that this intersection becomes possible on condition that the biochemical dimension of the substance and its cerebral alteration effects are not placed at the centre of the addiction par-adigm, which happens in the bio-medical paradigm of pathological addic-tions, A paradigm that, therefore, does not include eating disorders. In a psychoanalytical paradigm of pathological addictions, on the contrary, in line with Freud's teaching, the pivot of addiction is to be found in the circuit of jouissance, which pushes the subject to evade anguish, to disregard the loss of object, through a compulsive system of control practices that revolve around the body, a substance or a situation (e.g. gambling).

The definition of anorexia as addictive or drug-like behavior is more subtle. We find a formidable anticipation of this in Lacan's text *The Family Complexes*, where Lacan composes the series anorexia/oral addictions/gastric neuroses, indicating the common matrix in a fundamental nostalgia for the primordial maternal imago and for the archaic and totalizing, mythical jouissance that it entails.

The return to a full mythical jouissance, effect of a deficient crossing of the Oedipus complex, pushes the subject back toward the primary object of weaning. It is in the light of this reference that the addictive dimension at stake in anorexia and in the refusal that structures it becomes clearer. In fact, refusing food becomes for the anorexic the way to lose nothing of the mythical enjoyment of the object "nothing", embodied by the empty and often silent mouth. This is why we have defined the anorexic jouissance of refusal as a cannibal jouissance, a cannibalism of nothing. The counterpoint to such a full jouissance in anorexia is given, in the Lacanian language of *Family Complexes*, by a rejection of thought, by a non-mentalization, which allows the illusion of an uncontaminated jouissance to be maintained in relation to the signifier and the Other. This is why Lacan, as Ménard reminds us (Ménard, 1988, p. 25), defines anorexia as "mental". It is from this constitutive impasse – full jouissance/rejection of thought – that all the recurrent problematic articulations in the direction of the treatment – absence of demand, difficulty in the installation of a symbolic transference, push to the interruption of the cure – with anorexic subjects can be illuminated.

Brusset, who has greatly valued the relationship between anorexia and addiction, particularly around the dimension of enjoyment, has defined the conduct of anorexics as an "endogenous addiction" precisely because, as the most recent neurobiological research seems to reveal, anorexic refusal produces enjoyment effects that act at the intracerebral level by increasing the production of endorphins, with the result that the subject's arousal is amplified. In this sense, Brusset continues, "does the refusal of all dependence lead to a closed circuit addiction" (Brusset, 1998, p. 160).

I will try to illustrate what is at stake in this dimension from two cases that were treated in the past in the "La Vela" therapeutic community. The first is that of Marzia, a young woman of 40 who suffered from restrictive anorexia in her adolescence and who, after having spent two years in the community, began an analytical treatment in my office. The second is that of Lucy, a 30-year-old woman suffering from bulimia with vomiting and presenting self-injurious behaviors on her body – cuts, wounds – who stopped community treatment after about a year.

Marzia arrived in the community in desperate condition. She was referred to us through the psychiatric department specializing in eating disorders, after having been narrowly saved from a coma caused by excessive weight loss and being hospitalised in the clinical nutrition department of a large hospital in Bologna. Marzia was the only girl in a family of five children, and she quickly developed an identification with the position of "the outcast of the family", which she would repeat throughout her life. For her, this position entailed a substantial rejection of her feminine condition and a perpetual attitude of defiance toward her parents, in particular toward her mother: a sacrificing, over-motivated, depressed woman who had fixed the only daughter in the house in a position of support for her own solitude. During her adolescence, Marzia lived a parenthesis of her life with excess and a disordered sexual behavior. In retrospect, she would read this brief period of her life as an attempt to do the opposite of what her mother wanted her to do. Marzia responded, in fact, in a provocative and transgressive way to her mother's somewhat bigoted religiosity, to the mortification of pleasure. After this parenthesis, she lived through a very long period of restrictive anorexia, punctuated by a large number of hospitalizations, and the position of patient was affirmed within the family. In the community, she began a slow process of recovery, a recovery of a bearable body condition and, on her release, she regained the regularity of her menstrual cycle after more than 20 years of interruption. Finally, she would be able to reintegrate socially and become economically independent by obtaining a job.

Marzia's case is paradigmatic of a subjective position where, in anorexia, an addiction to extreme nothingness – Marzia was on the verge of death – and a structural functioning of a hysterical type are welded together. In her story, the less she felt her parents were listening to her subjective position, the more she radicalized her hysteria. For example, it was quite normal for her parents to decide everything for her, as though she were still a child. This was also reproduced in the therapeutic community between the family and the patient. Marzia's response, for a long time, was to conform to her parents' words and to radicalize the symptom. Her life was already mortgaged by the decisions made by her elderly parents: she should have taken over the delicatessen and continued the father's business activity. The patient was on a dead-end street. This is very often the feeling that many anorexic patients have about their fate. Faced with a family Other perceived as full, without fissures, the anorexic subject cannot find her own place of desire. And it is precisely in this condition that anorexia can become, in the hysterical subject as well, an addictive solution: no longer an unconscious demand addressed to an Other who does not listen and does not see, but an affirmative response of self-destructive jouissance. In Marzia's case, this reversal in the value of her anorexia was evident, and all the work done with her in the community and subsequently in analysis went in the direction of creating a place for her desire, highlighting the difference from that of her parents. This led her to publicly make decisions on leaving the community that conflicted with the parents' expectations: she did not return to work in their shop, she found another job; she did not return to live with them, she decided to continue the treatment with me, despite the parents' desire that she start psychotherapy with a well-known professor of psychiatry and customer of their shop. In this movement of hysterization, Marzia began to come regularly to Milan to have her sessions, each time facing a two-hour journey to get from her village in Piedmont to Milan, rather than satisfy the parents' request to start a "convenient" therapy, but deprived of the transference.

Lucy's case illustrates a variation of the addictive enjoyment of bulimia, where the massive features of perversion organize a structure that can be reconverted to the frameworks of ordinary psychoses, without being triggered. She is an intelligent young girl, holder of a master's degree in literature, obtained with honors, who immediately struck the team by the contrast between her initial calmness and the intractable behavior in relations with the doctors who had followed her in her previous hospitalizations. Her ferocious bulimia and her self-loathing tendency could not be treated during the previous hospitalizations. The coordinates of her family Other allow us to situate the girl's position. Lucy was the heterozygous twin of Jack, a young man with a history of drug abuse, particularly cocaine, that had never been resolved. Both were born in Australia, in a city where their Italian parents had emigrated in their youth to work as waiters. For this reason, the parents did not give their children Italian names. Lucy spent her entire childhood until the age of 12 in Australia and spent most of her time alone with her brother, as the parents were completely occupied with their work. There, Jack had his first experiences with drugs and Lucy started her bulimia. On their return to Italy, they settled in a well-known wine-gastronomy town in the Piedmont area, where the parents opened a restaurant and a few years later a hotel. Intra-family relations were strained, most evident in the violent discussions between Jack and his father, who reproached his son for not wanting to work and for dissipating the family money on drugs.

One feature that struck the team was the massive denial that characterizes the position of Lucy and her entire family. The brother's drug addiction was not communicated to us by Lucy or her family, but by Lucy's public service doctors. At the same time, we learnt that the parents were secretly passing large amounts of money to the girl in the community – thus violating a rule of living in the community – which enables her to gorge herself. In view of the team's firm stance, the parents verbally agree to stop supporting Lucy in the purchase of food, but the mother, unknown to the father, continued to pass money to her daughter. Lucy would react in two ways to the exposure of this situation. First, she would try to deny the evidence to the end; then, forced into real limitations with regard to money, she would lash out in anger to the point of breaking windows and objects in the community. This reaction revealed her inability to give up the limitless enjoyment of "food". Indeed, the surprising aspect of Lucy lies in the rigidity of this double position: on the one hand, the rigid mask, the empty, impersonal semblance of the patient to whom the access to the jouissance of "food" is not even touched; on the other, the unquestioning and unreserved anger at the introduction of a limit to her access to jouissance.

The anorexic as object-waste: masochism and superego in the clinic of anorexic refusal

Symptomatic jouissance in anorexia often takes the form of the subject being stuck in the status of the object-rejected, the object-refused, the object-waste (Ménard, 1992, pp. 6–7). The essential condition for this to happen is that the subject originally encounters the Other in the position of a refusing Other, which writes the refusal into the function of master signifier, of S1 of the subject. The original encounter with the Other thus becomes here the bad encounter with an Other that says "no" to the subject, that refuses him at the fundamental level of Freudian "*Bejahung*", i.e. that it is not there to receive him as a subject of desire in his coming to be. "Being the refusal of the Other" then becomes the destiny, the subject's drive programme. It is within this framework that the melancholic variants of anorexia are structured, studded in several cases by continuous self-injurious acts, by suicide attempts, by operations of disconnection from the Other that lead the subject adrift.

In the case of Luisa, a young woman of 30 years of age who was welcomed into the community for a year, this melancholic-auto-destructive dimension became clear very quickly. It came after a suicide attempt, carried out by swallowing a whole pack of psycholeptics. Her parents found her lying on the floor and rushed her to hospital. Since the age of 14, she had suffered from severe bulimia with vomiting, sometimes accompanied by alcohol abuse. As the second daughter in the family, she was the "unsuccessful" daughter. The older sister, married with children, had long since distanced herself from her sister and never contacted her during her stay in the community. Her parents were anxious about Luisa's leaving and return to the family; they preferred her to remain in the community.

In the parents' speech, especially the mother's, they had no hope of any change in their daughter's behavior, whom they considered to be permanently ill. Luisa, however, rarely let the desperate loneliness of her condition show. The addictive relationship with food and episodically with alcohol closed the space for her to speak about her despair. All the fundamental choices in her life had collapsed to a certain extent and had all ended in failure: moving away from her parents, her relationship with a young man who was not at all accepted by the family and described as "clueless and good for nothing", her work choices. Luisa's unconscious program was imposed with an absolute rigor that reduced to zero, each time, the possibility of introducing a subjective variation. The spontaneous effect that she produced in the community on the companions and on the staff was that of reproducing in them, because of her repeated transgressive behavior, deaf to the calls of the Other, the same parental judgment of condemnation. Luisa embodied the so-called hopeless case, without solution. Impotence and sadism were the imaginary variants that her way of being provoked in the Other. She left the emptiness of her discourse disarmed in relation to her own history – Luisa had worked for years as a clerk, she almost had a master's degree in philosophy – as if it were a history that did not belong to her. What prevailed in her discourse, on the contrary, was the desire not to repeat her transgressive behaviors – stuffing herself and vomiting, stealing food, drinking alcohol on the sly – in order to avoid conforming to them and thus feeding an unbearable feeling of guilt.

In the case of Monia, a psychotic anorexic patient with a strong self-alienating tendency, it was essential to intervene as a treatment team by introducing a regulation of her persecuting Other, which in the hallucinations took the form of the insulting father who ordered her to cut herself. She arrived in the community, accompanied by her father in his car, who told us: "I am only the driver. I leave her with you and I don't want to hear about it any more!". He never came to see her during her stay in the community, nor did he call her. The first operation that we carried out with her was that of putting ourselves between the subject and the insulting paternal voice, in fact, we said to her: "Don't worry, we're the ones who think about your father!". The second essential operation was that of symbolically punishing her every time she committed acts that violated the rules of cohabitation: in fact, if we did not punish her, she would give herself over to her self-destructive and self-eliminating thrust. Each time, she received our punishments – for example, not going out in the evening, or doing an extra cleaning chore – with a sigh of relief: for her, our law was much more sustainable than the merciless one of her archaic superego.

References

Ansermet, F. (1999), *Clinique de l'origine: l'enfant entre médecine et psychanalyse.* Laussanne: Payot.

Appeau, A. (1992), *Anorexie mentale.* Lyon: Césura Lyon Édition.

Bollas, C. (2000), *Hysteria.* London/New York: Routledge.

Brousse, M. H. (2002), Mort et resurrection de l'hystérie. *Mental,* no. 11, pp. 67–71.

Brusset, B. (1998), *Psychopatologie de l'anorexie mentale.* Paris: Dunot.

Cosenza, D. (1998), Il cibo e l'inconscio. Anoressia, bulimia e discorso alimentare. Recalcati, M. (Dir.), *Il corpo ostaggio. Clinica psicoanalitica dell'anoressia-bulimia.* Roma: Borla.

Cosenza, D. (2001), La comunità terapeutica come luogo della cura. Colombo, L. and others (Dir.), *La cura della malattia mentale. Vol. II. Il trattamento.* Milano: Bruno Mondadori.

Dewambrechies La Sagna, C. (1996), Un cas de toxicomanie du rien. *Mental,* no. 2, pp. 149–157.

Dewambrechies La Sagna, C. (2006), L'anorexie vraie de la jeune fille. *La Cause freudienne,* no. 63, pp. 57–70.

Kestemberg, E., Kestemberg, J., Decobert, S. (1981), *La faim et le corps: un étude psychanalytique de l'anorexie mentale (1972).* Paris: PUF.

Lacan, J. (2006), *The Direction of the Treatment and the Principles of Its Power (1958). Écrits. The First Complete Edition in English.* New York/London: Norton & Company, pp. 489–542; *La direction de la cure et les pricipes de son pouvoir. Écrits* (1966). Paris: Seuil.

Lacan, J. (1973), *Le Séminaire. Livre XI. Les quatre concepts fondamentaux de la psychanalyse, 1964.* Paris: Seuil.

Laurent, D. (2004), Inhibition, symptôme et angoisse aujourd'hui. *La Cause freudienne,* no. 58, pp. 56–60.

Ménard, A. (1988), L'anorexie mentale entre psychose et nevrose? Les anorexiques supposées sans demande. *Pas Tant,* no. 20, pp. 21–26.

Ménard, A. (1992), Structure signifiante de l'anorexie mentale. *Actes de l'ECF,* vol. 2, pp. 3–7.

Miller, J.-A., Laurent, É. (2005), *El Otro que no existe y sus comités de ética, 1996–1997*. Buenos Aires/Barcelona/Mexico: Paidós.

Naveau, P. (2001), La clinique du detail et l'hystérie. *Mental*, no. 11, pp. 72–92.

Schejtman, F. (2004), *La trama del síntoma y el inconsciente*. Buenos Aires: Del Bucle.

Soria, N. (2000), *Psicoanálisis de la anorexia y bulimia*. Buenos Aires: Tres Haces.

Soria, N. (2006). *Anorexia-bulimia, Associatcion Mundial de Psicoanalisis (AMP), Scilicet de los Nombres del Padre. Textos preparatorios para el Congreso de Roma (13–17 Julio 2006)*, pp. 23–26.

Chapter 7

The object nothing in the Lacanian clinic of anorexia

Return to the object nothing

In this chapter we will take up again, after the event, the questions regarding the Lacanian status of the object nothing at the heart of the clinic of anorexia nervosa, by returning to this notion after having gone through the itinerary followed up to this point. Our journey has led us to question the symptomatic status, typical of contemporary anorexia (chapter 1), to reconstruct the genesis of the concept of anorexia nervosa in the field of psychodynamic psychiatry (chapter 2), to indicate the two paths of contemporary post-Freudian psychoanalysis, in our opinion the most fruitful in their capacity to grasp the logic of its functioning (chapter 3) and to analyze in depth, in Lacan (chapter 4) and in the Lacanian orientation (chapter 5), the detailed construction of the perspective within which our research is progressing. In the previous chapter (chapter 6), we articulated the thread that supports our reading of the clinic of anorexia nervosa. It is the pivotal point of anorexic refusal, which is at the heart of Lacan's reading of anorexia and of which we have given a novel articulation by structuring its clinical essence in four different functional modalities of manifestation: as demand, as defence, as a modality of separation and as jouissance.

Punctuations on the object nothing in Lacan

As Dewambrechies La Sagna has pointed out, "it is the clinic of anorexia nervosa that leads Lacan to add the object nothing to the list of Freudian objects that are the oral, the anal and the phallic" (Dewambrechies La Sagna, 2008, p. 376).

This is not, as we know, Lacan's only addition to the list of Freudian objects: the voice and the gaze also find their central place among the objects of the drive, notably from *The Seminar*, Book X, *Anxiety*, as real innovations to the psychoanalytic theory of the drive. With these additions, Lacan introduces two objects that, in line with Freudian objects, open from two clearly identifiable edge zones, two openings of the body based on the

DOI: 10.4324/9781003318439-8

anatomical-physiological structure of the auditory and visual organ, as is the case with the mouth in relation to the oral object and the anus in relation to the excremental object. However, these are both objects which, by their structural characteristics and in the dialectical relation in which the subject constitutes itself in the field of the Other, present themselves rather as objects tied to the desire of the Other than as objects articulated to the demand of the Other, as in the case of the Freudian oral and anal objects.

For Lacan, the status of the object nothing appears as an object with a special status, or even, in certain aspects, unclassifiable or, in any case, out of step with the other objects of the drive. It is the most enigmatic of all the other objects indicated by Lacan, who gives us the list by including it in *Subversion of the Subject and Dialectics of Desire in the Freudian Unconscious*:

> "the mamilla, the feces, the phallus (as an imaginary object), and the urinary flow. (An unthinkable list, unless we add, as I do, the phoneme, the gaze, the voice ... and the nothing)".
>
> (Lacan, 2006a, p. 693)

In the first place, unlike the others, it remains problematic, in my opinion, to reduce it entirely to a precise erogenous zone. In fact, in Lacan's case too, it is not self-evident that we should necessarily reduce it to the oral zone as its exclusive object. Dewambrechies La Sagna also, in her reconstruction of the question of nothing in Lacan's teaching, only hypothetically relates nothing to the oral erogenous zone:

> "These objects that cause desire are the referents of discourse. One might therefore think that, in anorexia nervosa, it is the oral object".
>
> (Dewambrechies La Sagna, 2006, p. 65)

But it is a fact that Lacan distinguishes between the object nothing and the oral object. Lacan's nothing is rather, in our opinion, a "sui generis" object that gravitates in the drive body and that parasitizes the erogenous zones, certainly above all the oral zone, but more radically because it introduces itself into the root of the mechanism of functioning of the drive-itself.

It is probably for this reason that Lacan, in his teaching, does not attribute the function of the object nothing exclusively to anorexia nervosa, but also to hysteria (Lacan, 1994, pp. 136–144), phobia (ibid., pp. 244–245) and obsessive neurosis (Lacan, 2006b, pp. 327–337). As we shall see, Miller, in a clinical conversation at the ECF, clarified the status of the object nothing in a novel way, thanks to the role it plays in a case of ordinary psychosis (Miller, 2009a, pp. 169–170). These are, of course, different variations of the same object function. The fact remains that, for Lacan, anorexia nervosa has the merit of showing more precisely the function of nothing in its operativity and that, for this reason, he resorts to it several times in his teaching.

In this chapter, we will try to shed more light on the specific status of the object nothing, through the attempt to keep together the special status that Lacan attributes to the clinic of anorexia nervosa and the different declensions to which he refers, when he uses the object nothing in relation to different clinical structures.

We will try, in fact, to articulate our discourse by basing it on the cases where the anorexic symptom presents itself in different clinical structures, with the aim of showing, in this respect, the characteristic operativity of the object nothing in each of them.

Beyond the dualism of nothing

As we have seen so far, those who have worked most deeply on the clinical question of anorexia nervosa in the Lacanian orientation – first of all, Menard at the end of the 1980s (Ménard, 1989, p. 24) – have arrived at the identification of a double status of the object nothing at the heart of its functioning (Cosenza, 2008, pp. 29–31). On the one hand, the nothing is linked to the dialectic with the Other, in its status of object-in-desire-function, as the fulcrum of the subject's division, anchored to symbolic castration and coordinated by the phallic function. This is the side of the object-nothing that we find in the clinic of hysteria and which, for Lacan, is well represented by the Freudian case of the beautiful butcher's wife, where the nothing, interposed by the hysteric to the consumption of the desired food, has the function of preserving her desire by maintaining her dissatisfaction. This function of nothing is certainly present in hysterical anorexia and in its typical phallicization of thinness, which is at the basis of what has been called the metaphorical function of refusal as a demand for desire.

At the same time, the nothingness appears strongly in the clinic of anorexia as object-in-function-of-jouissance. A jouissance which, however, is not contained by the phallic mediation being out of speech, without limit or loss, total. Jouissance Une, which leaves the subject undivided and pushes him to refuse the relation to the Other, first of all to the Other who nourishes, often to the extreme risk of death. This side of the nothing is preponderant in the clinic of anorexia nervosa and, as a result, it situates this domain of the clinic beyond the phallic-oedipal coordinates proper to neurosis, imposing itself as more and more central in Lacan's teaching, in the clinical experience and in the conceptualization elaborated by the Lacanian analysts engaged in this domain. It is in this perspective that the action "I eat nothing", which, for Lacan, characterizes anorexia in *The Seminar*, Book XXI, as we saw in chapter 4, appears as the antithesis of a maneuver aiming to open up a lack in the Other, which was, in part, still attributed to him in *The Seminar*, Book XI in the dramatic form of: "Does he want to lose me?" The perspective of the 'Seminar, book XXI', the most advanced in Lacan's teaching on anorexia, allows us to liken the position of the drug addict to the anorexic action, more easily than the one, heroic in its own way, of the 'kamikaze of desire', which we can partly assimilate to the anorexic position of the Seminar, book XI.

The anorexic symptom appears, in fact, in "Les non dupes errent", as absolutely anti-heroic. Lacan photographs here the prosaic, de-subjectivized, enjoyment-ridden character of the anorexic rumination that precedes the encounter with food, all wrapped up around the problem "I will eat or I will not eat". The inevitable answer is, each time, "I won't eat anything" and, with such an answer, the subject closes the space of the Other each time, does not want to know anything about the desire to know. The anorexic action, here, does not aim at opening up a lack in the Other that could reveal whether the subject has a place, and what place, in the desire of the Other. On the contrary, the action "I eat nothing" is a movement of systematic closure of the space of lack. It is a refusal of unconscious knowledge that, according to Lacan, keeps the anorexic at a distance from the neuralgic point of knowledge, that is, the horror, the encounter with the structural lack of the Other and the hole in knowledge.

The object nothing as the only object *a* that is not the cause of desire: a recent contribution by Jacques-Alain Miller

Recently, Miller has made a decisive contribution to the clarification of the status of the object nothing. This contribution allows us, in my opinion, to better clarify the singular function of the object nothing, both in the general theorization around the objects a of the drive and with regard to the clinic of anorexia nervosa.

The context of reference for this Millerian contribution is given to us by the Conversation clinique des Sections Cliniques francophones whose title was *Situations subjectives de déprise sociale* and which took place in June 2008 in Paris. Miller's contribution on the object nothing was introduced during the Conversation in relation to a case of ordinary psychosis, presented by Jean-Claude Maleval, under the title *Déprise sociale paradoxale et clinique du désert* (Maleval, 2009, pp. 37–48; 150–170). The question of nothingness is at the heart of this subject named Charles and is expressed phenomenologically in a structural inertia that makes it impossible for him to do anything, be it working or building a relationship. This condition leads the subject himself to self-define as "a nullity". In this case, too, Miller asserts in agreement with Maleval, "one regularly encounters this *S0,* quite characteristic of ordinary psychosis, which should not be confused with the barred subject. This 'I'm useless' refers to another mode, much more radical than a simple attack on self-esteem. It is, as J.-C. Maleval has pointed out, the attraction of non-being, which is reminiscent of Heidegger's name. A relationship to nothingness is present in this subject" (Miller, 2009a, p. 150).

From this singular case, Miller returns to Lacan's notion of the object nothing, reformulating it in a new way:

"Thanks to this case, we capture something of this object a that is so subtle in Lacan's list of objects a: the object nothing".

(Ibid., p. 169)

Miller's argument on the object nothing is articulated here in five points:

- This case allows us to rethink the question of the object nothing beyond the classic psychosis/neurosis binomial.
- In dealing with a case of ordinary psychosis, "we need mathemes, reference points, instruments" (ibid.) that allow us to think the question beyond the classical binomial.
- S0 is a mathema that allows us to clarify the nothing as object a in ordinary psychosis: "S0 is one, which puts the object a as nothing back on the agenda in the approach to ordinary psychosis: it seems to be both attached to it and in a certain way to give it its status" (ibid., pp. 169–170).
- The articulation between S0 and the object nothing "does not give here a delusional anorexia", and "paradoxically designates the cause of her desire".
- The object nothing in the function of cause acts, in this case, as the object "cause of his' non-desire".

From this argumentation linked to the case, Miller manages to produce a general theoretical formulation that restructures, on a key point, the Lacanian doctrine of drive objects, to the point of isolating a special characteristic, proper to the object nothing in the function of cause, which is formulated as follows: "The object a as nothing would be the only one among the objects a that is the cause of non-desire and the cause of desert" (ibid., p. 170).

Some consequences for the doctrine of drive objects and for the clinical theory of anorexia nervosa

This clarification offered by Miller on the status of the object nothing goes in the direction of certain basic hypotheses that we want to formulate and that are related both to the foundations of Lacan's drive doctrine and to its implications in the framework of the differential clinic and, in particular, in our case, of the differential clinic of anorexia nervosa.

Rewriting the theory of the drive objects

Extraction of the object nothing from Lacan's list of objects of the drive

The operation here carried out by Miller clearly highlights the special status of the object nothing, first by extracting it from the list of drive objects, where Lacan had inserted it, and second by highlighting its special status. This is an operation already immanent, but implicit, in Lacan's teaching. This is why the nothing is both an object among the other cause objects (hence its insertion into the list by Lacan, along with the oral object, excrement, the voice and the gaze) but, in other places in Lacan's text, it acquires a special status. The object nothing is thus, in Lacan, both a causal object among the others and endowed with a unique function. Here we can schematize this operation that specifies the status of the object nothing:

Lacan		Jacques-Alain Miller	
Das Ding	mamilla	Das Ding	mamilla
	feces		feces
	voice		voice
	gaze		gaze
	nothing	nothing ←	nothing

In this diagram, we highlight the special status of the object nothing, in the relationship between the first mythical object of satisfaction, Freud's *Das Ding*, Lacan's *Chose* and the objects causing desire. We will now try to highlight the structural characteristics that give reason to this special status of nothing as an object.

The object nothing is the only object that cannot be located specifically and exclusively in a single erogenous zone of the body

Unlike breasts, excrement, the phallus, the voice and the gaze, which all have a precise libidinal location in erogenous zones of the body, the object nothing escapes this necessity and can only be identified, as the case may be, in different points of the body's drive organization, without having a pre-defined location. For example, in the clinic of anorexia nervosa, it can undoubtedly find its privileged place in the oral zone but without necessarily being limited to this erogenous zone of the body. In the case of Charles' ordinary psychosis, for example, it is not possible to locate the object nothing in a precise and exclusive erogenous zone but its action is exerted, more diffusely, on the impulsive body by reducing it to a fundamental inertia.

The object nothing is the only object a that functions as an object that is not the cause of desire

The action of nothing as a cause object is an action of inertia, devitalizing, anti-separative and anti-dialectic, a vector of a "regressive" negativity, of a return to the inanimate as in the Freudian Todestrieb, of an enjoyment of the One without loss, outside discourse.

The object nothing is the closest to the Das Ding among the a-objects, since it presents itself in the form of the absolute without limit of a non-partial object, as pure negativity

For this reason, it is the object that causes non-desire and the factor that pushes the subject toward cancellation in a jouissance Une, an echo, in the real, of the jouissance of *Das Ding* of which Lacan spoke to us in The Seminar, *The Ethics of Psychoanalysis*, while reading the *Entwurf* of the Young Freud (Lacan, 1986, pp. 27–102).

The object nothing is not only an object a among the others but also it embodies the anti-desire function, internal to the structure of the drive object

In this sense, the object nothing can parasitize the oral drive, the anal drive as well as the scopic or invoking one. This is what remains of the anti-desire function of the *Das Ding* in the structure of the drive object.

Re-articulation of the clinic of anorexia nervosa in the light of the status of the object nothing

Clinic of the phallus and clinic of the object nothing

The psychoanalytical clinic can be articulated, according to a recent bipartition of Dewambrechies La Sagna, by the distinction of a phallus clinic, based on symbolic castration, and an object clinic that does not find its pivotal point in the phallic signifier. We propose to situate the object nothing as object cause at the heart of this clinic of the object.

Anorexia between the phallus clinic and the nothing clinic

The phallus clinic is a clinic acting in the field of neurosis and within which it is important to situate, as far as anorexia is concerned, all those cases for which the anorexic solution is constructed, within the framework of a structure where the phallic signifier, signifier of the object of the lack of the Other, finds its place in the subject and orients, albeit precariously, his desire. In this framework, hysterical anorexia finds its fundamental place and the place that nothing occupies in it must related to the effect of signifying mediation operated by the phallic signifier. Where, on the other hand, the phallic signifier has not been inscribed in the subject's unconscious, anorexia nervosa becomes a solution concerning, in an extreme way, a clinic of the object nothing in its function of cause of non-desire. All cases of anorexia, beside neurosis, fully fit into this field, although each time with a singular modality.

A differential clinic of anorexia based on the function of the object nothing

This reformulation of the status of the object nothing allows us to rethink the differential clinic of anorexia, taking into account the relationship between the function of the object nothing and the domain of knowledge (*savoir*) in its structure. As Lacan himself has indicated to us on several occasions and especially in *The Seminar*, Book XXI, the function of knowledge is fundamental in determining the status of anorexia. It is therefore a question for us of proposing an articulation of the differential clinic that highlights the structural relationship between the function of jouissance, proper to the object nothing, and the structure of knowledge as it presents itself in the clinical case of anorexia.

The case of hysterical-neurotic anorexia

Between the clinic of the phallus and the clinic of the object nothing

In hysterical anorexia, which is female in most cases and manifests itself at puberty or post-puberty, the subject constructs her own anorexic response as a solution to the impasse she encounters in the assumption of her own sexual position. As we will see in more detail in chapter 9, especially in girls, anorexia is a possible response to the problematic, or even impossible, symptomatization of puberty. This symptomatization of the pubertal passage constitutes, according to Stevens' effective definition (Stevens, 1998, pp. 79–92), the very function of adolescence in the perspective of psychoanalysis. In the case of the anorexias that Dewambrechies La Sagna defines as "true" or mental and, even more radically, in the psychotic anorexias, this process of symptomatization has failed and anorexia is then presented as an alternative solution to this failure. In contrast, in hysterical anorexia, the anorexic symptom itself is an attempt by the subject to carry out this symptomatization. In hysterical anorexia, anorexia thus manifests itself as a neurotic symptom with all effects and the refusal to eat has a dialectical-metaphorical function of a demand addressed to the Other in the place that the subject itself occupies in the desire of the Other. The anorexic body of the subject thus presents a phallic side; it is inscribed in the phallic signification and it acts as a catalyst of the desire of the Other.

However, we do not share the hypothesis according to which hysterical anorexia could be entirely reconciled with a phallic type of logic. In most cases, indeed, the inscription in the phallic register proves to be precarious and weak for the subject; the work of hysterization does not produce its effects immediately, but it requires, for the activation of the signifying chain, a longer logical time than in a pure hysterical subject. On the one hand, in fact, the signifying chain is shown, especially afterwards, to be installed: the S1–S2 is structured and, however, the unconscious knowledge (of which the S1–S2 represents the elementary logical skeleton) appears to be inactive when the anorexia settles and takes root in the subject's life.

What has happened to them? Our hypothesis is that the appearance of anorexia brings with it, in the subject, the deposition of the object nothing in the point of interval between the signifiers S1 and S2, leading not to the impossibility but to the non-operativity, the deactivation after the fact of the functioning of unconscious knowledge. The following diagram represents an attempt to represent this passage:

T1	T2
S1 .... S2	nothing
S1	S2

In this perspective, especially in the early stages of the treatment, the anorexic solution presents, in hysteria, besides a phallic side, not always obvious at the beginning, a nirvanic-inertial side that manifests itself in the first instance. It is as if, in the work with hysterical anorexia, which should not be confused with a simple transitory anorexia, it were a question, fundamentally, of displacing the subject's libidinal economy from a condition where the action of annulling the object nothing deactivates the phallic function, to a condition where the relation is reversed and the phallic function carries out, insofar as it is possible, the giving of significance of the nothing by the elevation of its status to the pure signifier of the lack-to-be.

T1	T2
NOTHING	PHALLUS
-------------	---------------
PHALLUS	NOTHING

A clinical exemplification: the case of Clementina[1]

A tortuous preliminary

The case I am presenting to you concerns a young anorexic girl whom I followed for three years, in individual treatment, and to whom I have already referred briefly in chapter 6 about the first part of the treatment. I take it up here in a more complete way, until the resolution of the treatment. The treatment took place during the first year, in the context of the institution for the treatment of eating disorders of which I was the director at the time, and in my private practice during the following two years. At the time of our first meeting, the girl was 19 years old and had already been showing anorexic symptoms for four years. The treatment ended in September 2008 and lasted a total of three years.

I started seeing Clementina in May 2005. I agreed to meet her after she had interrupted individual psychotherapy at its very beginning with a colleague in the institution where I was working at the time. At the second meeting with the colleague, Clementina had limited herself to saying that she did not feel comfortable with her and that she wanted to be able to meet a male therapist.

When asked by the colleague why she was so demanding, she replied that for her it was a problem to talk to and deal with a man, while she had always been even too close to women, starting with those in her family (mother and sister). Before I met her, her case was discussed in the team; the colleague reported on the sessions with the patient and said that she was not willing to continue the therapy with the girl, suggesting a change of therapist to a male therapist.

From the three preliminary interviews for referral to psychotherapy carried out by another colleague according to the institution's usual procedure, no trace of psychotic functioning, underlying the anorexic symptom, had appeared. The diagnostic hypothesis of the first colleague was a restrictive anorexia in a hysterical type of personality structure, characterized, however, by a rather weak demand for treatment on the part of the girl and by a strong identification with the symptom. The motivation to change was not yet perceptible in the girl who, on the contrary, seemed proud of her own autonomous condition that the symptom gave her the impression of having. It was the parents who, as usual, had brought the girl to the institution to start treatment and they themselves had started a course of treatment before hers, led by a colleague from the institution, within a group of parents of anorexic and bulimic patients.

In the light of these reasons, according to the clinical logic followed at the time in the institution and after the failure of the start of individual psychotherapy with the colleague, the team had thought of inserting her in a group of anorexic-bulimic patients with neurotic functioning that I was co-ordinating at the time; it was thought that, in the modality of the small mono-symptomatic group with an analytical conduction, the group could function as a facilitator of the work of symbolization on the part of the patient.

I met her for the first time for an interview which was to precede her entry into the group and which would allow me to get a first idea of the patient in order to present to her in broad outline the functioning of the group's work. Clementina presented herself as a pale, very thin, tall, expressive girl with rapid, nervous gestures. What struck me immediately about her was the contrast between what she said and how she said it, between the content of her statements and her position in the enunciation. For example, in the content of her speech there was a reference to the indifference she said she felt for everything that she had been abandoning for a long time to withdraw into anorexia: friends, social life, the feminine treatment of the body. But what was striking about her was her curiosity about what was said to her, her lively eyes that lit up when she listened to something that impressed her. She did not show the anaesthesia typical of the more classic anorexics, while showing the symptomatic appearance typical of a case of anorexia: amenorrhoea, progressive weight loss, a problematic relationship with her body image, an urge to isolate herself and to get out of the social link. At this point, she had no idea why she had become anorexic, what the possible causes of her condition were. On the contrary, being anorexic was a value for her that she did not want to give up. She came to the institution for the anorexia treatment because her parents were worried and not because she wanted to be cured of the symptom. I pointed out to her that it would be impossible for her to achieve any kind of change without finding a motivation for the treatment.

The first group session was also her last: she spent the whole time in total silence, in an attitude of isolation from the other girls. After the session, she asked to speak to me and told me that she did not want to be in a group, that she had nothing in common with the others and that she wanted to start individual work with me. I was surprised by the modality she used in this circumstance. But I took the opportunity to point out to her that, although she continued to say that she had come only to obey her parents, there was something that she herself wanted and that it was not so true that she was so indifferent. I left the decision open for a few days and, after consulting the team, I informed her that we could start seeing each other for individual psychotherapy.

Being unique

During the first individual psychotherapy meeting, I asked her to say something about what had happened in the preliminary phase and to talk about the difficulties she had encountered there. She tells me that before she found herself in the situation in question, she did not know that she could not go into therapy with a female therapist: she found out once she was actually there and was not sure why. She had never tried psychotherapy before and had no idea what it meant. She had had the same experience in the group: she had consented willingly to try it, but once inside the group she had felt very uncomfortable, with the feeling that she did not belong. Hence the reaction of refusal and the quick decision she reported to me immediately afterwards: if she really had to start psychotherapy, then it would be with me and individually. I asked her why it was so important for her to see me alone and not, for example, in a group. She told me that her problem was not something she could or wanted to share with others and that her anorexia was something special that concerned only her. I told her that yes, I agreed, her anorexia has a singular value that, however, for the moment eluded us. And that if she wanted, our work would try to shed some light on this enigma that concerned her intimately. The fact of being special in the eyes of the Other emerged, from now on, as a characteristic trait of Clementina's personality, something that was, in truth, much older and more radical than anorexia. The fact of having grasped it and of having returned it to her during the session had a certain effect on her, a feeling of recognition that allowed her a first form of subjectivized attachment to the treatment, although it would remain undeclared for a long time.

In the course of the work, one of the fundamental operations would consist exactly in allowing her to extract her desire to be unique from the identification with the anorexic being within which it had remained condensed, thus allowing her to grasp its difference.

Clementina and the family

In Clementina's discourse, references to family were sparse and tended to be avoided, just as her childhood memories were rare. They were almost all linked to the summers spent in the holiday house in Sicily where she has always spent at least part of the summer period with the family. Her most beautiful memories are linked to this place, interrupted, however, by the onset of anorexia, which made this house a place of isolation for her. In this regard, she describes a watershed in her life, a clear detachment between before and after the symptom: before it, she had an intense social and relational life. Being, in fact, a very attractive and intelligent girl, many boys courted her. With the onset of anorexia, she began to withdraw gradually and to let go of the relationships she had built. The parents, too, according to what the colleague who was following them told me, confirmed this two-stage reading of Clementina's life and did not know how to explain it.

Clementina's parents appeared to be a couple devoted to work and the family, with the mother in the position of housewife and nodal point of the family bond. It was she who looked after the girls and started to worry about Clementina's conditions, asking for her daughter to be taken into care. The daughter experienced the mother as intrusive and clinging: she felt she was too much on her back and would like to be able to keep a safe distance. She was struck by her mother's ambivalence about her symptom: on the one hand, she was the one who had been most concerned about it, while on the other hand, she was struck by the fact that the mother had started a diet since she became anorexic.

In her family, Clementina was the second of two girls; her sister Giulia was two years older. They had very different characters: Clementina was more reserved and reliable, Giulia is more extroverted and enterprising but also wilder. Clementina said that she took after her father much more than her sister; like him, she was reserved and knew how to be self-sufficient, she did not depend on others and had a certain basic autarchy that had been pathologically amplified with anorexia. On the contrary, the sister appeared much more dependent on the object and excessive in her behavior. Giulia had always been more uninhibited in her sexual and sentimental relationships, as well as in the consumption of objects of enjoyment such as alcohol and light drugs, whereas Clementina's narcissistic-sacrificial side, linked to productivity, duty and hyperactivity, was more marked. For the parents, too, Clementina was the wiser of the two sisters.

However, there is a downside to this orientation that needs to be highlighted. Clementina, despite identifying with her father, had stayed away from his work, unlike Giulia, who had followed the same study path and started working with him in a company. Clementina seemed to want to follow a completely different path. She was enrolled in the Faculty of Pedagogy, but her real passion was the theatre, which had always fascinated her. For this reason, since she was very young, she had taken acting classes and wished to take part in a casting session to enter the most prestigious theatre school in her city. Thus the passion for theatre. "And how will you deal with this passion and the passion for anorexia?" I said to her as we finished a session. I thus introduced an element that would prove to be neuralgic in the treatment of this case: the impossibility of holding together the anorexic symptom and the practice of theatre beyond a certain threshold, for physiological-structural reasons. Not giving in to anorexia made the practice of theatre, which requires a certain amount of body functioning, infeasible in the future. I thus introduced, in fact, a basic concern that made Clementina divided and her relationship with the symptom a little less happy.

The either-or of the case: either anorexia or theatre

The girl, in any case, did not give up her intention to hold together the impossible, to perpetuate her anorexia combined with the theatre; she continued to eat very little, practically only fruit and vegetables, and in the meantime she registered for the casting session of the famous theatre school; she passed it and was selected. Now, after the euphoria of the first moments, a malaise mixed with anguish would invade her. Will I really be able to do this course I have so desired? Is this really what I want? With these questions also appeared the difficulties linked to the real experience of the theatre school, which absorbed her completely as and more than a full-time job: it made her encounter her own fundamental difficulties that she had previously tended to bypass and not want to look at. First of all, it was clear to her that the intimacy that was created within the relationships with the students and teachers of the school was a source of anxiety for her. It was particularly difficult for her to sustain the convivial, celebratory moments among students that often occurred at the end of lessons in the evening or after rehearsals for a performance. She felt deeply inadequate in sustaining the close experience of others, especially men, associated with the presence of food. Whenever she could, she withdrew but she realized that this was not always possible and that this condition limited her freedom. In the light of all this, I decided to propose to her that we increase the frequency of our meetings and move to two weekly sessions, outside the context of the institution, in my office. She accepted and, at the first session in the office, she gave me a very terse but important transference dream: we were both at her house with her parents. In the dream, she dreamt of the performance of L. R., the great director who runs the theatre school. I pointed out to her that I was appearing in her dreams for the first time and that this was something that carried weight in the work we were doing. From this moment on, the work with Clementina entered a new phase of reopening of the unconscious, characterized by a certain frequency of dream productions that challenged her. She began to be passionate about her question, even if for the moment the body remained immobile in its initial state. She had a feeling of greater vitality, but for the moment this was not matched by a transformation of the symptomatic condition. It would take two decisive passages to bring her body back into the process of transformation into action. The first passage was the re-proposal, in the experience of the theatre school, of the experience of the compulsory choice that I had pre-announced to her: one day a teacher of the school took her aside and told her clearly that in this physical condition she would not be able to continue to attend the school and that he would not assume the responsibility of making her continue if the condition of her body did not change. The intense dance and rhythmic movement exercises required muscle tone that she lacked because she was too thin. This intervention by the teacher had a significant traumatic effect and for the first time she started to cry during the session. "At this point you have to choose: either anorexia or theatre", I told her, putting the responsibility for her decision back on her shoulders.

The second passage was the reopening of Clementina's love and sex life. In the years of anorexia, she said she had avoided contact with men without feeling the sacrifice. Now, she felt precipitated into the problems that the relationship with them entailed. A meeting and courtship with one of her classmates, Luciano, led to a kiss that troubled her. She came to the session with a dream she had the night just after the kiss, which she read as her re-elaboration of what happened: she dreamt of a spider on her body; once she had eaten it, she was fine. The passage from fear to well-being was made by the act of eating the disturbing thing, the spider, which had landed on her body. This was a key passage which, for Clementina, was not so much about her relationship with Luciano, who turned out to be a transitory figure, but rather about her relationship to her own sexual desire in terms of a rediscovery. In September 2007, she returned from the summer break transformed: fitter and better groomed and decidedly less skinny. During the summer the cycle, which had disappeared at the beginning of the anorexia, also returned. She told me about the meeting with Giovanni, her boyfriend, with whom she had started a sentimental relationship that also included the resumption of her sexual life.

She started to eat again and agreed to introduce fish into her diet, in agreement with the nutritionist who follows her. She realized that she was still overly rigid with food and wished to be more flexible, but for the moment this was still difficult. However, she saw a significant change in this area as well. She asked at this point what sense it made to continue coming to see me, when so much seemed to have changed in her life. I told her that only she could decide, but that it seemed to me that we had not yet understood what had happened to her and that perhaps the attempt to say something about it would make her changes more solid. She agreed to continue the work for a short time and, in the meantime, her training at the theatre school was continuing better and more energetically. She now divided her time between the theatre and Giovanni with a new balance in her life, without giving up the moments of solitude she felt she needed to breathe. Two important knots would emerge in this final journey of her work. First, the context of the onset of anorexia, at the age of 15, became clearer. Her best friend, Giulia, with whom she had spent her childhood and early adolescence in a very close daily relationship, left for England for a whole year without informing her, except after the fact. Clementina suffered greatly from this, as though she had been abandoned without notice. The onset of anorexia occurred immediately afterwards. We can put forward the hypothesis that the break-up of the imaginary couple, represented for Clementina by her relationship with Giulia, had functioned as a conjuncture for triggering the symptom. The feeling of having been let down by her best friend had a triggering effect. On her return from England, Giulia would no longer be the same for Clementina: her original relationship had been irreparably broken.

Another traumatic memory, concerning something precious to Clementina, came to the surface: she had to undergo an operation on her vocal cords in early childhood because she was in danger of losing her voice. She suddenly recalled it during a singing lesson at school when, without knowing why, she experienced a particular emotion and started to cry. The memory came back during the session. She says that perhaps her passion for theatre, which puts voice and speech at the heart of the stage, was a way of reacting to this experience.

At the end of summer 2008 I saw her again for a final session. In the meantime she had finished school and was preparing to start her experience of working as an actress. She said she now wanted to finish our course, which she said she was satisfied with. I acknowledged her decision by recognizing the passages she had made and I pointed out certain aspects, which had remained somewhat in the shadows, from which, if she wanted, she could eventually resume her work.

Anorexia in classical psychoses

Anorexia when the nothing object is not drained by the phallic function: anorexic solution and holophrase

The situation is quite different when anorexia manifests itself in a subject for whom the structure of knowledge has not taken the S1–S2 form, typical of the signifying chain. In these cases, since the S1–S2 chain is not structured, there is no interval between the signifiers where the function of the subject as a divided subject ($) can be constituted. In these circumstances, it is clear that the anorexic solution cannot function as the subject's symptomatic metaphor, as in the case of hysterical anorexia: rather, it takes the form of a response to the failure of puberty symptomatization, of a "body event" that responds to the subject's failed inscription in the phallic register. In these cases, anorexia appears rather as a response in line with the holophrastic structuring of the field of the Other where the symptom does not function as a signifier of the subject for another signifier, but as a rigid identity sign, as an isolated and off-dialectic S1. The union between the S1 alone, as the holophrastic identification of anorexia, and the object nothing, as the cause, opens the way to forms of anorexia in psychosis. This structural condition where the rigid identification with the S1 of anorexia is married to an unbounded jouissance, provoked by the object nothing, presides over a varied phenomenology of the forms of psychotic anorexia. Here, the subject's body and the food function are subjected, on the part of the subject, to a delusional type of treatment that reinforces the refusal of food. In this context, the function of anorexia particularly accentuates the character of refusal as a defence against the persecuting Other.

In the most paranoid forms, it is the food object that embodies the persecutor object, in the form of poisoned or contaminated food from which one must keep one's distance by foregoing it. In the most articulated delusional forms, anorexia often takes shape within a religious construction. In these cases, the subject organizes his or her own construction of the refusal of food, around a framework with themes often borrowed from the mystical tradition or the precepts of the Bible, where the theme of fasting, as a practice of purification, is preponderant and important. It must be admitted, however, that it is rare to find highly articulated delusional constructs in anorexia and that these are paranoid schizophrenias rather than true paranoias. In most schizophrenic forms, anorexia has the function of holding together, in the anorexic holophrase, the structurally fragmented parts of the subject's body. In any case, in the most critical moments of the subject's life, when the presence of the persecuting Other becomes invasive, and in the structural absence of the regulating function of the phallic signifier, the function of the cause of non-desire, represented by the object nothing, begins to operate in the body in the direction of an unrestricted radicalization of the refusal leading the subject to risk their life. Also, in melancholic forms, this process appears evident in the moments of acuteness when the refusal of the Other changes its status from defence against an abandoning Other to the subject's existential condition: to be the refusal, the waste of the Other.

A clinical example: the case of Valentina

The beginning of the treatment

I began to see Valentina during a group session in an institution for the treatment of eating disorders where I worked and where I was the director for several years (Cosenza, 2005, pp. 71–82). Her journey was articulated in three stages: the monosymptomatic group therapy of anorexic and bulimic patients, which lasted for about two years; then, the entry into a therapeutic community that welcomed cases of anorexic and bulimic subjects; and finally, the start of an individual analytical treatment with a colleague from Parma, the city where Valentina was to go to live when she left the community.

On the occasion of her first group session, Valentina did not go unnoticed; on the contrary, she introduced a sort of change of scene into the group. When it was her turn to speak, after remaining silent for the whole time, she shut herself up for ten minutes in total silence, in front of the other participants, who asked her why she had come to the group. Her eyes were turned to the ground and she began to whistle something through her teeth in a strange tone of voice that was difficult to hear. The group gathered around her in silence so that they could hear what she was saying in that strange way. It was only some time later that some of the words Valentina hissed through her teeth would make sense. But the most important thing for her was to find a non-persecuting place in the group that could contain her despair and accept her as such. As time went by, she would be able to explain that she was going through a phase of withdrawal from the world, that she had interrupted her university studies, which she had started with great success, and that she spent her time locked up in the room of the university residence where she lived. Her appearance was very emaciated but she refused to see a doctor or take medication. In particular, it was impossible for her to be alone with male figures and she admitted that the very fact of coming in a group and knowing that the leader was a man had been very difficult, and that she had only decided to do it because she knew she would not be alone with me. At the root of this hostility toward men, she makes the revelation in the first session, anomalous in neuroses, of abuse suffered, at the age of 9, by her father's grand-father, whom she calls "old pig". She was certain of the fact, never described in detail; relating it never made the father react either in indignation or support.

The maternal mandate and the flight from the father

Valentina's relationship with her father has always been, even long before the story with the uncle, a radically disturbed one. He is a solitary and strange man who lives almost like a hermit, although he has financial resources and, in order to save money, forces the family not to use electricity and heating. Valentina and also her brother, as soon as they could, moved away from him, keeping up only remote communications with him. It took Valentina three years to agree to meet her father again, to resolve notary issues. Valentina's mother, a seemingly more worldly person to whom the daughter has always been closely related, died early of cancer when Valentina was a pre-teen. Her death triggered Valentina's anorexic symptom on the one hand, and imploded the family bond, creating a void around the father on the part of the sons.

The words that the mother said to her daughter on her deathbed, a few days before her death, were singular, and Valentina has inherited them as an order: "Don't have children and keep away from men!" This prohibition of her mother's would function for her as a kind of inexplicable S1 which, however, in fact, would organize her life like a law. In fact, for Valentina, the law is the maternal law, which, however, has not taken the form of a law in support of her desire, but rather that of an inexplicable superegoic order in which nothing functions as a third party between mother and daughter. This is why, when the mother died, the daughter would be faced with an abyss and be forced to find solutions.

Early anorexia and religious compensation

As we have said, the anorexic response was the first treatment modality invented by Valentina in response to the loss of her mother. Without her mother, Valentina felt at the mercy of the father, the object of the father's caprice, and this was unbearable for her. The anorexic response condensed a solution for her, on different levels. On the one hand, it was a concrete realization of the maternal mandate: you must not be a wife or a mother. Anorexia functioned as a barrier to both feminine desire and the desire to be a mother. At the same time, it was an attempt to put a stop to paternal madness through the construction of an illness of the body that kept it at bay. Valentina's anorexia thus appeared, at the same time, adorned with a whole self-self-harming symptomatology, made up of withdrawal from relationships and self-punitive gestures, such as cuts on the arms and body, which, however, never pushed the young girl toward a suicidal solution.

At the same time, in her history, the encounter with the Christian religion, in its radical version proposed by a fundamentalist current, was crucial; she devoted herself to it especially in the period of adolescence, in search of an unambiguous faith and a God who does not lie, which were different, for her, from the hypocrisy and ambiguity of Catholicism, practiced and defended by her family environment. In particular, in the biblical literalism of this religious community, she encountered something she had been looking for: the clinging to another whose word is clear and identifiable, written and unambiguous. In her God and in the sacred text, she thus found the mooring to a father on whom she could lean after the catastrophe of the mother's death. A father who told her what to do and what not to do, who forbade sexual intercourse before marriage and who, therefore, protected her from the relationship with sexual enjoyment. In fact, throughout her life, Valentina has avoided encounters with men and, where she has met them in the milieu of the witnesses of her religious community, she has always avoided the sexual approach, using the precept of religion to her advantage. On the other hand, she very effectively used the social network of the religious community as a support network for her movements and travel.

An oscillatory movement between withdrawal and euphoria

Valentina's case was also characterized by a subjective functioning in which the oscillatory movement between moments of withdrawal and phases of euphoria in which everything seemed wonderful was very strong. It is not just a matter of an altered perception of her condition. When she was in these moments of euphoria, Valentina, who is a very intelligent and capable girl, managed to act on reality for her own benefit with a certain efficiency. For example, in her studies, she was able to make a last-minute spurt to pass university exams without seeming to make a great effort.

It is exactly in these phases that Valentina also brought into action a surprising leadership capacity, also in relation to those around her, as happened with the other participants in the therapeutic group and with those in the therapeutic community. In these moments, she magnified the alliance with the carers to the extreme with disproportionate expressions of recognition and praise.

Erotomanic-persecutory ideation and anorexic response

However, in the work with her, it was in these same circumstances that any gesture that she might have interpreted as an interest on the part of the carers in her doing a certain thing caused a very delicate situation. In this situation, the effect on her was very sensitive and her position took on erotomanic or persecutory connotations, causing her to distance herself and weaken the therapeutic bond. Moreover, the same movement that occurred in her transference was repeated in all kinds of relationships with the other girls in treatment and the sisters of the religious community. The paranoid core of her position was manifested above all in the mechanism according to which any sign of interest on the part of the Other became for her the manifestation of an Other who wanted to enjoy her. And the response to this paranoid reading was the putting into play of the anorexic nothingness, in its most striking manifestations: refusal of food, social isolation, bodily self-harming practices, transformation of the voice from articulated speech to hissed speech that was difficult to hear. In these circumstances, the causal action of the object nothing destroyed the fragile constructions and progress in studies, broke up work situations, interrupted relationships and suspended or put a sudden end to therapeutic treatments.

Ordinary psychosis and anorexia nervosa

S0 + nothing: a formula for anorexia in ordinary psychosis

Having alluded to the function of the object nothing in hysterical-neurotic anorexia where the S1–S2 signifying chain is installed but the action of nothing temporarily deactivates it in its after-effects' functioning; and having highlighted the relation between the object nothing and the anorexic holophrase (S1 alone) in psychotic anorexics, we will now deal with anorexia in cases of ordinary psychosis (Miller, 2009b, pp. 40–51; Stevens, 2009, p. 65;

Zenoni, 2004, 75–77). To use Miller's formula in relation to Charles' case, these are situations where the signifier S0 shows us the emptiness of the subject function, the absence of a fundamental and structuring identification, capable of linking the subject's being to an S1 that can represent it. This is neither in the psychotic form of the holophrastic monolith, nor even less in the form of an S1 signifier that represents it as a subject for another signifier S2.

In the case of hysterical anorexia, the formula of the relationship between knowledge and jouissance, at the peak of the honeymoon phase with the symptom, can be written in this way:

$$\text{(nothing)}$$
$$\downarrow$$
$$S1 \ldots \ldots S2$$

where knowledge is articulated but the interval is occluded by the function of the object nothing which obstructs the movement of the aftermath. It will be the work of the treatment, as in the case of Clementina, to put back into function, for the subject, the signifying chain by the reopening of the relation of the subject with unconscious knowledge and the displacement of the function of the object nothing from the point of interval of the chain, where it rendered inactive the work of hysterization.

In the case of psychosis with anorexic symptoms, as in the case of Valentina, the key formula becomes:

$$S1 + \text{nothing}$$

where the anorexic holophrase is constituted as a defence against an Other who enjoys the subject and where nothing is the object of enjoyment around which the satisfaction of the psychotic subject is organized. Anorexia, in these cases, acquires a frankly delusional meaning or it functions in a delusional modality that finds its most usual manifestation in the aberrant relationship with food.

The question we need to ask, now, concerns the anorexias that settle in cases where the psychosis does not manifest itself in its classical and declared form but rather assumes the more discreet semblances of ordinary psychosis. In these cases, anorexia does not normally assume a special meaning for the subject, one that can be reconciled with a delusional construction; it is, in most cases, a silent condition that the subject experiences without making it his or her own identifying sign, but which is essential for the organization of his or her daily life regime. These cases appear as forms in which the anorexia, once installed, assumes less oppositional and more passive appearances that refer, in an obvious way, to the subject's identity void. For this kind of non-delusional psychotic anorexia, we feel that the formula proposed by Miller and commented on above is more appropriate:

$$S0 + \text{nothing}$$

In these cases, the central action of the object nothing as a cause presents itself, so to speak, without veils and in a more obvious way than in classical psychotic anorexias; the subject, in fact, is not in a condition to dress up his anorexia with "nothing" and the work of signifying construction proper to the delusion is reduced to a minimum, if not completely absent. Sometimes, in these cases, anorexia is established from a fundamental devitalization that is created by the effect of the fall of the imaginary identification, leaving the subject's place empty. Other times, on the other hand, it is impossible to find not only the point of discontinuity, typical of the triggering of the symptom but also the most discrete disconnection proper to ordinary psychosis: the anorexic condition thus manifests itself, in the history of the subject, as a continuum from childhood to adulthood.

A clinical example: the case of Emilia

A life organized around isolation

I saw Emilia, for about a year, in my office, after an analytically driven group psychotherapy with other anorexic and bulimic patients in an institution. She was referred by the group leader, after expressing the intention to conclude the therapy and eventually start an individual course. When I started to see her, she was a young woman of thirty-five, very thin, with an inexpressive face and a tendency to be taciturn. Her life revolved around two pivotal points: the elderly parents with whom she has always lived and her work as a university researcher in the biology department. Her parents' house and the laboratory have been the formula for her life for more than ten years now, since she began her university studies with the support of her professor, the head of the department. During the preparation of her Master's thesis on the brain structure of insects, her professor suggested that she continue to work with her and be part of her team, initially as a volunteer. After a few years, she took the research competition and passed. When asked what she was passionate about in this research work, she could not answer at all, except that she was a very regular worker, that in 15 years she had never failed to show up at the laboratory. The typical description of her work situation is as follows: alone, at her desk, in front of her computer, in the laboratory, near the refrigerated cell with the frozen insect samples ready for analysis. Her favorite times to work were early in the morning – she was the first one to arrive – and late in the afternoon – she was the last one, in fact, to leave the lab: when the other colleagues were not there, she felt better.

What was striking about Emilia was the description of a condition of radical isolation, especially because of the absence of suffering linked to this condition: her days were structured according to the perfect organization of a clock. There was time to sleep, time to work in the laboratory and, once a week, time to go swimming in the pool. But in all this rigid order, the common thread was the absence of real relationships. Moreover, Emilia avoided meeting others: she liked to stay in the lab when she was alone, she went to the pool at times when she knew she would not meet other people, she ate her meals in solitude both at work and at home.

Emilia's anorexia and the emptiness of her relationship with sex

She has been very thin since childhood and has had difficulties with eating from the start, especially with solid food in early childhood. She was not breastfed by her mother, who had no milk left after her older sister had been breastfed. Throughout her life, her diet would tend to consist of liquids and crumbled solid food, which she consumed in very small quantities. A whole piece of meat or fish is abhorrent to her. The tiny is the nearest thing to the acceptable: perhaps for this reason she has turned to molecular biology and the laboratory where the ordinary working instrument of the researcher is the microscope. Her early anorexia would always be treated as a strictly nutritional problem, without the parents feeling subjectively involved. Moreover, Emilia's very relationship with her difficulty in eating is manifested in her as desubjectivized and devoid of symbolization. The feature of anorexia, as a maneuver of challenge or provocation of the Other, would never appear in her words. Rather, it assumed the characteristics of a habitus, a modus vivendi and also a protective barrier against threats from the outside.

Her condition of extreme thinness made her lose the cycle right away, after its first appearance at puberty, without any return of cycle thereafter. However, for Emilia, the absence of the cycle does not represent a loss at all: she rather perceives it as an impediment, something cumbersome that she would not know what to do with. Emilia has never felt like a woman and the sexual question never appears in her speech as a problem. What is sometimes a problem for her is anything that may arise as a threat to the "clockwork" organization of her everyday life. It is to a situation of this kind, for example, that we owe the fact that Emilia was able to ask for a treatment that was not only nutritional in an institution, but that continued in short slices in the office with me. It was, in fact, the director of her laboratory who became alarmed at her extreme thinness and pushed her to seek help not only from nutritionists but also from psychotherapists, inviting her to take a period of leave. Faced with the anxiety of not being able to return regularly to the laboratory every day, Emilia agreed to seek help and started group psychotherapy, while at the same time intensifying the medical-nutritional controls.

Subjective emptiness and the construction of a supplementary device

Emilia's case seems to us particular since it shows us a situation where the S0 of the beginning, a condition which accompanied the appearance of anorexia from childhood, was followed, with the university, by a construction of a point of holding S1, structured around the work of university researcher in biology. This tempered, and in part resolved, the emptiness of the previous condition of S0 + nothing that characterizes her structurally. Basically, the work done with her in analysis was limited to supporting her in her relationship with the substitution linked to her work as a biologist, the sole point of subjective identification and the only brake on the deployment of the anorexic nothing. The sentence of her teacher: "Dear Emilia, if you don't cure yourself, I will be obliged to leave you at home" has indeed functioned for her as a limit, by distressing her and putting her in the position to better measure her anorexia.

Note

1   This case was presented at the 4th Seminar of the Mara Selvini School on "Il trattamento individuale della paziente con disturbo alimentare", in Milan, on 15 May 2010.

References

Cosenza, D. (2005), Les nouvelles forms du symptôme et l'ABA, *La Cause freudienne*, no. 61, pp. 71–82, novembre.
Cosenza, D. (2008), "Anorexie", Association Mondiale de Psychanalyse, *Scilicet. Les objets a dans l'experience analytique*. Paris: École de la Cause freudienne, pp. 29–31.
Dewambrechies La Sagna, C. (2006), L'anorexie vraie de la jeune fille, *La Cause freudienne*, no. 63, juin, pp. 57–70.
Dewambrechies La Sagna, C. (2008), "Rien", Association Mondiale de Psychanalyse, *Scilicet. Les objets a dans l'experience analytique*. Paris: École de la Cause freudienne, pp. 376–379.
Lacan, J. (2006a), *The Subversion of the Subject and the Dialectic of Desire in the Freudian Unconscious, Écrits*. The First Complete Edition in English. New York/London: Norton & Company, pp. 671–702; *Subversion du sujet et dialectique du désir dans l'inconscient freudien* (1960), *Écrits* (1966). Paris: Éditions du Seuil, pp. 793–827.
Lacan, J. (1994), *Le Séminaire. Livre IV. La relation d'objet*, 1956–1957. Paris: Le Seuil.
Lacan, J. (1986), *Le Séminaire. Livre VII. L'éthique de la psychanalyse*, 1959–1960. Paris: Le Seuil.
Lacan, J. (2006b), *Le Séminaire. Livre XVI. D'un Autre à l'autre*, 1968–1969. Paris: Le Seuil.
Ménard, A. (1989), Anorexie mentale et entrée en analyse, *Actes de l'ECF*, pp. 16–20, mai.
Maleval, J.-C. (2009), Déprise sociale paradoxale et Clinique du desert, Miller, J.-A. (Dir.), *Situations subjectives de déprise sociale*. Paris: Navarin, pp. 37–48.
Miller, J.-A. (Dir.) (2009a), *Situations subjectives de déprise sociale*. Paris: Navarin.
Miller, J.-A. (2009b), Effet retour sur la psychose ordinaire, *Quarto*, no. 94–95, janvier, pp. 40–51.

Stevens, A. (1998), Adolescence, symptôme de la puberté, *Les Feuillets psychanalytiques du Courtil*, Publication du Champ Freudien en Belgique, no. 15, pp. 79–92, mars.

Stevens, A. (2009), Mono-symptômes et traits de psychose ordinaire, *Quarto*, no. 94–95, pp. 61–65, mars.

Zenoni, A. (2004), Quélle réponse au mono-symptôme?, *Quarto*, no. 80–81, pp. 75–77, janvier.

Chapter 8

The teaching of infantile anorexia

The anorexic question in childhood

Our reading of anorexia nervosa, starting from Lacan, has highlighted a circuit of functioning where the refusal constitutes the anorexic action proper and the object nothing functions as a fundamental cause to support this action. In this sense, the anorexic refusal is another way of saying what Lacan defines as the anorexic's own action: "Eating nothing".

Depending on the case, we have specified that the anorexic refusal can respond to different functions and that the causative action of nothing can have an incidence, in different modalities, according to the structure of the subject's position in relation to their real nucleus and to the Other of knowledge, that is, in relation to unconscious knowledge (the signifying chain S1-S2).

In this chapter, devoted to infantile anorexia, and in the next one, concerning the beginnings of anorexia in adolescence, we will try to put to the test what we have formulated so far on anorexia nervosa, by taking into account these two essential times when the anorexic response takes shape in the subject's development.

Why not limit ourselves, like many psychoanalysts, also of Lacanian training, to dealing with the question by relying solely on the anorexia that begins in adolescence and which, for some, coincides with anorexia nervosa itself, true anorexia? First of all, I could say that Lacan himself pushes us toward infantile anorexia when he affirms, in *The Seminar*, Book XI, that the anorexic child eats nothing.

In several places, Lacan's thesis on anorexia in its key point, that they eat nothing, is also linked to the position of the child and not only of anorexic girls (as in the case, for example, of *The Seminar*, Book XXI, where it is the girl who is more in the foreground). This indicates to us that for Lacan there is something essential in anorexia that links in a continuum its form of infantile beginnings and that of its beginnings in adolescence, despite their undeniable and important differences. It will then be a question of testing this essential point of tension between continuum and discontinuity around the anorexic question, formulated in its structure of functioning.

DOI: 10.4324/9781003318439-9

In this perspective, it will be interesting for us to refer to Ansermet's thesis on anorexic refusal, contained in *Clinique de l'origine* (and developed in a recent article), where he proposes to "take up the question of anorexia in adolescence in the perspective of what early anorexia teaches" (Ansermet, 1999, p. 161).

Indeed, Ansermet continues, "early anorexia is a sign of an impasse in the emergence of the subject; in any case, it implies returning to the question of subjective constitution, based on the light shed by this pathology" (ibid.).

Logically, it is for this reason that he puts forward this hypothesis for clinical reflection on the relationship between early anorexia and adolescent anorexia:

> "Early anorexia could thus constitute a paradigm that would make it possible to identify what is also at play in adolescent anorexia: in this time of life (the second phase of sexual development, as we say), it is indeed the assumption of the subject that is at stake through the refusal that so strongly characterises the anorexic".
>
> (Ibid., p. 164)

The issue that we want to address here concerns the problem of anorexia, questioned in the perspective of its development and its different times of manifestation. Classically, in the literature of the psychodynamic psychiatry of childhood and adolescence, oriented by psychoanalysis, this problem is articulated above all around the question of continuity/discontinuity between eating disorders in childhood and adolescence and, particularly, around the relationship between infantile anorexia and the anorexia which begins in adolescence and which coincides, for various authors, with true anorexia. The issue was effectively framed by Widlöcher, in his "Preface" to Brusset's now classic book *L'assiette et le miroir. L'anorexie mentale de l'enfant et de l'adolescent*:

> "Two attitudes can be observed here. Some tend to emphasise the deep and archaic conflicts, postulating that the others constitute a cover, a screen, which the investigation during psychotherapy must overcome in order to establish the true cause of the syndrome. Others think, on the contrary, that the explanation of the symptom lies in the conflict linked to the emerging sexual identity, the refusal of the female body. They see proof of this in the fact that it is a rather specifically female pathology. This conflict is certainly superficial and linked to current problems, but it is reinforced and made pathogenic in many cases by more archaic childhood conflicts that are less accessible to consciousness. The first conception brings adolescent anorexia closer to that of the infant, the second insists on the differences".
>
> (Widlöcher, 1977, p. 10)

For this reason, our research will try, first of all, to develop, in a particular way, the question of anorexia in childhood and adolescence (around which it is also easier to find, compared to infantile anorexia, a more ample and reliable psychoanalytical literature).

Psychiatric, psychological and psychoanalytical literature tends to stress the difference and discontinuity between childhood and adolescent anorexia. What is especially emphasized, on the one hand, as a discriminating factor is the power that the sexual issue exerts on adolescence, which begins at puberty, and its predominant manifestation as a female syndrome affecting girls, in nine cases out of ten. This relationship appears, on the other hand, to be totally insignificant, from a statistical-epidemiological point of view, in infantile anorexia, which affects both males and females.

We will try to critically articulate here the status of this discontinuity, in the light of the structural coordinates, drawn from the Lacanian clinic, that we have isolated as the basis of anorexia nervosa: the particular relation of the subject in anorexia to the Other (characterized by a fundamental refusal) and their relation to jouissance (which we have defined as affirmative); both of which find in the refusal of food a paradigmatic embodiment. First of all, it will be necessary to develop what infantile anorexia is; second, if we can speak of a plurality of forms of childhood anorexia; and, third, if the supposed discontinuity between infantile anorexia and adolescent and adult anorexia turns out to be only a phenomenological discontinuity that the critical crossroads of development highlight, or if it is, at the same time, a structural discontinuity where the configuration of the subject's relation to the Other and to his jouissance takes on a different relational form and libidinal circuit.

We will try to answer these three knots by questioning, first of all, the most recent perspective of empirical-experimental research in the field of childhood psychopathology. We will place this recent perspective in a dialectically critical relationship with the most classic approaches of the psychoanalysis of anorexia in the development age (in particular in the work of Brusset), with a view to reading the question in the light of the most recent Lacanian contributions (Ansermet and Férnandez Blanco).

Classification of eating disorders in childhood, from the perspective of current psychiatric-descriptive classification systems

From DSM-IV to CD: 0-3R

Among clinicians, the most widespread reference for nosography in the developmental domain is represented by the Diagnostic Classification of Developmental Disorders in Early Childhood (DC: 0-3) of 1994. As Speranza and Williams point out:

"It is a multi-axial classification system that, positioning itself as comple-mentary to existing approaches such as the DSM-IV-TR (APA, 2000), focuses specifically on developmental issues".

(Speranza, Williams, 2009, p. 283)

The main difference between this classification and the DSM-IV is repre-sented first by the reformulation of the diagnostic frameworks, which involves a shift from a more classic perspective, focusing on the child in isolation from his or her context, to a more complex perspective that places him or her in his or her relational world and developmental period. Speranza further emphasizes:

"Traditional classification systems, in fact, tend to consider eating disorders as problems of the child as an individual, without taking into consideration either the evolutionary or the relational aspects within which these disorders manifest themselves".

(Speranza, 2009)

It is true that in the most up-to-date version concerning childhood, rep-resented by the DSM-PC (Diagnostic and Statistic Manual for Primary Care, AAP, 1996), the Manual has the novelty of introducing, among the char-acteristics of the eating disorder in childhood, a disorder "between the parent and the child". Nevertheless, this has not prevented specialists in the field, particularly under the influence of the new theories and methods of Infant Research and Developmental Psychopathology, from criticizing its complex categorical implementation and moving, more decisively, toward the CD: 0-3, particularly in its most up-to-date version, the CD: 0-3R (2005).

In its clinical description of the eating disorder of childhood and prepuberty, the DSM-PC presents a series of risk factors where the relational component comes into play: indeed, it not only indicates a difficult child temperament, coupled with aversive behavior toward food but also cites the presence of dis-rupted caregiver interactions and psychosocial stress in the family in addition to problems with attachment, autonomy, self-regulation and separation. However, its more psychodynamic-evolutionary critics point out that these features are only indicated as associated with the disorder itself. What is also criticized in the structure of the DSM is the *reductio ad unum* of the different subtypes of eating disorders under a single diagnostic category, in addition to a weak consideration of developmental factors (Chatoor and Ganiban, 2004; Speranza, 2009).

Irene Chatoor's classification of childhood eating disorders and the *CD: 0-3R system*

In the perspective introduced by the American researcher Irene Chatoor and subsequently accepted in the CD: 0-3R system, the definition of childhood eating disorders leaves the rigid and reductive categorical framework of the

DSM to be reformulated within the framework of a multi-factorial approach, centered on the relational and evolutionary dimension. It is not by chance that these disorders are classified here within Axis II: "Disorders of the relationship".

Development is understood here "as an interactive resolution of adaptive tasks, following an established epigenetic sequence" (Speranza, 2009, p. 12). In this context, infancy is characterized by the passage of the child through three fundamental developmental tasks requiring the mother-child couple to make a new adaptation at each passage:

> "The achievement of homeostasis, the construction of the attachment bond and the transition to autonomy (separation-individuation process)".
>
> (Ibid.)

Chatoor and Ganiban (2004) specifically investigate these tasks with regard to the child's acquisition of regulated internment feeding. They involve the acquisition of recognition and discrimination of hunger and satiety signals (0–2 months), regulated interaction between the child and the caregiver to support the child's self-regulation of feeding (2–4 months) and the child's transition to autonomous feeding after weaning (6 months–3 years).

Each task has a specific eating disorder, as indicated by the diagnostic classification CD: 0-3:

1 State Regulation Eating Disorder (homeostasis):

   a The child has difficulty being and remaining calm during feeding (e.g. the child is too sleepy, too agitated and/or too stressed by feeding).
   b Feeding difficulties start in the neonatal period.
   c The child is not gaining weight or is losing weight.

2 Reciprocal Feeding Disorder in the Caregiver-Child Relationship:

   a During feeding, the child does not give any appropriate signals of reciprocity with the caregiver, from an evolutionary point of view (e.g. eye contact, smiling, vocalizations).
   b The child has a significant growth deficit.
   c The growth failure and lack of relatedness is due to a physical or diffuse developmental disorder.

3 Infantile anorexia:

   a The child refuses to eat an adequate amount of food for at least one month.
   b Refusal to eat occurs before three years of age.
   c The child appears to have no hunger or interest in food but shows clear signs of interest in exploration, interaction with the caregiver or both.

d The child has a significant growth deficit.

e Food refusal does not occur as a result of a traumatic event.

f The food refusal is not due to a medical cause.

In addition to these three basic forms of eating disorders in childhood, the CD: 0-3R also indicates three other clinical settings: sensory aversions to food, eating disorder associated with a medical condition and post-traumatic eating disorder.

4 Sensory food aversions:

a The child refuses to eat food with a very characteristic taste, consistency, smell or appearance.

b Refusal of food occurs when a new food is offered.

c The child eats without difficulty when offered his or her favorite food.

d Food refusal causes specific nutritional deficits and/or delays in motor-oral development.

5 Eating disorder associated with a medical condition:

a The child starts feeding promptly but during the feeding, the child is uncomfortable and refuses to continue eating.

b The child has an associated medical condition that is considered to be the cause of the discomfort.

c Medical cures improve but do not completely relieve the discomfort.

d The child is not gaining weight or is losing weight.

6 Post-traumatic eating disorder:

a Refusal to eat following a traumatic event or repeated trauma to the oro-pharyngeal or gastrointestinal tract (e.g. choking, severe vomiting, naso-gastric or endo-tracheal tube placement, suctioning) triggering intense stress in the child.

b Severe refusal to eat in any of the following ways:

• refuses to drink from a bottle but may accept food offered with a spoon or in the hands;

• refuses solid food but may accept a bottle.

c The memory of traumatic events causes discomfort, which is manifested by one or more of these behaviors:

• he/she may show anticipatory anxiety when put in position to eat;

• he/she offers stubborn resistance when the bottle or food is approached;

• stubborn resistance to swallowing food in the mouth.

d Refusal of food represents an acute or long-term threat to the child's nutrition.

Childhood eating disorders in the PDM (*Psychodynamic Diagnostic Manual*)

The openness to the relational basis at play in childhood eating disorders is further emphasized in the PDM classification system, recently created in the United States and an expression of the psychodynamic orientations of the North American clinical milieu, in response to the need to go beyond a purely descriptive and rigidly categorical approach to diagnosis, as found in the DSM-IV. The framework of this Manual is the crisis of the DSM-IV and the attempt to hold together the rigor of empirical research with the competence of clinical experience which appeared to be sacrificed or lost, according to the authors, in the DSM's classificatory device. Faced with a self-declared a-theoretical approach, such as that of the DSM, the authors of the PDM respond with an explicitly psychodynamic perspective drawing, in particular, on psychoanalytic knowledge rooted in Anglo-American clinical culture. In its articulation, the work reproposes key concepts of psychoanalysis that recent editions of the DSM had discarded, such as the notion of neurosis, symptom, hysteria and subject. It is organized along three main axes (Personality Patterns and Disorders - P Axis; Profile of Mental Functioning - M Axis; Symptomatic Patterns: Subjective Experience - S Axis) and emphasizes a dimensional rather than a categorical approach in the diagnostic articulation.

The PDM also separates the classificatory frameworks on the basis of development, distinguishing between the "Classification of Mental Disorders in Adults" (Part I) and the "Classification of Mental Disorders in Children and Adolescents" (Part II) where a specific "Classification of Mental and Developmental Disorders in Infants and Young Children" also appears.

With regard to eating disorders, they are coded under Axis S ("Symptomatic patterns: the subjective experience"), in all three developmental classifications. The fundamental principle of PDM is that any symptomatic pattern or disorder (S-axis) cannot be a diagnostic factor if it is not related to the personality framework (P-axis) and mental functioning profile (M-axis) of the patient. This is also true for eating disorders, which therefore assume a different value and function depending on the personality, mental function and the time during development when they present themselves in the life of the subject and in the encounter with the clinician.

In the section on eating disorders in adults, the PDM uses the DSM-IV diagnosis of anorexia and bulimia, adding remarks on what results, in large part, from the accounts of clinicians working in this field (and collected with the SWAP-200 system of Westen and Shedler, 2003) around the most recurrent inner experience of the eating disorder patient. The Manual defines them, more precisely, as "descriptions of the inner and not immediately observable experiences of people with eating disorders, including emotional conflicts and concerns that, on the surface, have little to do with food"

(PDM, 2008, pp. 126–127). This section, as will be seen below, is divided into four clusters relating to affective states, cognitive patterns, somatic states and relational patterns, and is also considered valid in the Manual for the classification of eating disorders in childhood and adolescence, where anorexia and bulimia are defined as Psycho-Physiological Disorders (ibid., p. 311).

On the other hand, a few separate notes are specifically reserved for the classification of feeding disorders in infants and very young children, in a specific area of this developmental period called Infancy and Early Childhood (IEC). This is the age range that corresponds, more or less, to the classification developed by Chatoor and included in the CD: 0-3R. The PDM annotations on eating disorders in infants and very young children can be summarized in four points:

1 Feeding disorders (FD), as well as sleep disorders, can be symptomatic of many interactive disorders.
2 Eating disorders can represent a regulatory disorder with sensory hypersensitivities and oral motor difficulties.
3 ED (Eating Disorders) may reflect residual anxiety derived from unresolved biological problems (gastrointestinal difficulties, reflux and other pathologies) that had led to the anxiety and lack of pleasure in feeding.
4 EDs may depend significantly on the interactions between the caregiver and the child (ibid., p. 383).

    a Example: in the absence of adequate cures, there may be an over-reliance on food for relief and comfort.
    b Example: in the absence of symbolic expression, fear, anger or refusal may be expressed by refusing food.
    c In a family, the absence of adequate feeding patterns can alter the development of the child.
    d The presence of an eating disorder in a parent may facilitate the development of an eating disorder in the child.

Developments on anorexia in the most recent classification systems: DSM-5, DC: 0-5, PDM2[1]

The last decade has seen a renewal of the main diagnostic classification systems for mental disorders. Within this framework, we refer here briefly to what has been introduced with regard to childhood eating disorders and childhood anorexia in particular.

In 2013, the fifth edition of the DSM was released in the United States, which very recently, in February 2022, had its revision (DSM-5 Task Force, 2022, pp. 371–397). We will not elaborate here on the different approach in the classification of mental disorders that the DSM-5 has introduced compared to previous editions, marking more of a dimensional perspective and introducing a classification that is less rigidly categorical and more organized in a spectrum structure, which allows for greater appreciation of the range of internal variations in the course of the mental disorder. We limit ourselves to emphasizing that, notwithstanding these variations, the basic limits of the Manual, already underlined, remain: of the exclusion of reference to the functioning of the subject suffering from the disorder, of the little consideration of developmental times, of the undervaluation of the relational dimension in the constitution of the symptomatology (also underlined by Chatoor and collaborators), and of the absence of any reference to the modality of being in the therapeutic relationship.

With respect to the field of eating disorders, we find in the recent classification the unification in a common framework, the "feeding and eating disorders", of the disorders related to the relationship with food that the DSM-IV distinguished in two separate age-related categories: the feeding and eating disorders of childhood or early childhood (DSM-IV, APA, 1998, pp. 114–119) – including pica, rumination disorder and childhood or early childhood nutrition disorder –, and "eating disorders" (among which DSM-IV included anorexia, bulimia and eating disorder not otherwise specified) (ibid., pp. 591–603). From the point of view of the internal classification, the DSM-5 presents the greatest novelties, not so much for the frameworks mainly related to childhood, but for the eating disorders of adolescence and adulthood. In particular, they consist in the introduction of the Binge Eating Disorder, as a framework in its own right, and in the elimination of the criterium amenorrhae in order to be able to make a diagnosis of anorexia nervosa. The latter operation makes it possible to universalize the diagnosis of anorexia, extending it beyond the picture of women in their child-bearing period, thus including males and females in other phases of biological life. In the new organization proposed by the DSM-5 and confirmed in its recent revision, we therefore have seven diagnostic frameworks: pica, rumination disorder and food avoidance/restrictive disorder (which take up the legacy of the childhood forms of eating disorders in the DSM-IV), anorexia nervosa, bulimia nervosa, binge eating disorder and eating disorder not otherwise specified.

In 2016 a new classification was published in the United States, by the Zero to Three Task Force, which had already been engaged in the previous CD: 0-3 classification in creating a classification system that took the child's development into account, a new classification that extends the period to the pre-school age range, from birth to five years of age: the DC: 0-5 system. The centrality of the relational dimension in the framing of the child's symptomatology, already at the heart of the DC: 0-3, is here relaunched and extended "... not only to the relationship with primary caregivers but also to that relating to the extended growth environment" (Maestro, Muratori, 2018, p. XII). With regard to the field of childhood eating disorders, they are grouped around three disorders: overeating disorder, hypo-eating disorder and atypical eating disorder.

Overeating disorder, which cannot be found in children under the age of two years (because it requires a high degree of autonomy and verbal and motor skills to search for food), presents overeating or the urge to overeat, excessive pre-occupation with food, agitation of the child if he or she is hindered in this urge, the non-attributability of the disorder to other causes and significant impairment of the child's and family's functioning as a result of this disorder. It is often associated with the caregiver's chronic failure to respond to the child's nutritional needs, which not infrequently takes the form of excessive control over the child's feeding (Zero to Three, 2018, p. 130).

Hypo-nutrition disorder, on the other hand, is not age-specific and can occur from the first months of life. It is characterized by the following criteria: the child eats less than expected for his or her age; he or she exhibits one or more maladaptive eating behaviors within a series; these behaviors cannot be explained by medical condition or pharmacological effects; the symptoms of the disorder or the caregivers' adjustment to the symptoms significantly impair the child's and the family's functioning.

Finally, the atypical eating disorder groups three atypical eating symptoms: hoarding (the child hides food in unusual places), pica (habitual ingestion of inedible substances) and rumination (regurgitation and re-digestion of food).

In 2017, ten years after the first edition, the second edition of PDM, edited by Nancy McWilliams and Vittorio Lingiardi, was published in the United States. An abbreviated and updated version covering childhood and adolescence (the period from 0 to 18 years) was published in 2020 by the two editors of PDM2 together with Anna Maria Speranza. True to the "PDM philosophy", according to which every " classification of mental disorders must start from a complex view of mental health" (Lingiardi, McWilliams, Speranza, 2020, p. 4), the second edition, with respect to childhood and adolescence, provides a hierarchy of importance in the multi-axial system that (with the exception of early childhood, which provides its own multi-axiality) places the M-axis of mental functioning in first place in the diagnosis, with respect to the P-axis of personality and the S-axis relating to symptoms and subjectivity, since the personality of the child and adolescent is still in formation.

With respect to eating disorders in early childhood, the authors highlight the centrality of the parents' response to the child's refusal to eat, highlighting how a coercive or compensatory attitude based on a misreading of the child's emotional signals can contribute (as Hilde Bruch taught) to the onset and development of the eating disorder, both in a restrictive and a compulsive sense (Speranza, Mayes, 2020, pp. 20–21). Classified among the psycho-physiological disorders in childhood symptom patterns, nutrition and eating disorders in childhood "… are more food-centred" (Malberg, Rosemberg, 2020, p. 165). With respect to gender they are more characterized by selectivity in food choice in boys, and a greater tendency to develop anorexia and bulimia in girls. In any case "family factors play a fundamental role" (ibid., p. 165) in the genesis of the disorder. With regard to adolescents, Mario Speranza emphasizes the alexithymic dimension present in anorexia and bulimia, the different types of mental functioning that can be traced in these patients, the majority of whom are female, and the failure of the separation-individuation process (Speranza M., 2020, pp. 301–304). In general, empirical research tends to show, as Anna Maria Speranza points out, that "... the presence of eating problems in early childhood and/or adolescence carries a strong risk of developing an eating disorder in early adulthood" (Speranza, 2020, p. 352).

A child psychiatric approach to anorexia in children with an analytic orientation: the contribution of Bernard Brusset

Anorexia nervosa between an eating disorder and primary mother/child relationship disorder

We have briefly mentioned the main points inherent in recent psychiatric classifications of eating disorders in early childhood, based on empirical research data and sensitive to the relational-interactive dimension. It is opportune now to turn to the clinical investigation of psychoanalysis in its truest sense, in order to measure its distance from the more experimental and quantitative approaches. It is certainly not our intention here to systematically review all the contributions of psychoanalysts who have dealt with childhood eating disorders. What interests us more is to introduce the coordinates of a paradigmatic work of psychoanalytically oriented child psychiatry that can still represent, today, an essential reference for all those who deal with the clinic of anorexia in childhood and adolescence. This paradigmatic work should also function as a bridge between the psychiatric-descriptive classifications of eating disorders in childhood, as we have seen them, and the Lacanian approach to the question of childhood anorexia.

Brusset's work *L'assiette et le miroir. L'anorexie mentale de l'enfant et de l'adolescent* (1977), which has become a great classic, although more than 40 years have passed since its publication, remains one of the key references in psychodynamic approaches, in psychiatry and psychoanalysis, around the theme of anorexia nervosa in childhood and adolescence. His perspective would be enriched by the book he would write 20 years later, *Psychopatologie de l'anorexie mentale* (Psychopathology of Anorexia Nervosa), but the frame of reference concerning infantile anorexia will remain the one proposed in *L'assiette et le miroir*.

The fact of taking up, here, the most significant points of his theory of infantile anorexia already allows us to measure the scope and the internal limits of the most recent classifications of eating disorders in early childhood. First of all, it is important to bear in mind that, for Brusset, anorexia nervosa as such constitutes "an original mental organisation" (Brusset, 1977, p. 17): the form it assumes in early childhood and the one that appears in adolescence are reciprocally heterogeneous in several aspects but, nevertheless, they have at least one key point in common:

"The characteristic of adolescent anorexia, like that of infancy, is to associate disorders of both eating behaviour and family interactions".

(Ibid., p. 12)

The critical action underlying the recent psychopathological classifications of anorexia and which opposes the DSM-IV – i.e. the CD: 0-3 for infantile anorexia and the MDP – is nothing other than an attempt to rethink the eating disorder as a relational disorder, as Brusset has indicated and in line with the pioneers of the psychodynamic approach to anorexia: Bruch and Selvini Palazzoli. Brusset does a very careful job of distinguishing anorexia nervosa from organic anorexia, of showing its irreducibility to a loss of hunger or an alteration of appetite, or even of distinguishing, with Kreisler, Fain and Soulé (Kreisler, Fain and Soulé, 1974, pp. 130–174), the simple form of anorexia (reaction to an error in maternal attitude easily rectifiable by repositioning) from severe anorexia nervosa, which cannot be cured by simple therapeutic measures (ibid., p. 53).

In this work, Brusset provides us with a simple and rigorous definition of anorexia nervosa that allows us to insert, in the context of the mother/child interaction, the fundamental node that we have posed at the center of our clinical investigation.

Based on direct observation, *"we can consider anorexia as a refusal behaviour in the mother-child transaction"* (Brusset, 1977, p. 68).

Refusal in infantile anorexia and weaning anorexia

Brusset, therefore, does not emphasize either the loss of hunger or an alteration of appetite but the refusal as an operation characterizing the anorexia nervosa of the child and the adolescent. The question we are asking here is to know what characteristics refusal has in infantile anorexia and if it is possible to identify different forms of it in order to establish, in the end, what kind of relationship it might have with refusal in adolescence.

To begin with, it is interesting to highlight the fact that the diagnosis of childhood anorexia, formulated by Brusset and also defined as "weaning anorexia", coincides (and not only as a temporal framework) with the diagnosis of childhood anorexia formulated by Irene Chatoor and inserted in the CD classification system: 0-3R:

"In the usual form, it is an infant in the second half of its first year, awake, showing much curiosity about its surroundings and appearing to be in advance in its development. More or less abruptly, he/she begins to refuse the food presented to him by his/her mother. Given the most frequent age of appearance of this behaviour, it has been defined as weaning anorexia, the transition to a solid and varied diet being incriminated. But let us say straight away that this triggering factor is not necessary".

(Ibid., p. 51)

We encounter here, in the most typical form of infantile anorexia, the double-sided feature, also recurrent in many cases of adolescent anorexia and which takes the form of hyperactivity: a basic vitality, united with a marked and sudden refusal of food.

Oppositional anorexia and anorexia of inertia

Brusset also recovers, in this respect, a classic distinction between anorexia of opposition: reactive, vital, oppositive and active, and anorexia of inertia: passive and, at least in appearance, devoid of intentionality and conflict. These would be mutually irreducible modalities by which the anorexic child manifests the refusal of food:

> "We have tried to oppose anorexia of inertia and anorexia of opposition. In anorexia of inertia, the child appears satiated from the beginning of the meal, and remains without crying, without agitation. This anorexia only occurs in the middle of the meal, for certain meals intermittently or permanently. It may be limited to certain foods. Oppositional anorexia is an active behaviour in which the child shows obvious hostility as soon as there is a question of making him/her eat, even though he/she is otherwise very alert and very friendly. Vomiting may be associated with this. Whatever the descriptive relevance of such a distinction, the question arises as to its theoretical basis".

> (Ibid., p. 61)

Inertia anorexia and autism: an open question

We could put forward the hypothesis that oppositional anorexia, in which we think we recognize the paradigmatic form of anorexia nervosa, corresponds to the framework of infantile anorexia that Chatoor situates from the sixth month onwards; here the problem of weaning comes into play to the same extent as the passage, in time, to the child's autonomous feeding. In this context, the oppositional and power value toward the Other who takes care of the child (first and foremost the mother), which the child stages by orchestrating the game of the refusal of food, is evident. Even before any evaluation of the personality structure, we are dealing here with an act of the child, the refusal of food, which appeals to someone else and thus establishes an outline of a dialectical relationship.

On the contrary, in the typical settings of the so-called anorexia of inertia, we could perhaps hypothesize the presence of forms of early anorexia, more easily identifiable in settings situated, according to Chatoor, between the first two and fourth months of life (respectively, state regulation eating disorder and reciprocity eating disorder in the caregiver-child relationship). Here food refusal seems to acquire a different value for the child, in the form of apparent indifference and non-investment in food substances. In this context, we can identify the proximity and, in many cases, the intersection between forms of early anorexia and child psychoses where the dimension of withdrawal and closure, of inertia and apparent passivity are predominant. As we will try to explain better later on, when addressing the Lacanian elaborations on early infantile anorexia, the hypothesis we could put forward here is that, in these settings of passive early anorexia, we need to recognize the primary function of refusal as a defence against the dis-being (distress) that life implies. Many of the cases reported by Brusset fall within the frameworks of what he defines as severe anorexia nervosa, where the simple modification of the inadequate position of the caregiver is not sufficient for treatment and where, quite often, one is obliged to resort to pharmacological support and hospitalization of the child. Among these settings, Brusset points to anorexia involving anaclitic depression in infancy and early infantile psychoses (ibid., pp. 54–55), close to autism, of which he gives as an example the case of John, described by Bettelheim in *Truants from Life*.

Childhood anorexia and personality structures: perverse and psychosomatic frameworks

Brusset's clinical perspective leaves open, in any case, in a plurality of forms the question of the relationship between infantile anorexia and personality structure. In the spectrum of structurally severe forms of anorexia, alongside these more frankly psychotic settings, Brusset also indicates the setting of a perverse anorexia nervosa, characterized by a perverse use of the eating symptom in the unrestricted power struggle between the child and the mother, where the structure of the relationship ends up taking on a sado-masochistic form, with the risk of becoming part of the structure of the child's character (ibid., p. 55). Brusset also points out psychosomatic forms of anorexia where the child's activity seems to be reduced and the disorders do not manifest themselves so much on the behavioral level as on the physio-pathological level (ibid.). For Brusset, in any case, whatever the framework of the personality, infantile anorexia nervosa is an issue solidly linked to the difficulties of the mother, in her being, for the child, the Other who is able to welcome and support him in the process of symbolization of the states of the body and of the relationship to the object. In this sense, a treatment of anorexia that does not take into account a treatment of the position of the maternal Other is not possible. It is therefore necessary to take into consideration the specificity of this position and to allow the mother to overcome her anguish in relation to the child and its feeding. This applies to both the so-called simple and the severe forms of anorexia:

"A typical example of the maladjustment of the mother-child relationship, anorexia nervosa in small children is often nothing more than a refusal that will give way as soon as the mother has modified her attitude; but it is sometimes a symptomatic behaviour, the meanings of which are multiple and can only be understood by a dynamic study of the organisation of mother/child transactions".

(Ibid., p. 89)

The Lacanian perspective on infantile anorexia

Lacan and the refusal of the anorexic child as an action: eating nothing

The orientation of Lacan's School, unlike the copious and fertile production on anorexia that begins in adolescence, offers only rare significant theoretical-clinical contributions on infantile anorexia. This is not at all justified on the basis of Lacan's lack of interest in early infantile anorexia or the sole emphasis in his conception of adolescent anorexia which, for some Lacanian authors such as Dewambrechies La Sagna, is synonymous with anorexia nervosa or anorexia vera. However, the key thesis that Lacan formulates in *The Seminar* of 1964, *The Four Fundamental Concepts of Psychoanalysis*, "in anorexia nervosa, what the child eats is nothing" (Lacan, 1973, p. 102), obliges us, at the very least, to question this reading. In this statement of Lacan's, in fact: (a) anorexia nervosa is explicitly referred to the child (and therefore we cannot affirm that it concerns only the clinical setting of the adolescent girl); (b) the anorexic child actualizes the structural operation that, for Lacan, designates anorexia nervosa as such, beyond the moment of its appearance in the framework of development: eating nothing. In the previous chapter, we tried to probe in detail the clinical value of this operation and the particular status of the object nothing in Lacan's teaching and, in the specific case, its function in the clinic of anorexia nervosa. What is worth underlining, in any case, as a significant aspect, is that Lacan reads the essential operation of the anorexic child as an action, their refusal of food as an act, as a subjective decision. What sustains such a radical decision in the child represents the real enigmatic question of infantile anorexia. To think of the child as a subject, as Lacan does, means to think that, although it appears in the field of the Other, it is not completely in the hands of the Other but can, on the contrary, implement an operation that individualizes it. In this sense, Lacan posits weaning in the child more generally as an active operation of the subject in the process of formation and thereby revives the idea of a "desire for weaning" in the child, as he had formulated the previous year in *The Seminar*, Book X, *Anxiety*. Here, in fact, Lacan clearly affirms that weaning is something that the child puts into action and not something that he undergoes Lacan, 2004, pp. 379–380). This allows us to find, in Lacan, a conception of the child as an active subject from infancy, in line with the most advanced experimental discoveries on early childhood (in particular, the non-existence of an original autism as the starting point of development, the heart of the theory supported by

Frances Tustin); discoveries developed, first on the qualitative level, by the Infant Observation (see especially the writings of Ester Bick and Marta Harris (Francesconi, Scotto Di Fasano, 2009)) and, in the last decades, on the level of experimental-quantitative research by the "Infant Research", in particular in Daniel Stern's research on the early mother/child interaction.

In Lacan, the child's anorexia nervosa is also presented in the form of an action and yet, in our opinion and as we shall see, it is not oriented in line with the child's "desire to wean" nor does it simply go in the direction of an effective maneuver of separation from the object of the very first satisfaction.

As we have tried to demonstrate, at the heart of the paradox of the anorexic maneuver, animated on the one hand by a dialectical-separative type of inclination, is the anti-separative nucleus where the object nothing does not function, in the subject in anorexia, as a cause of desire, but rather as a thrust toward inertia and as the jouissance of the One without the Other, as nothing for the Other. This is the fundamental node from which the contribution of the Lacanian orientation can shed another light on the question of infantile anorexia, not only in relation to current international psychiatric nosographies but also in relation to Brusset's masterly reading.

The contribution of Manuel Férnandez Blanco

The unconscious stake of the anorexic subject: digging a hole in the real through his own death

We refer here, in particular, to the contributions of Manuel Férnandez Blanco and François Ansermet, trying to articulate a Lacanian perspective in the clinic of early anorexia. Both argue their theses from clinical experience in hospitals, neonatology, paediatrics and neuropsychiatry: Férnandez Blanco in La Coruña and Ansermet in Lausanne and Geneva.

Férnandez Blanco, in a recent conference entitled "Clinical theory of infantile anorexia", sets out his conception structured around certain fundamental theses, the first of which seems to us to be coherent with the core of Brusset's conception: "In infants and in early childhood, anorexia represents an expression of massive refusal, internal to the maternal-filial relationship" (Férnandez Blanco, 2011, pp. 176–195).

It is in relation to the function of this refusal in the mother/child relationship that Férnandez Blanco introduces, in relation to the framework highlighted by Brusset, the elements characterizing a Lacanian approach to infantile anorexia. First of all, he deduces, from Lacan's references combined with his own clinical experience, a feature characterizing the maternal-filial bond in infantile anorexia:

"If we were to find a common denominator in Lacan's references, we could say that he relates anorexia to a maternal-filial bond of asphyxiating saturation in which the child must take on the separation, the weaning, on its own, although to do so it must reach the point of embodying [itself] the object lost in the real".

(Ibid.)

In other words, we could say, on this point, that the child's anorexia embodies here, in its paradoxical movement, the genesis of refusal in its (attempted) separation function; it has to come close to death, by incarnating it in the reality of the body, in order to be able to separate itself from this flawless Other, which does not leave it its own place. Thus, Férnandez Blanco continues:

"This is the unconscious stake of the anorexic subject: to dig in the Other a hole in the real by their own death since he believed he could not do it with his life".

(Ibid.)

With these premises, the author takes up, from clinical cases treated in hospitals, the classic distinctions of psychiatric nosography on early childhood anorexia. He thus underlines the distinction between early essential anorexias, of the inert and passive type, which begin very early and evolve severely, and oppositional anorexias which develop from the sixth month. He also points out certain more clearly neurotic forms where anorexia manifests itself as a symptom in the classical sense of the term, through which the child questions the desire of the Other toward him.

Saturating maternal asphyxia, deficit of the paternal function

Fernandez Blanco also highlights certain common characteristics in cases of infantile anorexia, where we can find elements that are in continuity with the characteristics of adolescent anorexia: (a) in the mother, a posture of annulment and negation of the child's subjectivity and demands, combined with a focus on her physical needs; (b) a limited presence of the father figure in the maternal desire, which leads to a difficulty of the father in functioning as a mediating third element in the mother/child relationship and therefore leaves the child in an unmediated relationship with the maternal drive. This aspect, linked to a fundamental deficit of the paternal function, constitutes, perhaps, the most characteristic feature of Lacanian-oriented readings of anorexia nervosa, while being little valued, neglected or absent in readings from other orientations.

Massive refusal of the Other and symptomatic refusal: a principle for the differential diagnosis of infantile anorexia

While it is true that these traits seem to bring together the anorexias of early childhood, it is no less essential to distinguish them in their function in the personality structure of the subject. For this very reason, Férnandez Blanco proposes to divide the field of infantile anorexia into two groups, based on the characteristic "refusal position" of the anorexic child. In this respect, he distinguishes between cases where we are dealing with "a massive refusal of the other's request, referring to a psychotic structure" and cases where "the refusal is symptomatic and refers to a neurotic structure". This is, in fact, the classic perspective of the Lacanian structural-differential clinic, amply used by most Lacanian authors who have dealt with adolescent and adult anorexia, in order to clarify the question of diagnosis.

Early childhood anorexia between autistic-psychotic forms and neurosis

According to Férnandez Blanco, the elements on which a diagnosis of psychosis in early childhood anorexia is based are the following:

- We are clearly faced with clinical phenomena that show a difficulty in separating the child, as a differentiated other, from the mother.
- For this reason, according to the author, one cannot speak of symptoms in the strict sense of the term, as in the neurotic forms.
- In these cases, anorexia is a response of refusal, on the part of the child, which takes place in the reality of the body, without mentalization or symbolic mediation.
- Since it is a symbiotic bond of undifferentiation between mother and child, where it is difficult, if not impossible, to establish a symbolic separation, a similar problem occurs when food is introduced as a differentiated object (especially with the switch to the spoon): the child may perceive it as something foreign and this may trigger refusal.
- For these reasons, in a setting of severe early anorexia, it may be one of the first manifestations of autism or childhood psychosis.

As for what happens, on the other hand, in neurotic forms of infantile anorexia, the author points out the following:

- The disorders manifest themselves later when the child has already begun to differentiate and separate from its mother.
- At this time, the child refuses food and opposes the mother's request in order to push the mother's desire beyond basic care.
- In their successive evolution, these patients remain fixed to a mode of relationship with the other of the oppositional type, which maintains a posture of reproach, protest and latent rebellion.
- These are children with difficulties in the mental elaboration of psychic conflicts and who resort to somatization.
- In many cases, anorexia extends to the school register and the children show, at the beginning of schooling, an attitude of inappetence or refusal of knowledge.

The contribution of François Ansermet

François Ansermet's contribution *L'anorexie du nourisson. Oralité et constitution subjective: détresse du nourisson et anorexie precoce* ("Suckling's Anorexia. Orality and subjective constitution: Distress of the infant and early anorexia") (Ansermet, 2008, pp. 37–47), appears to us as an original work in which (a) the author seeks to develop a differential theory of early infantile anorexia, by articulating the classical difference between active and passive early anorexia in the light of clinical experience in neonatology, oriented to psychoanalysis; (b) he expresses important remarks concerning treatment; (c) in the opening of his article, he finally puts forward his hypothesis on the difference between early infantile anorexia and adolescent anorexia which, in our opinion, deserves to be questioned and discussed.

The dialectical-hysterical paradigm of adolescent anorexia and the question of early anorexia

We will start from exactly this third point, which represents a premise to Ansermet's theses: the difference between infant anorexia and adolescent anorexia. He articulates it from an initial presupposition: according to Lacan's classic indication in *The direction of the treatment* (ibid., p. 37), adolescent anorexia would be fundamentally structured around the dimension of desire and the refusal/desire circuit. In our reading (but also in different authors of the Lacanian field such as Ménard, Soria, Recalcati, Fernandez Blanco, Dewambrechies La Sagna ...) this reference appears to be non-exhaustive in the field of adolescent anorexia, since it leads the latter fundamentally back to the framework of hysterical anorexia. We could add that, on the basis of chapter 4 of this work, the reference to Lacan is only limited to a time of his teaching, which is not his last word on anorexia, i.e. to the classical phase, linked to the primacy of the symbolic and desire. According to a recent distinction made by Dewambrechies La Sagna, anorexia based on desire, that is to say on the refusal/desire structure (we would say, on refusal as a function of demand) constitutes the framework of hysterical/neurotic anorexia and revolves around the clinic of the phallus. In this it differs from the "real" anorexia of the girl, where the refusal of food has no metaphorical structure but is a phenomenon "outside discourse, in fact" and is situated within the framework of a clinic of the object. Although we do not share this thesis of anorexia nervosa as an independent structure in itself, we agree with Dewambrechies La Sagna, when she affirms that to attribute adolescent anorexia, as it is most often manifested, to the hysterical structure and the function of desire represents a forcing linked to a classical reading, in Lacanism, that the current clinic of anorexia in adolescence no longer allows us to carry out. Nevertheless, a sector of the clinic of anorexia nervosa in adolescence remains, which is not predominant in my opinion, which is however attributable to the paradigm of hysteria.

Early infantile anorexia as a clinic of the "emergence of the subject"

However, although this premise is debatable, Ansermet's theses on early anorexia are interesting. First, he elaborates a difference between the "dialectic of desire" and the "emergence of the subject", claiming that early infantile anorexia, that of the infant, is not so much about the former (typical of adolescent anorexia) as the latter:

> "In infant anorexia, I think the term anorexia coupled with infant is problematic. We are not yet really in the dialectic of desire: in any case, this does not seem to be the main axis for thinking about what happens in the eating disorder at an early age. This should rather be seen in the coordinates of what is at stake in the emergence of the subject".
>
> (Ibid.)

Early infantile anorexia as a defence against distress

Ansermet questions the basis of the problem of the emergence of the subject which is at the root of what is called, in his opinion in a debatable way, infantile anorexia. He arrives at an original formulation based on the phenomenon of neonatal inappetence:

> "Anorexia at an early age would be a response of the baby against the distress that inhabits him, a first attempt at subjective establishment, of construction of a defence in relation to a primordial jouissance, and to the en-trop of the living".
>
> (Ibid.)

Ansermet thus introduces an important definition: early infantile anorexia as a primordial defence against a jouissance (also primordial) in excess. In this sense, primordial inappetence, the original refusal to eat, eventually takes the form of defence rather than that of the demand inherent in desire.

A question arises in this regard. Is it not possible to recognize, in several cases of anorexia that begin in adolescence, the re-emergence of this very nodal point: the refusal to feed as an extreme defence against an invading power, which testifies to the structural impasse of the subject, as Soria has emphasized, in the constitution of the object (a) as lost and, consequently, in the construction of a phantasm and in the phallicization of the sexed body? This would imply a complexification of the clinic of anorexia in adolescence, from the point of view of structural variations close to psychosis, both in its classical manifestations and in the forms of ordinary psychosis.

Active and passive early anorexia

The most significant aspects that characterize Ansermet's conception of active anorexia praecox are the following:

- Active anorexia is food refusal. The child says no, or manifests it, turning their head away, refusing the breast, pushing the spoon away. This is a very frequent symptom;
- In active refusal, desire is at stake.
- It is therefore a form that is similar to classic anorexia.
- It is a clinic where a subject manifests themselves, in their vitality, through an opposition.
- It is a symptom in the proper sense of the term, linked to the place of the child in relation to the desire of the mother, of the father, to the conditions of its coming into the world.
- It is often a manifestation related to the child as a symptom of the parental couple.
- In this form, it is a very frequent symptom, with sleep disorders and oppositional behavior.
- In this clinic, we rely on the refusal to open a way out, between the father and the mother, but also between the woman and the mother (ibid., pp. 37–38).

In this conception of early active anorexia, Ansermet performs two operations: first, he reconstructs, through the reading of refusal in the young child as a function of desire, a line of continuity between early active anorexia and the anorexia of the adolescent as animated by the dialectic of desire. On this point, therefore, the discontinuity classically underlined between early anorexia and adolescent anorexia finds a crucial exception and objection in the structure of the active refusal/desire function that ties together its forms of anorexic manifestation in the course of development. Second, it converges active anorexia praecox, read in the light of the refusal/desire structure, as Lacan thought of it for anorexia nervosa in 1958 (paradigmatically attributable to hysterical anorexia) with Irene Chatoor's descriptive diagnostic framework of infantile anorexia, with its characteristic of oppositional vitality and whose onset is from the sixth month.

Let us see, on the other hand, what Ansermet's framework of passive precocious anorexia consists of (ibid., pp. 38–40)[2]:

- It is an anorexia where the child shows no appetite.
- They do not show anything in the exchange.
- They do not institute the oral object, they do not do anything to take this object from the other, to make it their own. More exactly, they have not subtracted the oral object that the drive could resolve around, to go and look for it, to aim at another object that takes its place, for example food (ibid., p. 38).

- The clinic of precarious passive anorexias gives the feeling that the functions of need, in order to be put in place, should be supported by an appetite which should already be there (ibid., p. 40).

In passive anorexia, something enigmatic occurs, like a melancholic process from the start (a kind of early melancholy: a shadow that falls on the subject from the start without a problem of loss) (ibid.).

The enigma of passive precocious anorexia: two open questions

Ansermet also offers for reflection to further, unresolved problems about the status of passive anorexia praecox, which, according to him, turns out to be a clinically enigmatic issue in itself.

First of all, the problem Ansermet raises is whether, in this passive anorexia praecox, one should read the absence of a point of emergence of the subject as a kind of continuum without any discontinuity, or whether one should not recognize, already in this very early and non-oppositive form of anorexia, a primordial manifestation of a refusal, of a defence against distress (ibid., pp. 41–42).

Is early passive anorexia, therefore, an absence of cutting or a defence against primordial distress? As Ansermet himself says, unlike what the passage of weaning implies for the child, "in the case of passive anorexia, there has been no cut. [...] Unless anorexia is a defence, a defence against distress".

The second problem that Ansermet poses concerns, on the other hand, the relationship between passive early anorexia and autism. Should we not recognize this as a very serious form of autism?

One could also ask whether massive early anorexia in infants is not ultimately a very serious form of autism (ibid., p. 43).

Ansermet defends the plausibility of this thesis in these terms:

"This is what is at stake in autism: no babbling, no primary processing of jouissance, no S1. The autistic person is the one who has not been able to complete the path of the drive and who has not been able to treat the jouissance in excess. The same may be true of passive precocious anorexia. In any case, there is no hallucination of satisfaction, no representation of desire, no Wunschforstellung [...], no more representation of desire than anticipation of the desire of the Other; no anticipation of pleasure, either".

(Ibid., p. 44)

Concluding remarks on the anorexia of early childhood

While it is true that Lacan taught us, in *The Seminar*, Book XI, guiding us along this path, that the child, in anorexia nervosa, eats nothing, the digressions made in this chapter on early infantile anorexia have shown us that there are at least two different ways of eating nothing. These two modalities correspond to active early anorexia, otherwise known as oppositional or weaning anorexia – which manifests itself from the sixth month and before the third year – and passive early anorexia, also known as inertia anorexia, which appears, on the other hand, between birth and the first six months of the infant's life. This classic distinction, in child psychiatry studies, is however taken up again and radically reformulated, as far as its concept is concerned, in Lacan's perspective. It allows us, in fact, a structural distinction between the two forms, starting from the function of the object nothing in relation to the field of the Other and its fundamental signifiers.

In the case of passive anorexia praecox, the mathema formulated by Miller S0 + nothing could give us the specificity of the problem: the subject function reduced to a minimum; when the child is One with the primordial jouissance of the living; the absence of a minimal point of attachment to the field of the Other, necessary for the exercise of the vital and primordial function of the satisfaction of the need to feed. In this context, it is obvious that the anorexic refusal is not inscribed in the register of the demand on the Other (the refusal as a metaphor of the demand), nor in the register of the attempt to separate from the Other (the refusal as an attempt at separation); and this is because the Other has not been installed as such for the subject who is alone, too, in the larval state of S0 and is one with the nothing as an embodiment of the real of *Das Ding*. This refusal of food represents here only the function of pure jouissance of the *Thing* and, possibly, also, as Ansermet mentioned, a primordial defence against distress.

In the case of active early anorexia, the general formula could be written in the form of S1 + nothing, according to which the subject in anorexia still has a point of attachment to the Other and is in relation to it (albeit in an oppositional and conflictual way); it is thus possible to contain the causative action of the object nothing in its most devastating effects. I believe that the thesis that the frames of active early anorexia should all necessarily fall within the framework of hysterical-neurotic structures should be discussed. I think that the forms of infantile hysterical anorexia undoubtedly fall within the framework of oppositional anorexia, but this can also include, within it, non-neurotic forms characterized by a link with the Other, albeit precarious and imaginary. One could put forward the hypothesis that the forms closest to autism could be reconciled with the passive early anorexias and that the spectrum of oppositional anorexias could be broadened to include not only neurotic forms but also, in various cases, forms of infantile psychosis (Férnandez Blanco, 2011, cit.)[3]. In the perspective of psychoanalysis, this seems essential to us, first of all as a question of method: not to reduce, in a too marked a way, the structural question of the subject in anorexia to the phenomenology of his behavior.

In any case, the framework of active early anorexia, which, according to current international psychiatric classifications, corresponds precisely to the diagnosis of infantile anorexia, includes the operational function of refusal as a separative maneuver and, in the hysterical-neurotic forms, undoubtedly brings into play the metaphorical function of refusal as a demand that goes beyond the plane of need, in order to go to call out to the parental Other at the level of its desire for the subject.

Notes

1 This paragraph has been added as an update in this English edition of the book.
2 Marie's case, a severe precocious anorexia from birth, is in the middle of this article by Ansermet.
3 See, in this respect, the case of Laura, an anorexia of the second semester, with oppositional behavior, but not at all reducible to a neurotic framework of functioning, in Férnandez Blanco, 2011, cit.

References

APA (1996). Diagnostic and Statistical Manual of Mental Disorders. Fourth Edition. Prymary Care Version. Washington DC: American Psychiatric Publisher.

American Psychiatric Association (APA) (1998), *DSM-IV. Manuale diagnostico e statistico dei disturbi mentali.* Milano Parigi Barcellona: Masson; (1994), *DSM-IV. Diagnostic and Statistical Manual of Mental Disorders.* Wasinghton DC: American Psychiatric Association.

American Psychiatric Association (APA) (2022), *Diagnostic and Statistical Manual of Mental Disorders. Fifth Edition. Text Revision. DSM-5-TR.* Wasinghton DC: American Psychiatric Association Publishing.

Ansermet, F. (1999). *Clinique de l'origine: l'enfant entre médecine et psychanalyse.* Laussanne: Payot.

Ansermet, F. (2008), L'anorexie du nourrisson. Oralité et constitution subjective: détresse du nourrisson et anorexie précoce, *Cahiers de la clinique psychanalytique,* vol. 13, pp. 37–47.

Bettelheim B. (1955), Truants for Life: the Rehabilitation of Emotionally Disturbed Children. Glencoe, IL: The Free Press.

Brusset, B. (1977), *L'assiette et le miroir: l'anorexie mentale de l'infant et de l'adolescent.* Paris: Privat.

Brusset B. (1998), Psychopathologie de l'anorexie mentale. Paris: Dunot

Chatoor I., Ganiban J., Surles J., Doussard-Roosvelt J. (2004), Physiological regulation and infantile anorexia: a pilot study, American Academy of Child & Adolescent Psychiatry, 43 (8), pp. 1019-1025.

Férnandez Blanco, M. (2011), Teoria e clinica dell'anoressia infantile, *La Psicoanalisi,* no. 50, luglio-dicembre, Roma: Astrolabio, pp. 176–195.

Francesconi, M., Scotto Di Fasano, D. (dir.) (2009), *Apprendere dal bambino. Riflessioni a partire dall'Infant Observation.* Roma: Borla.

Kreisler, L., Fain, M., M. Soulé, M., (1974), *L'enfant et son corps. Étude sur la Clinique psychosomatique du premier âge.* Paris: Presses universitaires de France.

Lacan, J. (2004), *Le Séminaire,* Livre X, *L'angoisse,* 1962–1963. Paris: Le Seuil.

Lacan, J. (1973), *Le Séminaire,* Livre XI, *Les quatre concepts fondamentaux de la psychanalyse,* 1964. Paris: Le Seuil.

Lacan J, The Seminar. Book XXI, Les non dupes errent, 1973-1974, 9th of April 1974, unpublished.

Lingiardi, V., McWilliams, N., Speranza, A. M. (2020) Introduzione, Lingiardi, V., McWilliams, N., Speranza, A. M. (a cura di) (2020), *Manuale Diagnostico Psicodinamico. PDM-2 0/18. Infanzia e Adolescenza*. Milano: Cortina, pp. 1–8.

Maestro, S, Muratori, F. (2018), Introduzione all'edizione italiana, Zero to Three, *DC: 0-5 TM. Classificazione Diagnostica della salute Mentale e dei Disturbi di Sviluppo nell'Infanzia*. Roma: Fioriti, pp. XI–XIV.

Malberg, N., Rosemberg, L. (2020), Profilo del funzionamento mentale nell'infanzia – Asse MC, Lingiardi, V., McWilliams, N., Speranza, A. M. (a cura di), *Manuale Diagnostico Psicodinamico. PDM-2 0/18 infanzia e adolescenza*. Cit., pp. 145–197.

PDM Task Force (2008), *PDM. Manuale Diagnostico Psicodinamico*. Milano: Cortina; *Psychodynamic Diagnostic Manual* (2006). Alliance od Psychoanalytic Organisations.

Shedler J., Westen D. (2007), The Shedler-Westen assesment Procedure (SWAP): Making personality diagnosis clinically meaningful, Journal of Personality Assessment, 89 pp. 41-55

Speranza, A. M., Williams, R. (2009), Fare diagnosi nell'infanzia e nell'adolescenza, Dazzi, N., Lingiardi, V., Gazzillo, F. (2009), *La diagnosi in psicologia clinica: personalità e psicopatologia*. Milano: Cortina.

Speranza, A. M. (2009), Disturbi dell'alimentazione da 0 a 3 anni, Piccolo, F., Speranza, A. M., Cuzzolaro, M. (2009), *Disturbi dell'alimentazione e del peso corporeo da 0 a 14 anni*. Bologna: Carocci.

Speranza, A. M., Mayes, L. (2020), Classificazione della salute mentale e dei disturbi dello sviluppo nella prima infanzia – Asse IEC 0-3, Lingiardi, V., McWilliams, N., Speranza, A. M. (a cura di), *Manuale Diagnostico Psicodinamico. PDM-2 0/18 infanzia e adolescenza*. Cit., pp. 11–87.

Speranza, A. M. (2020), L continuità omotipica ed eterotipica nella psicopatologia dello sviluppo, Lingiardi, V., McWilliams, N., Speranza, A. M. (a cura di) (2020), *Manuale Diagnostico Psicodinamico. PDM-2 0/18. Infanzia e Adolescenza*, pp. 337–364.

Speranza, M. (2020), Pattern sintomatologici in adolescenza: l'esperienza soggettiva – Asse SA», Lingiardi, V., McWilliams, N., Speranza, A. M. (a cura di) (2020), *Manuale Diagnostico Psicodinamico. PDM-2 0/18. Infanzia e Adolescenza*, pp. 271–331.

Widlöcher, D. (1977), Préface, B. Brusset (1977), *L'assiette et le miroir. L'anorexie mentale de l'enfant et de l'adolescent*, p. 10.

Zero To Three (2005), Diagnostic Classification of Mental Healt and Developmental Disorders of Infancy and Early Childhood (Revised). Arlington, VA: Zero To Three/National Center for CLinical Infant Programs.

Zero to Three (2018), *DC: 0-5TM. Classificazione Diagnostica della Salute Mentale e dei Disturbi di Sviluppo nell'Infanzia*. Roma: Fioriti; (2016) (*CD: 0-5 TM. Diagnostic Classification of Mental Health and Developmental Disorders of Infancy and Early Childhood*. United States: Zero to Three).

Chapter 9

Anorexia nervosa in adolescence

From child anorexia to young girl anorexia nervosa

We have seen that three fundamental factors unite, despite the obvious differences, childhood anorexia and anorexia of the young girl: the refusal of food, the deregulated maternal-filial relationship and the passion for nothing. The first two aspects have already been highlighted by the tradition of contemporary psychodynamic psychiatry; the third is represented by Lacan's most original contribution to the anorexic question. In our digressions on early anorexia, we wanted to identify two possible declinations of the child's relationship with nothingness: in passive early anorexia, which can appear from birth and concerns, in any case, the very first months of life, nothingness occupies the very place of the subject, becomes one with them and interposes itself as an obstacle in their relationship to the living as such. Here nothingness is what holds the infant back in its jouissance of the One; it is the anchoring to Das Ding, the refusal to put itself into play as an enjoying substance (*substance jouissante*) in the world of life. It is the refusal of the *Lebenswelt*, as the phenomenological psychiatrists would say. It is the radical refusal of the se-partition of which Lacan speaks, of the original loss of that piece of the body – represented by the placenta for the infant, by the amniotic fluid and the umbilical cord – which allows the entry into the world and the emergence of the subject. Refusal of lalangue, from its very first whispers, from the first echoes of the voice.

In active early anorexia, of opposition or weaning, which can manifest itself from the sixth month onwards (a condition which determines the recognition of the diagnostic framework of infantile anorexia by official psychiatry), the child actively poses the nothing between the Other and themselves, in the attempt to be able to act on the Other, without being acted upon by it: to wrest from the Other a quota of jouissance without losing anything is a structurally impossible operation in which the anorexic remains trapped. It is the refusal of the Other as the Other of language, as the Other of signifying alienation, as the Other that provokes, for the child, the loss of the breast as a piece of its own body that merges with the mother's body.

DOI: 10.4324/9781003318439-10

Infantile anorexia of opposition is the refusal of the signifying cut on the subject's body.

The first is thus a response of the subject to the trauma of coming into the world, to the trauma of birth. It is a refusal to come into the world. The second is a response to the trauma of weaning.

The passage from infantile anorexia to anorexia of the young girl, a condition where the diagnosis of anorexia nervosa proper is recognized, is essential, at this point of our work, not only to reconstruct the characteristics of the syndrome that we have spoken about at length in the previous chapters, but above all to try to answer certain fundamental questions. First, why does anorexia nervosa occur mainly in adolescence? Second, why do the vast majority of cases involve young girls? Third, how does the object nothing act in this context, and toward what is the anorexic refusal in adolescence oriented? In this chapter, we will try to answer these three questions.

The bifurcation of the subject facing the denouement of puberty: the path of the symptom or the path of refusal

In the *Three Essays on the Theory of Sexuality*, a work in which he offers us his theorization of the psycho-sexual development of the human subject, Freud poses the question about which we are asking ourselves in the chapter on the "vicissitudes of puberty". The question of adolescence is thus conceived, by the father of psychoanalysis, from the drive denouement of puberty: from the problem of the relationship to one's own body in transformation and from the libidinal-drive restructuring that runs through the radical biological changes that the young person experiences. In this process, during which we witness the development of secondary sexual characteristics, the growth of the body in proportions that will remain the same in adulthood, the change in the voice and the massive investment of the genitals on the part of the libido, the adolescent subject is radically challenged and questioned on the issue of choice and decision. There is probably nothing like the passage to puberty to highlight the impact of the transformations of the body on the subject but also, at the same time, the irreducibility of the subject to these very transformations. That is to say, to paraphrase Lacan's famous thesis, in this passage the young person discovers both having a body and not being their body, not coinciding with their own body. They also discover that they have a body which, contrary to what they might have imagined at the beginning, is not subject to their control, since events occur in it that do not depend on their will. This does not only concern the biological transformations that take the young person by surprise: the appearance of the cycle in the girl and the first ejaculations in the boy. It also concerns what happens during sleep during dream activity, in the formation of the unconscious through the dream which begins to be populated with scenes where the relationship of the young person with sex and death, and the encounter with the sexual partner, come into play. Lacan would attribute a fundamental importance, in the process of sexual initiation in the adolescent, to this dreamlike appearance which raises the sexual relationship to the status of an unconscious question. This means that, in the sexual experience of the young person, both the drive awakening that crosses their body and the unconscious construction of the scene that organizes and orientates this awakening in a singular way are essential. The young person will therefore be called upon to confront this drive awakening that imposes itself on them, in the intimacy of their body, and the enigma concerning the cause of this drive awakening, that is to say what functions for them as the cause of their desire.

The psychoanalytical clinic of adolescence teaches us, however, that this passage of the adolescent toward a recognition, toward an assumption and a subjectivation of what moves him or her in desire, we have said, is problematic and often does not lead him or her toward an assumption of his or her own impulse choice but, rather, toward its refusal. In the process of subjectivation, it is a crucial passage, and never without difficulties, to accept or refuse the transformations of the sexed body, acted upon by the sexual impulse and by the push toward the partner, both in the auto-erotic-masturbatory ideation and in the search for the sexual encounter. One could say, however, that the adolescent is, at this point, at a crossroad where they are called upon to choose between two possible directions: the path of the symptom, as psychoanalysis understands it, in the strict sense of the term, and the path of radical refusal, as a rejection or rupture of the subject's own relationship with sex.

The path of the symptom, classically conceived, is the neurotic path to the sexual life of the formation of the compromise, where the subject, while keeping a fundamental ambivalence with regard to sexual desire, agrees to enter the game of love life and to inscribe their drive in the field of the Other, in search of a partner. This is the paradigmatic case of hysteria where the subject, although implementing a refusal of sexual satisfaction and of her own body as the locus of the drive, does so paradoxically through appeal and seduction, constructing a form of jouissance that feeds on dissatisfaction. This is a typical oscillation of hysteria, which shows us, in a direct manner, the subjective division that runs through it in its relationship to what causes its desire.

The path of radical refusal, on the other hand, is a treatment of the pubertal passage that does not pass through the gateway of sexuation, that does not lead the young person to assume his or her sex, that takes the path of the rejection of symbolic castration and the non-access to phallic jouissance. This path leads us to the field of psychotic foreclosure or, more precisely, to the "rupture of the marriage with the phallus". A formula that Lacan used to define, in this regard, the position of the drug addict in relation to jouissance, but which we could also use to define, provisionally, the position of many anorexic girls, in their way of facing the question of puberty. It is true, as the young Lacan wrote, that in anorexia the presence of "phallic fantasies" is a constant and yet, as Férnandez Blanco pointed out, "the anorexic does not make the phallic fantasy the symptomatic feature of her jouissance" (Férnandez Blanco, 2010, unpublished).

The young person who completes a treatment of the passage of puberty through the symptomatic path specifies their position as that of a divided subject, subject to the laws of the unconscious and of symbolic castration; they agree to pay the price of an enjoyment in loss (such as is permitted by phallic 'jouissance), in order to be able to enter the dialectic of love life and to assume a sexual position, even if ambivalent, in the sexual relationship with the partner.

On the contrary, following the path of radical refusal as a way of treating the passage of puberty involves anchoring the young person to a position of undivided subject and to a modality of full and autistic jouissance, without a dialectic with the Other and an alternative to sexual jouissance.

Adolescence as a symptom of puberty

Stevens has summarized the essential question at stake in adolescence in the perspective of Freud and Lacan: adolescence is the symptom of puberty (Stevens, 1998, pp. 79–92). This is to say that, in a subject, the essential function of adolescence corresponds to the process of symptomatization of the pubertal passage. This symptomatization serves to construct, for both boys and girls, the singular mode of each to face, frame, find a context, put into perspective, signify and appropriate the drive that moves them. In this sense, adolescence is a work of symbolization around the most radical knot that directs the subject's desire: the object that causes it. In this perspective, we can perhaps read the definition of puberty as a logical time, which Lacan presents to us in The Seminar, Book X, *Anxiety*, a logical time that would be "a function of a link to be established of the maturation of the object a" (Lacan, 2004, p. 300).

We can put forward the hypothesis that adolescence functions as this logical time necessary to produce this "link to be established of the maturation of the object a" which is precisely the object cause of desire. The drive awakening of puberty radically brings into play for the young person the object a, the lost object that causes their desire; it is now necessary to reposition its function for the subject within a new link with the drive, with respect to childhood. In this sense, adolescence turns out to be a logical time when there is something that returns from childhood, something that is repeated. This is what Freud highlighted most: adolescence as a time when the child's oedipal question is reactivated in the terms in which it was elaborated in childhood and left behind by the mechanism of repression, in the latency phase. At the same time, adolescence is also a logical time when something new has to happen for the subject to effectively go through it. It is therefore not only a question of repetition of the past, of inheritance from childhood, but also of invention in the present, capable of opening up the subject's perspective in the future.

It is only in this perspective that defining adolescence as a logical time of separation can be justified. It is only justified on condition that the subject's relationship with their infantile heritage, and in particular with the object a, is repositioned in a new and sustainable framework for them in adult life. If, in fact, childhood can be seen as a time of alienation where the child is, generally, in the position of an object in the hands of the Other, adolescence is the time when they will be able, as a subject, to relate both to the field of the Other and to the object that causes their desire. In this passage, the ethical dimension, at stake in adolescence, takes shape: it is the possibility of recognizing and assuming the desire that inhabits the subject and of acting in accordance with it.

This passage requires a triple effect of transformation of the subject around the three registers that, for Lacan, constitute its experience. First of all, at the level of the real of the drive, it is necessary to resituate the function of the object a, an effect of the se-partition where the child loses a piece of themselves (by birth at the beginning and by weaning thereafter), through their cession to the field of the Other and their localization in the body of the Other sex. This is the effect of the drive restructuring that occurs through sexuation where the very partner is put by the subject in the position of object a, that is the object that causes their desire.

Second, at the symbolic level, the adolescent is in search of a new language and a personal way of naming themselves in their being within the social bond; in this process, they are in search of an Other who is able to recognize them in their exceptionality and to say yes to their original invention that is not already written in the code. This Other always functions, in adolescence, in the way described in The Seminar, Book V around the function of the father, as the one who gives in the third stage of Oedipus. This is exactly the key function of the Ego Ideal that Freud had already defined in *The Decline of the Oedipal Complex* and that he had already developed, in '*On the Psychology of the High School Student*' (Freud, 1984, pp. 227–231), around the function of the master, a substitute figure for the father in adolescence.

At the imaginary level, it is a matter of reconfiguring the adolescent's relationship to their body image and to their own identity, in the light of the work and effects of drive restructuring and symbolic re-naming of their very being. Around the fact of being male or female and the desire for a particular path rather than another, a reinvention of his or her image will occur for the subject, which will never be fully consistent with the real of his or her being.

The logical time, necessary for the adolescent subject to go through this transformative journey from the drive reemergence during puberty to the time of separation from their position in childhood, is a time crossed by a problematic trajectory where the adolescent experiences the crisis: the identity that was formed in childhood is no longer able, in an obvious way, to respond to the desire that now runs through them. It is in this "delicate transition", as Lacadée defines it (Lacadée, 2001, pp. 87–107; Lacadée, 2004), between puberty and the achievement of separation, that we must situate the time of crisis in adolescence. A crisis that classically implies the opening up of all the fundamental questions of existence: am I male or female, alive or dead, does existence have a meaning or is it meaningless?

The process of sexual initiation of the adolescent and its logical times

It is important for us to go into the details of what is at stake for the adolescent in the process of symptomatization of their puberty. This is essential in order to try, later on, to read the anorexic solution in relation to the question of adolescence and to question the status of contemporary adolescence and its relationship to anorexia in the young girl.

As we have recently tried to show, it is Lacan who offers us the keys to enter the question of the treatment of the passage from puberty to adolescence. Lacan does this through the door of the sexual initiation of the adolescent.

In his "Preface" to Wedekind's *Spring Awakening*, he indicates, according to what we thought possible to isolate in the text, two logical times around which the initiation of the adolescent subject is structured. The first logical time is given by the dream representation of the sexual relationship of the adolescent subject with a partner. Lacan, in fact, writes that "boys would not even imagine what it would be like for them to make love to girls [...] without the awakening of their dreams" (Lacan, 2001, p. 561).

This is the time when, for the adolescent, sex becomes an enigma about what it means to make love between a boy and a girl. This passage is essential since it raises sex to the level of the unconscious, making possible, in the imaginary form, a phantasmatic or phantasmatizable representation of one's relationship to sex. This is the logical *time of the veil*, as we have defined it (Cosenza, 2009, pp. 46–50; 2014, pp. 24–30), which makes the sexual relationship exist for the adolescent subject. Second, Lacan clarifies the concept of the real knot that this initiatory experience reveals to the adolescent, defining it as the true principle of initiation, "the veil lifted [on the mystery of sexuality] shows nothing" (Lacan, 2001, p. 562), which is another way of saying that sexuality makes a hole in the real (ibid.).

The second logical time is given to us by this encounter, in adolescence, of what makes a hole in the real and which Lacan defines as the true principle of initiation: behind the veil covering the mystery of sexuality, there is nothing.

If, in the first logical time, the adolescent structures sex as an enigma in the locus of the Other, thus allowing the existence of the sexual relationship, in the second logical time, which we could call the *time of trauma*, the adolescent encounters, in his or her first sexual experiences, the non-existence of the Other, the irreducible heterogeneity of the partners' enjoyments. They discover, in short, that the sexual relationship does not exist. In the first stage, it is the unconscious as the locus of the Other that structures the adolescent's relationship to sex; in the second stage, it is the unconscious as real that is at the center of their experience.

This second stage, where the adolescent discovers in sexual experience that histheir jouissance is irreducible and unrelated to the jouissance of the other, the time of "there is no sexual relation", is structurally related to the first stage where, on the contrary, the sexual relation exists and is representable for the subject, since it functions as an unconscious veil around the hole of non-relation. It is in this dialectical tension between the push to make sexual intercourse exist (T1) and the traumatic encounter with its non-existence (T2), between the time of the veil and the time of the trauma, that the process of sexual initiation of the adolescent is structured.

The third time (T3) of the process of sexual initiation, the time that sanctions, for the subject, the exit from adolescence, is represented by the assumption and subjectivization of the symbolic castration that establishes that "there is no sexual intercourse" and therefore by the decision to enter under these conditions, without losing one's own singular construction around sex, into the game of love life. We could call this *time of decision* the third time, when the adolescent's relationship to sex is caught in the oscillation between the unconscious phantasmatization that they produce and the recognition of symbolic castration.

Elements for a differential clinic of the symptom in adolescence

In this sense, adolescence as unconscious work of phantasmatization on the drive is, like the transference in analysis, a process of essential construction of something that is destined to reveal its unconsciousness – the subject supposed to know attributed to the analyst, the phantasmatic veil on the non-sexual relationship for the adolescent. Yet, without this construction, there could not be, in analysis as in the formative experience of the adolescent, any effective change that is supportable and symbolizable for the subject. The theme of initiation historically refers us to this type of transformation: to become adults by crossing the enigma of the relationship to sex which implies, in the experience with the partner, the encounter with eros as well as with thanatos. Clinical experience with adolescents clearly shows us, moreover, that the passage to T2, to the time of the trauma of the non-existence of sexual intercourse, proves to be difficult to sustain and subjectivize if the adolescent has not been able to pass through T1 beforehand, that is to say, through the time of the veil as the logical time of construction of a subjective phantasmatization of sexual intercourse. Without this preliminary work, the encounter with symbolic castration appears to the subject as an abyss, as a ruinous and unbearable passage, to which the adolescent tends to respond by withdrawing or acting out.

Now, our clinical hypothesis is that it is possible to outline the framework of a differential clinic in adolescence, following these indications given by Lacan, by distinguishing:

• cases where the subject finds their own fundamental impasse in the T2 of the encounter and the crossing of the trauma of the non-sexual relationship, while having been able, nevertheless, to elaborate their own phantasmatic construction in T1;

- cases where the phantasmatic construction in T1 is already deficient or absent, which makes the young person's passage to the T2 of the encounter with castration untenable and often ruinous.

In the first typology of cases, we can recognize the frameworks of a clinic of the construction of the neurotic symptom in adolescence. In the second typology of cases, the territory of the clinic of adolescence beyond neurosis opens up to us, where the young person is not able to construct a symptom in the Freudian sense of the term, since, for them, the process of symptomatization of puberty has proved impractical. They may, then, eventually find another kind of adjustment to their precarious condition, which may be closer to a solution or, in the best of cases, closer to a symptom, without taking the form of the symptom considered neurotic.

Anorexia as a failure of the symptomatization of puberty

As far as anorexia nervosa in adolescence is concerned, our fundamental thesis is, first of all, that it is configured, with the exception of the hysterical-neurotic forms of anorexia, as a failure of the process of puberty symptomatization. Anorexia, therefore, as a result of the failure of adolescence itself in its essential developmental task: to bring the subject to make their encounter with the drive in puberty a singular construction, more precisely a symptom. It is thus a formation of compromise between the law of the Other and the subject's desire, between symbolic castration and the drive. Perhaps Lacan was alluding to this passage in The Seminar, Book X, when he associated with puberty the link to be established in order to make the "maturation of the object a" effective. In the neurotic symptom, in fact, it is not so much a question of mediating between the urges of the law and those of desire, since the latter shows us, by its very structure, that, as Lacan affirms, "there is no desire without law". Or, as Jacques-Alain Miller pointed out in Silet, for Lacan "castration is the shoehorn of the object a".

This is quite the opposite of what happens in anorexia nervosa where an absolute superegoic law – without desire, or a pure and absolute desire, independent of the Other, which ends up being transformed into an absolute will to self-domination and a death drive – tends to dominate.

In the case of Luciana, one of my anorexic patients, welcomed into the therapeutic community, life was about having to or, above all, not having to depend in any way on the Other. In her case, this thesis, which accompanied her anorexia from the beginning, when she was a young girl, was pushed to the extreme, to the point of leading her to oppose for a whole year the slightest contact between the community workers and her parents, under the threat of leaving the community if they were contacted or met. Her problem was the demand that she herself be the only one responsible for her illness, the only one to bear the burden and the blame, without involving anyone else, especially her family. This position did not take an explicitly persecutory form with her; rather, she said that she did not want to give her parents any worries because she saw them as fragile and in difficulty. So she did not want to be an extra burden for them.

In her case, the ethical principle of subjective responsibility was perverted and became a paroxysmal and superegoic way of covering up a push for absolute control of the treatment and the refusal of any involvement of the Other in it.

In this sense, anorexia generally presents itself as a solution where the essential aspects of the classical symptom, for example hysterica (Férnandez Blanco, 2011), are missing.

I limit myself here to indicating three of them: the *metaphorical function* of the symptom in anorexias – except for hysterical-neurotic anorexias – appears to be absent or deactivated: the unconscious function of the symptom, as a message addressed to the Other embodied in the body by the illness, does not appear as such, as happens, on the contrary, with the somatizations of the hysteric.

There is no *enigmatic dimension* to the symptom that provokes in the neurotic, beyond the demand to be cured, the demand to know the meaning of what happens to them.

The *egodystonic effect* that the classic symptom always brings about, by hurting and dividing the subject (the counterpart of the underlying phantasmatic) egosyntonia, does not appear in anorexia, especially in the early stages, the time of the honeymoon with anorexia, which, in certain aspects, is analogous to that experienced by the drug addict with drugs.

For all these reasons, we cannot define anorexia as a symptom in the classical sense of the term, and this is also true for drug addiction.

The impasse of contemporary adolescence: loss of veil on sex and decline of the father

It is essential, in our opinion, to define the framework of contemporary adolescence, in order to better understand the anorexic issue in adolescence and the impasse that especially girls encounter in the process of symptomatization of puberty. This is first of all because – as we pointed out in the first chapter – in the last 50 years, anorexia in girls has been transformed from a rare phenomenon to a significant epidemiological phenomenon. It is therefore crucial for us to understand whether, in this historical period, the fundamental role that psychoanalysis has recognized in adolescence, for the development of the subject, has undergone transformations and encountered impasses in its process of realization in the concrete experience of contemporary young people.

Our hypothesis is that in the contemporary era, characterized by a decline in the symbolic function and by the rise of the objet petit a to the social zenith (as Lacan indicated to us in *Radiophonie*) (Lacan, 2001, p. 414), the response to the passage from puberty to adolescence no longer takes, for many young people, the classic form of crisis. Contemporary adolescence seems to be, in fact, as many specialists of adolescence think, both in the sociological and psychological field, like an indefinite time that seems to have lost its function of cut, of discontinuity between the past and the present, between childhood and adulthood.

There is a whole psychological and psychiatric literature, produced by the Anglo-American area, in the last 20 years, which aims to discuss, with the help of empirical-epidemiological research, the crucial valence of the crisis of adolescence and of the generational conflict between young people and their parents and, more generally, the world of adults; at the same time, the aim is to reconcile the so-called adolescent crisis with the Romantic myth of the *Sturm und Drang* (Offer, Shonert-Reichl, 1992, pp. 1003–1013). From this line of research emerges an image of the contemporary adolescent as a subject not at all in crisis but, on the contrary, relatively serene and adapted to the social and family context of reference. From our point of view, the greater apparent conformism of contemporary adolescents opens up another kind of reading: disagreement has not disappeared but its dialectical manifestation, its transformation into conflict, has reached an impasse. This phenomenon does not seem strange to us in an era where the Other does not exist and where it is increasingly difficult for the adolescent to find an Other against whom to fight and who accepts to be the recipient of his or her demand for change while keeping his or her position. If the young person in disagreement has difficulty in finding the dialectical path of conflict to be able to express themselves, they then seek, by other, non-dialectical ways, a modality to deal with the intensity and urgency of their situation. In any case and from our perspective, contemporary adolescence encounters specific impasses and solutions that are also specific and that transform its processes in relation to the classical form.

And this is not only in the obvious sense of the difficulty of the contemporary adolescent in getting out of adolescence, for economic and social reasons that are at the origin of the noted phenomenon of prolonged adolescence. Today, we are convinced that the entry into adolescence, as a symptom of the passage through puberty, also represents a problem.

Second, the contemporary adolescent's relationship with sex cannot fail to be affected, in its functioning, by the loss of the veil around the enigma of sexuality. Lacan underlines this by pointing out the public dimension, typical of today's world, of the "lifting of the veil" around the question of puberty. The effect of this operation, which is one and the same to the decline of the paternal function, is found – as the sociologist Lipovetsky (Lipovetsky, 2006) underlined and Cottet (Cottet, 2006, pp. 67–75) reaffirmed – in the "disenchantment of sex", in the "trivialization of sexual intercourse", in the "indifference" and "apathy" in love present in most contemporary adolescents. This difficulty of sex to represent an enigma for many contemporary adolescents testifies to an impasse in the process of symptomatization of puberty, seen by psychoanalysis as a fundamental issue in the experience of adolescence.

We can, in fact, see in it, first of all, a difficulty of the contemporary adolescent in situating themselves in the T1 of sexual initiation, that is to say, in the subject's encounter with sex as an unconscious enigma that can be represented on an "other sscene" (eine andere Schauplatz). The first level of difficulty of the contemporary adolescent is precisely to make the sexual relationship exist, to make an Other of the Other exist, in a world characterized by an essential closure, a refusal, of the unconscious. This condition does not allow sex to acquire an enigmatic value for the subject. It is thus a transformation, the social elimination of the veil around the enigma of sex, which is one and the same, in the contemporary world, with the decline of the father and the loss of value of the symbolic Other. In fact, the decline of the father at the beginning, rather than as the final result of the process, makes it even more difficult for the young person to constitute an Ego Ideal, for which they have to displace the father with another adult, given that the person who embodies the Ego Ideal is, for the young person, an object of admiration and at the same time an enigma. This is what happens, in a classic way, in Wedekind's play *Spring Awakening*: the figure of the Masked Man embodies, for the adolescent, the enigma of the desire for a man with whom he can be in a relationship of identification which, by virtue of the enigma, makes it necessary for him to carry out a subjective work of phantasmatization and interpretation.

The unveiling of sex, which is done from the outset, today, for the adolescent, makes the passage to T1, to the time of the veil as a time of agalmatic phantasmatization around sexual intercourse, even more problematic and, in some cases, unbearable. The experience of sexual initiation immediately becomes less agalmatic, less fantasized and less the effect of a singular unconscious construction.

But, this absence of structuring of sex as an unconscious representation is detrimental to the modality of the adolescent's encounter with the T2, the time of initiation as an encounter with the trauma of the non-existence of an Other of the Other. Indeed, as Miller points out, there is no subjectifiable trauma without a veil and an ideal (Miller, 2005, p. 40). In a condition such as the present, where the non-existence of the sexual relationship and the absence of the Other as a guarantee represent the starting point, spread throughout society as a shared truth typical of present-day nihilism, how can the adolescent find a way back to their own subjective initiation?

The refusal of the drive body

The clinic of anorexic beginnings is a clinic of the sudden and unassimilable irruption of jouissance. This can take the form of a sudden trauma following the loss of someone, the betrayal of a friend, the encounter with sexual jouissance, the unassimilable word or silence of a parent, the unsatisfied judgment of a teacher; but also, more banally, an accident, a body that falls and collides with something, an injury or the emulation of an admired other. All of this can function as a conjuncture that triggers the anorexic response.

The fact that the beginnings of anorexia are mainly verified shortly before the passage of puberty indicates to us, however, the particular importance, in the young girl, of the relationship between the pulsionalization of the female body and the anorexic response. Even when the triggering conjuncture occurs following an episode that seems to have nothing to do, directly, with the sexual question, for example a fall from a horse, the anorexic response shows us, afterward, in the subject, a fundamental non-acceptance of the state of her own body as a feminine drive body. This non-acceptance finds, in the conjuncture of the triggering of the anorexia, an occasion on which to lean and deploy its refusal of the female body.

This consideration already allows us to sketch a first definition of anorexia nervosa in adolescence, which clearly distinguishes it from the forms of infantile anorexia. If early passive anorexia is the infant's refusal to enter the world, if oppositional anorexia is a refusal of weaning, often charged with ambivalence on the part of the child, anorexia nervosa is, first and foremost, a refusal of the drive body and, in particular, a refusal of the young girl to possess a feminine body, a female body.

The clinic of anorexia nervosa in adolescence is therefore a clinic of refusal of the sexed body, a refusal of the drive body. It is essential, however, to manage to articulate a differential framework within this clinic, taking into account the logical times that structure the process of symptomatization of puberty in adolescence, in order to understand what form of adolescent anorexia we are dealing with.

And this is all the more so because, as we know, psychoanalysis originates, basically, from the question of the refusal of the female drive body, brought into play by the hysteric, which Freud testified to as early as his first Studies on Hysteria. Refusal of the body in hysteria, to which Lacan would return on several occasions, and in which Miller has emphasized a double status: as a refusal of the sexed body (of the woman) and as a refusal of the reproductive body (of the mother) (Miller, 2000, pp. 40–41). Hysteria often expresses, moreover, the refusal of the body *sub specie anorexiae* through the semblances of the anorexic symptom. For this reason, it is essential for us to distinguish the modalities of the refusal of the body in the anorexia of the young girl, in order not to confuse its status and its function in the differentia differential clinic of the anorexia of the young girl.

Differential clinic of the girl's anorexia

The refusal of the body in hysteria

If the clinic of hysteria configures, as Lacan affirms in The Seminar, Book XVII, a clinic of the "refusal of the body", it is thus essential to see how this refusal manifests itself and what it aims at, what moves it. In the hysterical woman, the refusal of the body appears, first of all, as a refusal of the sexual body as a body subjected to the domination of the Other. It is thus an insubordinate body that resists mastery on the part of the Other, that does not allow itself to be reduced to the object position of the jouissance of the Other but subtracts itself from it as an object of full satisfaction. Yet, in hysteria, this refusal of the sexual body presents a stake that aims at the heart of the Other: it aims at arousing the desire of the Other, at stimu-lating the lack in the Other. In this logic, the refusal of the sexual body in the hysteric is in no way an adialectical, autistic operation but, on the contrary, it is an operation oriented to have an incidence in the field of the Other. In the perspective of the hysterical woman, the refusal of the body, the path of the deprivation of jouissance and the anchoring to dis-satisfaction, becomes the modality from which to try to call into question the lack of the Other and to be the cause of the Other's desire. The lesser jouissance that the hysterical woman unconsciously imposes on herself, in the bodily symptoms she produces and in her way of being in her bond of love, is translated in her experience by the demand for more desire in her way of being the cause of desire. The refusal of the sexual body in hysteria is thus an operation fundamentally inscribed in the dialectic with the Other: it is not a refusal of the Other as such but, rather, a refusal-in-function-of-desire. This is the hysterical's way of trying to be unique for the Other. In this sense, it is fully inscribed in the logic of the phallus, in phallic signification and in the modality of jouissance – phallic jouissance $J\varphi$ – that revolves around the phallic function, where jouissance is structurally cut off from the signifier and regulated by the law of castration, which presides over the link between the two sexes. "To be the phallus for the Other" is the goal that the hysteric aims at through her refusal of the sexual body as a maneuver to cause the desire of the Other.

If we take into consideration the logical times of the process of sexual initiation in adolescence, as we have drawn them from Lacan, we are con-fronted, in the case of the hysterical girl, by a subject who constructs in T1 a phantasmatic veil around sex; this very veil orients her position and desire in the encounter with the partner. The problems of the hysterical girl occur, eventually, in the passage to T2, the encounter with the trauma of symbolic castration which, in a particular conjuncture, shows the structural impasse of the phantasmatic position ("being the phallus") in which the subject had situated herself in relation to the desire of the Other. The problem in which the hysterical woman struggles, in this conjuncture, is that of how to assume the structural fact that the phallic universal with which she has identified herself (which is the Lacanian way of translating into logic the virile identi-fication of Freud's hysterical woman) does not recognize her position as woman. In fact, for Freud as for Lacan, for the woman there is no signifier in the unconscious; this is why Lacan affirms that the Woman does not exist, whereas the Man exists as a universal and that the phallic signifier alone regulates, in the discourse, the relationship between man and woman.

On the side of the symptom, hysteria is a non-assumption of this structural datum that obscures the feminine specificity, linked to the uniqueness of each woman. For her, in the perspective of the Seminar, book XX, *Encore*, what is worth it is (no longer only) the Oedipal logic of the exception and of the universal law, proper to phallic jouissance, but (in the specific), the logic beyond the Oedipus of seriation, proper to female jouissance.

The refusal of the body in hysterical anorexia

The clinic of hysterical anorexia is an internal version of the clinic of hysteria as such. The same structural elements, also at play in the hysteria of the young girl, are valid here: the effectiveness of the paternal metaphor in childhood and the inscription of the subject in the phallic logic, the construction of the phantasmatic veil around the enigma of sex, the refusal of the sexual body united to its phallicization in the function of cause of desire, the use of the veil as a semblance in the game of feminine masquerade.

Hysterical anorexia as a response to the trauma of castration

Our fundamental thesis implies that, in the girl's hysterical anorexia, the encounter with the T2 of the trauma of castration produces a symbolically unsubjectifiable effect in the conjuncture of her advent; the girl then responds with action, by refusing food and structuring the anorexic symptom. What vacillates, precisely, in this conjuncture, is the ideal that the girl embodies as a unique being for the Other: this ideal comes to be lacking by the effect of the emergence of the real that makes the subject topple from the imaginary place that she thought she occupied for the Other.

In the case of Clementina, for example, the conjuncture of the triggering of the anorexic symptom coincided with what she experienced as the "betrayal" of her best friend with whom she had shared, in the first years of puberty, the exploration of the male world and the seduction of boys. As she was very attractive and seductive, she had created a close solidarity with the friend: they went out every night together, always with boys who alternated, in occasional relationships, with each other. What remained stable was the relationship between the two girls, their complicity which never took the direction of an acted homosexuality. When they went out in the evening, "they went hunting for boys" and in this they found satisfaction in seducing and conquering them. Clementina had constructed a way of relating to the object of love that consisted in identifying with it while keeping her distance: she had done this with the father, whose determined character she had taken on and whom she resembled physically but whom she loved from afar, refusing, for example, to follow his career in the bank, as he would have liked, in order to devote herself to the theater instead. She loved him without serving him, which is typical in hysteria. She seems to have structured a similar solution with her best friend in her pre-adolescence: to be unique for her and to give herself to men without loving them. The conjuncture for the triggering of the anorexic symptom occurred when Clementina, after returning from the summer holidays, learnt from her sister that the friend had left for England for a year, without telling her anything. From then on, she began to refuse food, to close herself off, to lose weight visibly until the beginning of our meetings.

A clinic of the phallicization of thinness

In hysterical anorexia, the thinness of the body acquires a phallic value, the thin body metaphorizes, for the subject, the phallus as signifier of the object of lack of the Other. For many hysterics, anorexia functions as a kind of phallic reserve to which they have access in critical passages, after the encounter with the trauma of castration, which presents itself in their love life by the exacerbation of the passage from thinness to symptomatic severity. It is not, therefore, in any way a manifestation of an exit from the phallic logic but, on the contrary, an attempt to remain in it by other means and by the reduction to the bone of the hysterical equation body = phallus. The equation that hysterical anorexia brings into play does not replace the hysterical equation but rather represents a differential distribution of its internal value. According to this distribution, which conforms, among other things, to the system of bodily values of contemporary society (Cosenza, 1998, pp. 129–179), below a threshold that does not exceed the extreme limits of undernutrition, the new equation is "lean body = phallus". For hysterical anorexia, in fact, the equation becomes "very thin body = phallus", according to which the decrease in body weight would increase its phallic value, i.e. its desirability.

In Teodora's case, the sudden anorexia at the age of 18 condensed, at the same time, a response to a critical conjuncture where she had been radically disappointed in her father's love, and the phallic recovery linked to the libidinization of the thin body as a signifier of desire toward the woman on the part of the father. Teodora's life followed the thread of love for the father, which for her, however, would take the form of a love from a distance, made up of missed expectations and appointments, of broken promises. When she was about ten years old, the father, who was in constant conflict with his wife, decided to leave home and go to live abroad. He moved his industrial business there, gradually going bankrupt and reducing his assets to a minimum. With his only daughter, he had an epistolary relationship and occasional but passionate meetings, during which he hinted to Teodora at the possibility of going to live with him. In the meantime, Teodora's mother had become involved with an important, widowed entrepreneur who already had a daughter. She eventually decided to marry him and, after the divorce was granted, to move into his large house with Teodora. There, Teodora found herself with a stepfather and a stepsister and, despite her and her stepfather's best efforts, she ended up feeling second-class.

As time went by, she increasingly developed the fantasy of going to live with her beloved father, trusting in the half-promises he had made to her on the occasion of their sporadic meetings. What would precipitate the traumatic event, however, was the gradual realization of the father's new relationship with a foreign woman and his decision to move in with his new partner and daughter. This precipitated Teodora's identification with the "family out-cast", both on the father's and the mother's side. The encounter with the father's partner and daughter took the aggressive form of rivalry, and in the face of the hostility of his new partner toward Teodora, the father was forced to abandon the promise he had made to his daughter about their life together and to reduce the number of encounters with her, which became increasingly fleeting and clandestine.

Teodora's anorexia was a sudden, acute response to the failure of her life plan with the father. It would also lead to her being hospitalized in specialized clinics for the treatment of anorexia. The symptom would, however, become a lifeline for her. She structured it on the basis of a paternal signifier central to the choice of love object: thin women represented the common denominator of the father's wives, the element that could not be missing for him to desire them. This was how it had worked for Teodora's mother, and it also worked for the father's new, younger companion.

This produced a double effect on Teodora. On the one hand, the emergence of her condition would function, for the father, as a summons to her. This was the function of refusal as a call, as a metaphor for the demand for love, which had been amply demonstrated: I eat less until I starve myself, in order to be more the cause of your desire, the key to your love. On the other hand, this would direct the choice of object toward a partner obsessed by thinness in women.

Knowledge (savoir) as an enigma in hysterical anorexia

A key point in hysterical anorexia lies in the subject's relationship to knowledge. This is an aspect of capital importance, since it is surely one of the most nodal points that allow a separation between hysterical anorexia and anorexia nervosa in the strict sense of the term. If it is true, indeed, that the development of the anorexic symptom, especially in the honeymoon phase with anorexia, also has the effect of closing the unconscious and freezing the signifying chain in the symptomatic response, it is also true that at the heart of the subject's relation to knowledge, there is the enigma. In hysterical anorexia, the passion for anorexia and the enigma cohabit, coexist, for a certain period of the subject's life, even if the enigma is structural for the hysterical subject, whereas anorexia is an acted response by the subject to their question that circumvents the enigma. All the resources of the treatment of hysterical anorexia are concentrated, first of all, in work of detachment, in the subject, between the passion for the enigma and the passion for the anorexic answer. This operation is far from simple insofar as, when the symptom settles down and offers the subject its secondary benefits, it produces as an effect, also in the hysterical subject, a tendency to close the enigma, at least temporarily. To play, in the subject, hysteria against anorexia means, in fact, in these cases of hysterical anorexia, to oppose the hysterical passion for the knowledge that divides the subject to the anorexic passion for the frozen and empty knowledge. This also means positioning the enigma in the place of the interval between the signifiers S1-S2, where anorexia would tend, on the contrary, to eliminate this interval holophrastically, to purge the enigma from the field of knowledge, to put, at the heart of knowledge, an absolute certainty outside the signifier, a petrification of the jouissance represented by nothing.

The refusal of the body in anorexia nervosa

A clinic of the rupture of the veil

In the anorexic forms of adolescence that cannot be reconciled with the hysterical-neurotic frameworks, we observe, to varying degrees, a failure of the subject's entry into adolescence, already in the T1 of the construction of the phantasmatic veil around the sexual relationship. In other words, we see the radical impasse of the sexual initiation of the adolescent, which will prevent an effective assumption of their sexual position and a subjective inscription within the phallic logic. This has the effect of a fundamental nonstructuring of the symbolic equation body = phallus and a substantial deprivation of the enigmatic value of sexual and love life.

The issue becomes particularly significant for the girl, insofar as the function of the veil assumes a central value in the construction of the female position within the phallic dialectic between the sexes. The function of the veil is, in fact, the pivotal point that allows the girl, lacking the phallus in her body as a visible organ, to enter as a protagonist into the feminine masquerade, giving the male partner a glimpse of her own phallic value as a woman, in order to cause his desire. In the dialectic between the sexes, this can push the male, through the virile parade, to want to give the girl what she does not have and the girl will be led to want to be for him what he lacks.

The construction of the phallic veil, produced by the subject's signifying work around the body, is a key operation that finds, from the time of puberty, the most important moment of consolidation and completion. This is one of the fundamental reasons why, in our opinion, anorexia nervosa is above all a female pathology, because it suffers more radically from the devastating effects of the disappearance of the veil around the enigma of sexuality in the contemporary world. The veil, in fact, functions as a kind of symbolic organ in the woman's body and as the product of a singular construction work of each woman. This symbolic organ is essential for love life. Its absence is devastating for the subject because it prevents a signifying treatment of the Other and a mediation with the desire of the Other in the relationship between the sexes.

In the clinic of non-hysterical anorexia nervosa, we observe, in fact, a structural lesion of the function of the veil; even in the most serious cases, a true psychosis, a total absence of the veil.

This condition does not allow the girl to enter the game as a protagonist and to assume her gendered position as a woman, in the dialectic of love life. This does not necessarily mean that the anorexic girl will not be able to have a sexual life or be in a couple. But, even where the subject keeps open a space for sexual life or life in a couple, this space will appear as devoid of phallic value, absent of agalma and will not be the expression of a singular phantasmatic construction. The relationship of the anorexic girl with her partner will rather be characterized, fundamentally, by a narcissistic-specular demand for support. This demand is always supported by a mimetic need for inclusion that makes the girl feel more in line with the parameters of social life of young people of her age.

In Alessia's case, in the account of her early sexual life as a girl struck us as having felt only annoyance, and not even a little attraction, for the boy of her first experience: she just had the conviction that she had to do it because girls her age did it. Faced, then, with the first advance she received, she consented to have her first sexual encounter. No construction, no expectations or curiosity, no exploratory demands, no satisfaction around the event of the first sexual intercourse: only the certainty of a duty to assume as a girl like the others. In place of the veil of castration, we have here the deployment of a superegoical order that must be obeyed in order to be a young woman. As we have already seen in this case, Alessia's anorexic beginnings coincided with the girl's response to the father's call to occupy the place of the unexpectedly dead mother.

The lack of veiling of the driving body in Alessia would become evident on the occasion of her psychotic decompensation when, unexpectedly, while she was kneeling down to put the clothes in order in the shop window where she was working, she met the gaze of a group of boys on her behind. She remained locked in her room for a whole month, not going to work or university, terrorized by this encounter with someone's gaze. The therapy with me continued by phone, before we could meet again.

The phenomenology of sexual and love life in anorexia nervosa is presented as devoid of desire; where it still exists, if not abruptly interrupted by the onset of the illness, it is characterized by an anaclitic and supportive aspect. The partner is often the one who cares for the subject, takes care of his or her needs and often colludes with the illness. The partner does not antagonize the anorexic symptom, but rather often finds his or her place exactly within the girl's anorexia nervosa symptomatic system. In this way, it reinforces the symptomatic omnipotence instead of introducing a symbolic limit capable of chipping away at it.

Failure of the equation body = phallus

We thus witness, if not a rejection, at least a rupture of the equation body = phallus in the girl's anorexia nervosa. In certain respects, this is something reminiscent of the rupture of the marriage with the phallus that Lacan talks about when he tries to define the jouissance of the drug addict. Indeed, a good definition of anorexia nervosa is that it consists of a refusal or rupture of the marriage to the phallus.

Indeed, the failure of the equation body = phallus, in neurotic anorexias, is more easily made clear if we take into account the subject's marriage to the image of her own body as a 'marriage without veil'. It is a devastating, persecutory and unmediated encounter with the mirror, precisely because the subject has been deprived of the measure of the phallic veiling of the body. This measure is introduced into the subject's experience by the desire of the Other, through the sign of love that the Other gives in the regime of lack and symbolic castration. In the girl at puberty, this sign has the power to double its effect of bodily unification that the child has experienced, in the mirror stage, thanks to the word of the Other, usually the mother, who orients the child's identification with her body image. This repetition, however, is not a simple repetition, since it introduces sexual difference into the girl's identification with her body: it is the identification with the female body that the girl will obtain through the passage to the stage of the veil. We could say that the mirror stage allows the child to pass from the experience of a fragmented body to the experience of a unified body, while the stage of the veil, at the beginning of puberty, allows the transformation of a unified body into a sexually oriented body, able to enter into the dialectic of the love life between the sexes:

Structuring of the body in the subject's neurotic development
| Stage of the mirror | Fragmented body | Unified body |
| Stage of the veil | Unified body | Sexed body |

In hysterical anorexia, the subject structures these passages in her development, but she encounters a difficulty in fully supporting herself, in her sexual position, at the critical moment of the encounter with the trauma of castration. In this way the girl can support herself, as a woman, only in the position of refusal that anorexia allows her and which produces this metaphor:

Anorexia

Woman's body

The clinic of non-neurotic anorexia nervosa is a clinic in which the failure of the process of "corporization" of the signifier, a process that Miller defined in *Biologie lacanienne et événements de corps* (Lacanian Biology and Events of the Body) (Miller, 2000, pp. 57–59), is noted. This process libidinizes the subject's body by organizing it symbolically and orienting it at the level of the drive. It is essential to distinguish between cases of psychosis, where the structural failure that is already visible in childhood is revealed at puberty although contained by the anorexic solution, and cases of anorexia, where the process of signifying corporization takes root in the subject's body, both at the passage of the mirror stage in childhood and at the stage of the veil at puberty.

	Psychosis	Neurosis
Mirror stage	Fragmented body	Divided body
Veil stage	Anorexic solution	Anorexic symptom

In the psychotic type of anorexic solution, the passage of puberty reopens the structural conditions of the splitting up of the subject's body by the revelation, after the fact, of the failure of the mirror stage. In these cases, anorexia nervosa is the subject's response to the re-recognition of the structural fragmentation that inscribes in the girl's body the rigid phallic armor in place of the phallic veiling that has proved impossible.

An outsized jouissance: perverting the "not-all" in the limitless anorexic

The lack of access to phallic jouissance condemns the anorexic girl to a disproportionate jouissance, without limits, which is directed at her body and devastates it. The fact that this happens in anorexia nervosa much more in girls than in boys is also justified on the basis of an element that is specific to women in their relationship to jouissance. This is a differential factor which, as we have already emphasized, is at the basis, today, of many female pathologies of excess, declined in particular from deprivation (Francesconi, 2007; Eldar, 2009). In this context, we can undoubtedly include, alongside anorexia nervosa in women, the clinic of female depression.

In The Seminar, Book XX, Lacan emphasized that women, unlike men, have the possibility of direct access to a jouissance that is not reducible to phallic jouissance, which he calls Other jouissance, and which is characterized by the fact that it is situated beyond Oedipus and castration. It is a non-meaningful and supplementary jouissance that puts the woman in direct relation with an absolute otherness (Lacan, 1975, pp. 92–93). This is why Lacan pointed out its proximity to the mystical experience where the subject's relationship to God is without any mediation.

Authors such as Geneviève Morel have underlined the destructive weight of feminine jouissance in the new symptoms, particularly in serious cases of anorexia-bulimia with a hysterical structure, where the subject is divided in the experience of jouissance (Morel, 1997, pp. 33–36; 1999, pp. 15–20) and disturbed by the devastation of the relationship with the mother (Brusa, 2004). But the question remains open about the forms of anorexia and bulimia beyond the framework of hysteria and the neurotic symptom, in particular in the perspective of Lacan's last teaching (Eidelberg and others, 2003, p. 13).

In fact, we have to ask ourselves what happens to this "other" dimension of jouissance in the woman's body when its inscription in phallic jouissance fails or when the girl's marriage with the phallus breaks down. In other words, what about the typically feminine experience of the "not-all", when a woman refuses or breaks the marriage with the phallus?

According to our hypothesis, it is precisely in this domain, united to the theme of the lesion of the veil that we have addressed, that psychoanalysis could perhaps provide a specific answer to the question: why does anorexia manifest itself above all in young girls and, more generally, in women? Our reading of the problem specifies that a radical distortion of the relation to additional jouissance occurs for the woman, where the marriage with the phallus is weak, refused or broken.

In this distortion, the not-at-all of female jouissance is transformed into the limitlessness of anorexic jouissance, while limitless jouissance stagnates and devastates the girl's body. The body itself becomes a fetish object, suppressed by the subject itself through incessant superegoic practices of hyper-control and deprivation, or even, quite often, lesion, cut, devastation (Dewambrechies La Sagna, 2006, p. 68). In these practices, the hyper-control turns out to be only a superegoic delusion of anorexia, which is directed, on the contrary, by a structural loss of control, by a radical excess that makes it run without brakes toward death.

Our hypothesis is therefore that:

- anorexia nervosa manifests itself above all in young girls because it is in feminine jouissance that the limitless finds a structural place;
- where the girl refuses or breaks the marriage with the phallus, the phallic "not-all" side of feminine jouissance acquires the aberrant and malignant physiognomy, in the body of the anorexic, of a jouissance of unlimited deprivation;
- this unlimited jouissance is practiced, in a perverse way, by the anorexic on her own body, which is assumed as a fetish of adoration and devastation.

The clinical and paradigmatic exemplification of the limitless anorexic is represented by all the cases of anorexia nervosa where, without the limit introduced by the caring Other and, often, by the compulsory hospitalization, the announced marriage of the anorexic with death would have been realized. Indeed, we could say that the anorexic girl refuses or breaks the marriage with the phallus to become, without wanting to, a bride of death. Death does not function here as a symbolic limit but, on the contrary, is a limitless real. In anorexia nervosa, the subject does not normally have suicidal intentions, they do not seek death, toward which they are indifferent, although they often end up finding it. It is their passion for nothing that causes their enjoyment, that annihilates desire and blinds them to the point of dying for it.

The object nothing in childhood anorexia and in young girl's anorexia

It is important to distinguish the function that the object nothing plays in the girl's anorexia from the role it plays in early infantile anorexia. One enlightening way of doing this consists in relating infantile anorexia, in its different forms, to the equation that psychoanalysis considers essential in the child's relationship to the maternal function, i.e. child = phallus. Similarly, we will try to relate the anorexia nervosa of the girl to the equation body = phallus, which psychoanalysis considers essential in the sexual structuring of the subject and, in particular, of the woman, within the dialectic of love life. On the basis of this differential correlation, we will try to show what specific function the object nothing covers in the different cases.

First of all, we can affirm that, in infantile anorexia, the function of nothing must be thought of in relation to the failure or deregulation of the equation child = phallus. It concerns, therefore, the child's relationship with the desire of the primordial Other, which, for him, is the Desire-of-the-Mother. On this subject, the clinic of early anorexia identifies at least three fundamental variants.

The first is represented by the early anorexia of the infant, where we witness – as in many cases of infantile autism – the failure from the start, the abortion of the phallicization of the child. Mother's desire is not there waiting, as vital lymph, when the child comes into the world, but appears as a dead desire. Precocious passive anorexia is thus a primordial refusal of life, a primary devitalization that keeps the child below history, in an original jouissance without loss, which leaves no place for the Other. The nothingness occupies the place, left empty, of the phallus and radically marks the child's destiny, their refusal of an existence inserted in time and in history, in a form that could be written by a paradoxical equation:

$$Child = nothing$$

In active precocious anorexia, we find, on the other hand, two other structures in which the object nothing plays a different role. The infantile anorexia of opposition or weaning presents, in fact, two structural variants, irreducible to each other. In both cases, the equation child = phallus and the infant's encounter with the Mother's desire take place. However, there is a first class of cases where the Mother's desire phallicizes the child, without passing through the symbolic castration. It is, therefore, an adialectical phallicization of the child, which produces the child as the real object of the mother's jouissance, thus contravening the structural principle of phallic logic, the principle of castration. Here the mother phagocytizes the child, as in the metaphor of the crocodile's mouth, used by Lacan in The Seminar, Book XVII (Lacan, 1991, p. 129): she makes the child an exclusive object of her jouissance as a mother, without giving it the status of a gift of love to be offered, as a woman, to the male partner, the child's father. In these cases where the paternal metaphor fails, where the Name-of-the-Father does not intervene to regulate the Desire-of-the-Mother, the child finds themselves to be, in the real, the phallus of the mother, the object of a desperate two-way link where the madness of their jouissance condenses. In these cases, inherent to the field of psychosis, the development of the child's anorexia nervosa introduces a somatic limit (in the absence of the symbolic limit) between the child and the madness of the maternal Other; it is a defense against this Other who wants to enjoy them without limit. The object nothing is situated, here, between the child as subject and the mad desire of the mother, as a primordial defense of the anorexic child against the possibility of being a real and exclusive object of maternal jouissance:

Child/nothing/maternal jouissance

Oppositional infantile anorexia also presents a third form where the paternal metaphor manages to be inscribed in the child, albeit weakly, and where, as a result, the equation child = phallus takes on a transmissible form in the phallic logic, organized by symbolic castration. In this way, the child includes the father within the writing of this equation and can thus encounter something of the maternal castration and the desire for woman in the mother. In these cases, we are dealing with a neurotic child, who develops an early anorexic symptom. We are talking here about a symptom in a strictly analytical sense since the child, in these cases of infantile anorexia, functions as a symptom of the parental couple, of the link between the father and the mother, and not only as a factor of contention of the maternal jouissance. We are therefore in the framework of an oedipal logic where the child develops a symptom, stops eating, in order to transmit something unheard-of to his parents. Whereas, in psychotic infantile anorexia, the child's anorexia functions as a brake on the deregulated jouissance of the maternal Other, in neurotic infantile anorexia, the anorexic symptom acts on the desire of the parental Other (Lacan, 2001, pp. 373–374): it questions it, provokes it, causes it anguish, but with the aim of operating a subjective rectification in them.

More precisely, in the anorexia of the neurotic child, the anorexic symptom aims at dissipating, in the parents, the confusion, of which they are not aware, between taking care of the child and giving him love. In other words, it aims at repositioning the family bond on the vital axis of the primacy of desire, mortified by the sensible reasons of need and by the invasion of jouissance. In this context, the child's anorexic nothingness aims at the heart of the parental Other's desire, but in a radical form where, in the most serious cases, it is trapped in the absolute position of pure desire, for which the principle of "either desire or death" is valid. This is why the anorexic child, in order to awaken his parents' desire for him, is willing to play with his own death and to make what Lacan calls in The Seminar, Book XI, the threat of disappearance, act through a hunger strike. For him it is better to die than to live without the desire of the Other. This is the radical side of his fundamental action: eating nothing.

Child/nothing/desire of the parental Other.

How does the object nothing act, on the other hand, in the girl's anorexia nervosa? As we have said, in the anorexic girl, its functions revolve around the vicissitudes of the symbolic equation body = phallus.

Only in hysterical-neurotic anorexia does this equation show itself in its effective structuring and operativity, thus allowing the girl to access the phallic dialectic between the sexes and to sustain the female masquerade for the male partner. The anorexic symptom is established, at puberty, in a critical conjuncture where a contingent experience reactivates, in the subject, the encounter with the trauma of castration and makes the subject fall from the imaginary position where he was, in relation to the desire of the Other. The holding of the equation body = phallus requires at this point, for the girl, the introduction of an additional element of phallicization, represented precisely by anorexia, to be able to continue to function for her. The production of the anorexic symptom transforms, in these cases, a condition of weakness into a test of strength; it accentuates the phallicization of the body in the sense of thinness and acts as a factor that pushes the desire of the Other, whether it be the partner or the parents, to awaken and make room for the subject.

Young girl/skinny body = phallus/desire of the Other

In these cases, the function of nothing has a double aspect. On the one hand, it functions as a signifier; it is thus inscribed within the phallic logic and coordinates with the dialectic of desire and its structurally metonymic movement. Nothing becomes, in this framework, that signifier which declares the impossibility of defining which object causes the subject's desire. In this sense, and particularly in hysteria, nothing condenses in itself an enigmatic and allusive value and coincides, to some extent, with the locus of the enigma.

And yet, at the same time, in the hysterical anorexia of the girl, especially in the honeymoon phase with anorexia, we also find the real and adialectic dimension of nothing, as a point of condensation of a jouissance unrelated to the signifier, foreign to the phallic logic, symbolically intractable. In the clinic of hysterical anorexia, these two aspects of nothing coexist together and, in the most acute moments of the symptom, the jouissance of nothing produces the effect of obscuring the function of nothing as an enigmatic signifier, to the point of occluding the interval between the signifiers S1-S2. The direction of the treatment will strategically go toward highlighting the difference between the enigmatic dimension and the dimension of pure jouissance, which the nothing condenses here, and also toward the contradiction that inhabits the subject in relation to his or her own symptom, which will put the mechanism of the signifying chain back into operation. In other words, it will be a question of highlighting, in the discourse of the young girl, the hysterical passion for nothing as an enigma, her position as a divided subject, in order to make her work against the anorexic passion for nothing as a full jouissance that refuses the signifier.

Hysterical anorexia
it is characterized for the 2 aspects of the nothing: as
enigma and as jouissance

Nothing = enigma   *Nothing = jouissance*

In the non-neurotic forms of the girl's anorexia, as we have seen, the equation body = phallus is not structured, the formation of the phallic veil over the body does not take place or is interrupted during its course; the object (a) is not extracted from the body and fails to constitute a fundamental fantasy. For the girl, the appearance of anorexia thus becomes a way of digging a gap between herself and the Other, since everything that comes from the Other to her takes the form, for her, of a persecuting and devastating jouissance. It is the nothing that represents, for the girl, this impassable gap between self and Other, between what causes the full jouissance of anorexia and her rejection of desire.

Young girl/nothing//jouissance of the Other

The anorexic nothing here aims to extirpate desire at the very root of the drive, to transform the girl's body into a body without desire, asexual, inhabited only by the death drive. In this very movement, we witness, in the most critical moments, the transformation of the anorexic nothingness: from a defense operator against the invading jouissance of the Other, it becomes a causative factor that pushes the young girl to the limitless jouissance of anorexia, to the race toward death, to an aberrant perversization of female jouissance.

Anorexia nervosa
it participates of the 2 dimension of the nothing: defence against
the jouissance and cause of jouissance

Nothing = defense against the   Nothing = cause of jouissance
jouissance of the Other   without limit

Here we see a kind of paradox emerging around the operativity of the object nothing in the girl's anorexia nervosa: nothing functions in the anorexic refusal both as an extreme defense against the invading jouissance of the Other and as the cause of an unbounded jouissance that ravages the girl's body, bringing her close to death. Defense and devastation together.

References

Brusa, L. (2004), *Mi vedevo riflessa nel suo specchio: psicoanalisi del rapporto tra madre e figlia.* Milano: Franco Angeli.

Cosenza, D. (1998), Il cibo e l'inconscio: anoressia, bulimia e discorso alimentare, Recalcati, M. (Dir.), *Il corpo ostaggio: clinica psicoanalitica dell'anoressia-bulimia.* Roma: Borla, pp. 129–179.

Cosenza, D. (2009), « L'initiation à l'adolescence: entre mythe et structure », *Mental,* no. 23, pp. 46–50, octobre; (2014) « Initiation in Adolescence: between Myth and Structure », *Lacunae. Lacanian Journal of Psychoanalysis,* v. 4 (Issue 1), pp. 24–30.

Cosenza, D. (2014). Le refus dans l'anorexie. Rennes: Presses Universitaires de Rennes.

Cottet, S. (2006), « Le sexe faible des ados: sexe-machine et mythologie du cœur », *La Cause freudienne,* no. 64, pp. 67–75, octobre.

Dewambrechies La Sagna, C. (2006), L'anorexie vraie de la jeune fille, *La Cause freudienne,* no.63, pp. 57–70, juin.

Eidelberg, A. and others (2003), *Anorexia y bulimia: síntomas actuales de lo femenino.* Buenos Aires: Del Bucle.

Eldar, S. (Dir.) (2009), *Mujeres, una por una.* Madrid: Gredos.

Férnandez Blanco, M. (2010), Trastornos del comportamiento alimentario en la adolescencia", Giornata di Studi "I disturbi alimentari in adolescenza, Istituto Freudiano, Roma, 20 febbraio, unpublished.

Férnandez Blanco, M. (2011), Teoria e clinica dell'anoressia infantile, *La Psicoanalisi,* no. 50, luglio-dicembre, pp. 176–195.

Francesconi, P. (Dir.) (2007), *Una per una. Psicoanalisi e femminilità.* Roma: Borla.

Freud, S. (1984), *Sur la psychologie du licéen* (1914). *Resultats, idées, problèmes.* Paris: PUF, pp. 227–231.

Lacadée, P. (2001), « L'adolescence, une délicate transition », *Mental*, no. 9, pp. 87–107.

Lacadée, P. (2004), *L'éveil et l'exil: enseignements psychanalytiques de la plus délicate des transitions, l'adolescence*. Nantes: Cécile Defaut.

Lacan, J. (2001), *Note sur l'enfant* (1969). *Autres écrits*. Paris: Le Seuil, pp. 373–374.

Lacan, J. (2001), Préface à *L'éveil du printemps* (1974), *Autres écrits*. cit., pp. 561–563.

Lacan, J. (2001), Radiophonie (1970). *Autres écrits*, cit., pp. 403–447.

Lacan, J. (1991), *Le Séminaire. Livre XVII. L'envers de la psychanalyse*, 1969–1970. Paris: Le Seuil.

Lacan, J. (2004), *Le Séminaire. Livre X. L'angoisse*, 1962–1963. Paris: Éditions du Seuil.

Lacan, J. (1975), Le Séminaire. Livre XX. Encore, 1972–1973. Paris.

Lipovetsky, G. (2006), *Le bonheur paradoxal: essai sur la societé d'hyperconsommation*. Paris: Folio.

Miller, J.-A. (2000), « Biologie lacanienne et évéenement de corps ». *La Cause freudienne*, no. 44, pp. 7–59, février.

Miller, J.-A. (Dir.) (2005), *Effets thérapeutiques rapides en psychanalyse*. Paris: Navarin.

Morel, G. (1997), « Des symptômes et des femmes: boulimie et féminité », *La lettre mensuelle*, no. 16, pp. 33–36, septembre.

Morel, G. (1999), « Féminité contre identité », *Feuillets psychanalytiques du Courtil*, no. 17, pp. 15–21, mars.

Offer, D., Shonert-Reichl, K. A. (1992), « Debunking the myths of adolescence: findings from recent research », *Journal of the American Academy of Child and Adolescent Psychiatry*, no. 31, pp. 1003–1013.

Stevens, A. (1998), « L'adolescence, symptôme de la puberté », *Feuillets psychanalytiques du Courtil*, no. 15, pp. 79–92, mars.

Chapter 10

Guidelines in the treatment of anorexia nervosa

Diagnostic issue: structure and position of the subject

The last chapter of this book is devoted to a brief presentation of the main points of orientation in the treatment of anorexia nervosa, as they can be deduced from the perspective of Lacanian psychoanalysis and as they have been sedimented in the course of our personal clinical experience. In many of these points, we can also recognize decisive contributions from sources beyond the Lacanian horizon, which can be found both in the great authors of psychiatry and in essential contributions in the field of contemporary psychoanalysis, psychotherapy (especially in the systemic-relational approach) and psychiatry.

We had the opportunity and the good fortune to develop our experience in different therapeutic contexts, for several years and over a wide range, on the clinic of anorexia nervosa – which allowed us to treat anorexic subjects in the context of real analyses, in individual consultations in institutions, in small monosymptomatic groups and in team work in therapeutic communities, and even to follow patients' parents. The indications given here are the direct fruit of this experience, sifted through by a careful elaboration a posteriori that takes into account the results of the treatments, what worked and what, on the contrary, proved useless or wrong.

The first problem I would like to address here concerns diagnosis. This is, as many authors have noted, a thorny issue, especially as soon as one considers the problem of a diagnostic framework at a level that is not only descriptive but also inherent to the structure of the subject. The intrinsic and specific difficulties of the clinical experience in the encounter with the anorexic patient, together with the internal plurality of the diagnostic and nosographic debate on anorexia nervosa, add to and complicate the matter.

We do not wish to revisit this debate here, but only to isolate some significant key points in relation to the clinical orientation of the therapist dealing with the diagnosis of these patients.

The thesis we put forward here is that a true diagnosis must succeed in isolating three levels of the subject's functioning: an essential descriptive level

DOI: 10.4324/9781003318439-11

of the symptomatology, a level inherent in the structure of the personality and, finally, a level that concerns the subject's position in the present moment of treatment and in relation to the real of their own symptom. As far as anorexia nervosa is concerned, the recurrent elements in the symptomatic constellation essential for a descriptive diagnosis are known: "significantly low weight" (APA, 2022, p. 381) linked to the refusal of food with the subsequent weight loss, "intense fear of gaining weight or of becoming fat" (ibid.), disturbed perception of the body image. Possible phenomenological variations from the restrictive form of anorexia, such as purging anorexia where food consumption is accompanied by vomiting or other forms of evacuation (laxatives or hyperactivity), do not alter the achievement of these three pathological outcomes essential to the formulation of a descriptive diagnosis of anorexia. Similarly, the difference between this overall descriptive framework and cases of malnutrition, including those of a psychogenic nature, is evident. This level of diagnosis can be formulated without major problems, once the patient has benefited from a scrupulous medical examination and a knowledgeable psychiatric consultation. Clinical experience in this area shows that many patients tend to "cheat" on weight at the time of the medical visit by drinking large amounts of water beforehand.

Eating disorder is not a diagnosis in its own right

It is obvious, already at the level of a descriptive diagnosis, that eating disorder does not constitute a diagnosis in its own right. Indeed, even a diagnostic orientation limited to the *DSM-4* domain can only more and more rarely lead the psychiatrist to simply formulate a diagnosis of eating disorder on Axis I. The most common practice in the psychiatric field is to combine a diagnosis of anorexia, bulimia or binge eating disorder on Axis I with an indication of a personality disorder on Axis II. Among these, some frameworks seem to prevail over others, if they are associated with eating disorders. Selvini Palazzoli and her pupils indicated, through a retrospective use of the *DSM*-4 nosographic categories and in the light of the results of one of their research studies, a transformation in progress in the field of eating disorders, in the past few decades and in comparison with the 1960s and 1970s: in the past few decades, there has been a shift from restrictive anorexia, largely associated with addictive and obsessive-compulsive personality disorders, to a prevalence of purging anorexia and bulimia, mostly associated with borderline and narcissistic personality disorders (Selvini Palazzoli and others, 1998, pp. 175–195). This transformation seems to be accompanied, with the historical mutations internal to the society of advanced capitalism and their propagation by the mass media, by the passage from sacrificial forms to forms adhering more to the imperatives of consumption and to the compulsive-narcissistic drifts that characterize them. As far as the *DSM*-5, including its recent revision, is concerned, we can emphasize that the general change of perspective in classification and its shift to a more dimensional spectrum organization has not changed this basic orientation to associate the diagnosis of an eating disorder with other related diagnoses. This is emphasized both in the differential diagnosis criteria and in the comorbidities of the individual syndromes classified among the eating disorders.

Beyond the personality disorder: the structural diagnosis

The descriptive diagnosis of a personality disorder in a patient suffering from anorexia nervosa should not, however, be confused with a structural diagnosis. Indeed, the latter, unlike the former, is not formulated in the light of recurrent traits and characteristics in behavior, but aims to isolate, in relation to everything that emerges within the subject's discourse, the nodal point around which their existential functioning is structured. In Lacan's formulation of it, wanting to be very faithful to Freud on this point, the diagnosis of structure fundamentally aims to isolate: (a) the subject's dominant relation to the Other; (b) the subject's dominant relation to jouissance. As far as the subject's relation to the Other is concerned, it must be understood above all as the subject's relation to the symbolic dimension: their relation to language, their own history, the law, the signifier. This is why Lacan writes Other with a capital A for the French word Autre: exactly to emphasize that it is not a question here of the relation with a similar person, with another man (otherwise, he would have written "other" with a small a), but of the relation with something dissimilar. On this point, Lacan is Freudian in his diagnosis, since he aims to isolate the fundamental symbolic mechanism around which the subject's discourse is organized: repression (*Verdraengung*) at the basis of neurosis, forclusion (*Verwerfung*) at the basis of psychosis and denial (*Verleugnung*) at the basis of perversion. As far as the subject's relationship to jouissance is concerned, it constitutes the most singular and irreducible dimension of the diagnostic process, that is, the isolation of the subject's own libidinal core, of his way of jouissance that makes them different from any other subject; this dimension is not identifiable if we place ourselves only at the symbolic level of structural diagnosis. The Freud-Lacan approach to the diagnosis of structure is presented as an alternative to the one that is dominant in post-Freudianism and in contemporary psychoanalysis and that refers, essentially, to the model proposed by Otto Kernberg. While it is true that Lacan emphasizes, in the diagnosis of structure, the relationship of the subject to the unconscious dimension, to what Freud called "the core of our being" (*das Kern unseres Wesen*), Kernberg's perspective emphasizes more the centrality of the ego and its relationship to reality in the process of diagnostic framing. It is, in fact, around the triad "structure of the Ego/defense mechanisms/examination of reality" that Kernberg's diagnostic grid is constituted, proposing an alternative structural tripartition to that of Freud by introducing, alongside psychosis and neurosis, the borderline personality organization and dropping the structural framework of perversion.

However, apart from the fact that one makes the choice, which is ours, to orient oneself toward Freud's or Lacan's approach or, on the contrary, toward Kernberg's, the formulation of a true structural diagnosis, for a subject suffering from anorexia, remains much more complex and problematic. First of all, it is a diagnosis that, in most cases, becomes clearer in a wider arc of time than the descriptive diagnosis. This temporality is not reducible, in most cases, to the range of preliminary interviews, but remains open for a large part of the treatment. Second, structural diagnosis places at the center of its operation a crucial factor that descriptive diagnosis excludes: transference. It is only under the effect of transference, in the light of the transference relationship between patient and therapist, that the essential elements for the formulation of a diagnosis can emerge from the discourse in progress in the place of the treatment. In the light of this, we can understand the efforts of psychoanalytically oriented psychiatrists to re-include the transference in the *DSM*-4 diagnostic system, as is the case of Gabbard in his *Psychodynamic Psychiatry in Clinical Practice*; just as we can understand, in the same direction, the construction of a psychodynamic classification system integrated into the *DSM*, such as the recent *Psychodynamic Diagnostic Manual* (PDM), now in its second edition.

The diagnosis of structure in anorexia nervosa: inclusive and exclusive version in the Lacanian orientation

But the first factor that makes a diagnosis of structure with these problematic patients is the anorexia nervosa itself. While it is true, indeed, that a diagnosis of structure can only be given under the effect of transference, the subject who suffers from anorexia nervosa nevertheless constitutes a challenge to the diagnosis of structure since they present themselves, when at the peak of their illness, as a subject without demand and in the absence of transference. In other words, in anorexia nervosa, the subject tends to efface himself in his own symptom, to become one with it. This is why the time of a structural diagnosis dilates at least to the point of producing a transference effect.

The recent position of Dewambrechies La Sagna, attributing to anorexia nervosa an independent diagnostic framework, irreducible to psychoses as well as to hysterical-neurotic forms, does not change the substance of the problem, even if it reverses its perspective. From her perspective, it is a question of excluding the psychotic or neurotic-hysterical functioning of the subject, before being able to formulate a diagnosis of "anorexia vera". In the most classical and widespread perspective in the Lacanian world, anorexia nervosa does not constitute a framework in its own right, and therefore the time of the diagnosis coincides with the time of the revelation of the structure in the subject's discourse, which takes place through the opening to the transference. It is, therefore, the time of the inclusion of the symptom in the structure of the subject who carries it. We can therefore distinguish between an exclusive version, in the diagnosis of anorexia nervosa (the one proposed by Dewambrechies La Sagna, where anorexia nervosa is a diagnosis in its own right, which is deduced by exclusion from the psychotic and hysterical frameworks), and an inclusive version (where, on the contrary, the problem is to inscribe anorexia nervosa in a structural framework).

The anorexic closure as an obstacle and a resource for the diagnosis

We have seen, therefore, that on the one hand the specific characteristics of the anorexic symptom hinder the formulation of a structural diagnosis. The ego-syntonic nature of anorexia, the absence of an effective request for a cure, the difficulty in developing a transference, even the fundamental refusal of treatment combined with the lack of knowledge of one's own condition as a patient, all these elements constitute, on the whole, a constellation that makes it difficult not only to start a treatment but also to clarify the structure of the subject we are dealing with. Indeed, the symptom, as a whole, has the effect of obscuring the structure (Eidelberg and others, 2003, p. 109). It closes, therefore, the subjective division in the neurotic forms of anorexia nervosa and repairs, by compensating for it, the psychotic fragmentation. It is, for all that, thanks to a flaw produced in the compensatory solidity of the anorexic symptom that we owe the opening, within the subject's discourse, of the elements that can allow us to frame the structure and the specific function that anorexia exercises in their life.

On the other hand, the same symptomatological characteristics of anorexia nervosa orient the diagnosis in a positive way, showing us the presence of a psychopathological constellation characterized, at least, in the absence of a structural autonomy of its own, by a specificity all the more marked, as it is able to provide the subject with a greater stabilization in the symptom with which he identifies and from which he derives an extreme satisfaction. This aspect of the question of diagnosis in anorexia is essential for us since it allows us to identify the strength of the subject's link to their own symptom, that is, the position of the subject in relation to their anorexia. This position is normally characterized, in the first consultations where it is rather the family and not the anorexic who ask for treatment, by a massive and exclusive identification.

Indicators of change in the subjective position

From the first clinical encounter with a potential anorexic patient, two crucial points are essential in the diagnostic identification: the conditions of the body, which can be analyzed by a thorough medical examination, and the position of the subject carrying the disease, which can be identified in one or more interviews oriented analytically by the psychiatrist or psychologist. Identifying the position of the subject in relation to his or her symptom does not mean formulating a structural diagnosis, which requires more time for its adequate formulation. This identification is essential insofar as it provides, through certain clinical indicators, the state of the subject's relationship with his or her own symptom, which can be analyzed at different moments in the therapeutic process. The changes in the subject's position in relation to the symptom thus become passages that testify to an ongoing transformation, throughout the process of the treatment. Two important clinical indicators, according to our clinical experience of anorexia nervosa, are represented by the degree of egosyntony in relation to the anorexic symptom and by the level of subjectivation of the pathogenic condition that this involves. When the subject enters anorexia nervosa and begins the so-called "honeymoon" with the anorexia, their egosyntony in relation to it is at the maximum level; and the subjectification of their pathogenic condition is at the minimum level, or even totally absent, since the subject sets up a fundamental unawareness of the illness.

Honeymoon with anorexia	Maximum egosyntonia	Minimum recognition of the illness

This is the typical condition in which we begin to see young anorexic patients, accompanied by their parents, in the clinical consultation. In fact, for them, anorexia is much more a solution than a problem. It is clear that this initial state makes any treatment project practically impossible and only serves to make the subject survive, until something intervenes and allows the change of their position of confinement around the symptom. It is only when the anorexic solution begins to prove insufficient to treat the subject's suffering, to show that it is precarious and beyond the subject's control, that the necessary conditions for the change of the subjective position and the beginning of the therapeutic treatment are created.

Beginning of treatment	Emergence of an egodystonic point	Beginning of the recognition of the illness

This passage is accompanied by a feeling of loss of control over the symptom itself, which can allow the anorexic subject to emerge from their state of anhedonia and mortifying indifference toward the world.

The state of the body and the problem of hospitalization

A prerequisite for talking to an anorexic patient is the verification of their physiological condition by a careful medical examination. If the patient's physiological values, first of all the body mass index (BMI), are below the threshold indicating a condition where survival is at risk, it becomes counterproductive to even begin psychotherapeutic work: the therapeutic indication that is needed is hospitalization in a clinical nutrition ward. Quite often in these cases, a stay in a psychiatric hospital becomes necessary, when the patient's refusal to be hospitalized, often driven by a delusional blindness to their physical condition, puts their life in danger. Hospitalization is, in these cases, not only a medical priority but also a necessity for eventual talk treatment, be it psychotherapy or analysis, and it can only be started or restarted after an effective hospitalization that brings the body's values down to an acceptable minimum. This is true for at least three essential clinical reasons.

The first reason is represented by the following observation: when an anorexic patient reaches physiological values below the minimum threshold, an effect occurs on the psychic level that we have called eclipse of the subject. The subject disappears, their speech is completely emptied of value, their relationship with others becomes non-existent and their position is out of discourse with respect to what is happening around them. In short, a double structural effect occurs in which the subject eclipses itself by becoming an object full of jouissance.

In this condition, the state of anorexia nervosa as a "de facto outside-discourse" being, of which Dewambrechies La Sagna speaks (Dewambrechies La Sagna, 2006, p. 67), reaches its peak. It is vital that the clinician involved with the anorexic in psychotherapy recognizes and acknowledges this condition, by becoming a therapeutic partner in supporting the need for hospitalization as a condition for resuming psychotherapeutic work. The second reason lies in the avoidance of the risks of reverse hypnosis, often carried out by these patients, and sometimes by their families, toward the therapist, to convince themselves that the treatment of speech with them, and not hospitalization, will bring the patient out of her state of risk. Giving in to the patient's flattery in this situation means falling into the trap of what Racamier calls "narcissistic seduction" where a devastating alliance is created, with many possibilities of leading to death, between the therapeutic omnipotence of the carer and the uncontained omnipotence of the anorexic symptom. From a Lacanian perspective, this also means not taking into account the fact that, in this case, the power of speech is deactivated by an unbounded jouissance and that it is therefore impossible in these conditions to treat this extreme state of the subject through speech and the laws of the signifier.

The third reason lies in the fact that, for the therapist, supporting the hospitalization of their patient in these conditions becomes the only way to reintroduce a limit in the therapeutic relationship to the unlimited devastating development of the patient's symptom. It is, on the other hand, important to reason clinically about the ways in which the therapist or the family prescribes the patient's hospitalization, in order to allow this hospitalization to be revealed as an encounter with not only something that keeps her alive but also a real symbolic limit. Our experience of this kind of situation, both as a professional analyst and as a psychotherapist in the institution, has led me to believe that the most effective hospitalizations, that is, those from which the patient returns not only physically healthier but also in a different subjective position from before the hospitalization, require certain preliminary conditions at the time of referral. In other words, a hospitalization that has the effect of transforming the patient's subjective position, in relation to the jouissance that binds her to their symptom, requires on the part of the one sending the actuation of a non-expulsive modality that does not have as its starting point a situation of impotence. The powerlessness of the sender is specular and feeds the pathogenic omnipotence of the patient's anorexia. The subjective position of the carer, in the act of hospitalization, is effective if we manage to situate ourselves on the level of the impossibility of doing otherwise; it is a question of taking note of the fact that, if the patient has entered the tunnel of anorexia without limits, we must introduce the missing limit through the suspension of the work of speech, which is impossible in this condition of the subject. This operation is essential to allow the patient to encounter castration, in the other who takes care of her, not as a real deprivation on the part of the other of something that belongs to her but as the presentification of a universal symbolic limit. This is the most difficult operation to accomplish with the anorexic who, as Lacan says in The Seminar, Book XI, avoids the encounter with symbolic castration by their constant reversal, in the relationship with others, into the register of the deprivation, by the other, of something real. What, in other words, as Ménard has well pointed out, the anorexic does not manage to accept is the impossibility that anyone can deprive her of what she already lacks in a structural way (except for psychoses), and that her problem lies rather in the assumption of this structural castration (Ménard, 1992, pp. 3–5).

A guideline: the quadripartite grid on anorexic refusal

An aid to the diagnostic and treatment process that we propose is represented by the quadripartite grid of the four functions of anorexic refusal, identified and discussed in Chapter 6. Since it is the strategic core around which the anorexic position is structured and which we have taken as the common thread of our reading of anorexia nervosa in the footsteps of Lacan, the fact of analyzing the specific function (or functions) of refusal in the anorexic subject with whom we are involved in the treatment and its possible variations of function or intensity, at the different moments of the treatment, can constitute a useful orientation compass for the clinical work. The first function of the anorexic refusal introduces the refusal as a demand function. It is necessary to verify if this functional level of refusal acts or not in the anorexic patient with whom we are engaged. In the hysteric-neurotic forms, we almost always encounter the demand function active in the refusal. What remains to be clarified each time is what the subject is asking for, in most cases without knowing it, and whom he asks for it. It will be useful to try to answer this question case by case. In hysterical anorexics, desire is the object of refusal as a demand. As Lacan taught us, by refusal the anorexic consults the desire of the Other, embodied by the parents or the partner of the moment, to verify if their own place in the desire of the Other exists and what it is. In psychotic forms, we cannot always identify a demand function in the refusal. When this is possible, the refusal has no relation to the desire of the Other but is rather a demand to limit the invasion of the Other, a demand that is often addressed to the carers. The effectiveness of this can be verified a posteriori when this reading allows the carer to regulate the invasion of the parents, which produces a reduction in the girl's restrictive closure in her position.

The second function of the anorexic refusal concerns the refusal in its defensive function. In the hysterical-neurotic forms, the object of the defense is, in the final analysis, the subject's own desire in its drive component. In psychotic forms, refusal as a defense acts as a limit to the invasion of the Other. Whereas in neuroses the emergence of refusal as a defense protects the subject from their own division, in psychotic forms it protects them from fragmentation (in schizophrenia), from persecution (in paranoia), from the sensation of feeling let down by an abandoning Other (in melancholic-depressive forms). The third function of refusal in anorexia nervosa concerns refusal in its function as a separation maneuver. It is an active movement of the subject toward the Other that intends to go in the direction of an autonomy but that, in anorexia, spontaneously acquires the form of a solely imaginary liberation from the Other. This is insofar as, contrary to the logic of anorexia, there cannot be here a total autonomy from the Other, a construction of one's own position within the symbolic field of the Other and its laws. This is the reason why we prefer to speak of anorexic pseudo-separation from the Other, referring to the imaginary autonomism present in the discourses of anorexic patients, and of a symbolic separation when it happens from a "yes" that the anorexic subject can manage to say toward the Other, because of the effect of therapeutic work that has an incidence on their position and that modifies the status of the Other by making it a habitable field where it is possible to find one's place. In neurotic forms, refusal in its separative function is structured, therefore, around a process articulated in two stages. The initial time is that of refusal as an imaginary autonomization in relation to the Other, which is one with the symptomatic egosynthony of the honeymoon period with anorexia. The time that the therapeutic process aims at is the one that leads the subject toward a more dialectical use of refusal, which allows him to say no to an omnipotent Other who decides in his place, in order to be able to say yes to an incomplete Other who lets him occupy his own place. In psychotic forms, the subject cannot produce a symbolic separation on his own since they cannot take responsibility for a decision that is his own. The symbolic separative maneuver can occur especially in the form of the intervention of a third actor who can be the therapist or the care team, capable of regulating the Other of the psychotic subject by preventing it from being invaded. Finally, the fourth function of anorexic refusal is represented by refusal in its function of jouissance. In relation to this aspect, which is the most enigmatic knot of the anorexic position, we must first distinguish the modality of jouissance on which the scaffolding of the anorexic symptom is based. It will thus be necessary, on this subject, to keep quite separate a hysterical-neurotic jouissance of dissatisfaction or deprivation from a nirvanic-affirmative jouissance, with almost addictive features, which we find in the forms of "true anorexia". In the former, the refusal has the function of keeping the lack open and feeding the desire. In the latter, quite differently, refusal is a practice of active and irresistible enjoyment, unhooked from the dialectic of desire and aiming at obtaining an autistic and self-destructive satisfaction. In the most clearly psychotic forms, this autistic jouissance is related to the delusional construction that the subject has produced in their relation to the Other and consists in their way of being able to remain in this relation.

The question of the treatment of parents and the family

Beyond the systemic-family approach: anorexic jouissance

As we have already pointed out, the centrality of the parents' involvement in the therapeutic treatment has been further highlighted by the systemic-relational school, especially in the systemic-familial approach to anorexia nervosa of Selvini Palazzoli's Milan school. In this perspective, in fact, it is the family system of the anorexic patient that constitutes the network of transactions where the trap of the double bond is triggered, locking the girl patient into the position of victim designated by the family. Exactly for this reason, in Selvini Palazzoli's classical systemic approach, it is the family system as a whole that becomes the object of treatment, with the aim of revealing to the family members the altered communicative circuit within which the girl's anorexia has found its place. The analytical approach oriented toward anorexia as a symptom built around a singular jouissance of the subject, while accepting the centrality of the family discourse in the determination of the position of the anorexic subject, does not believe that the girl's anorexia can find a solution in a work of symbolization of the deformed communicational structure, internal to the functioning of the family system. Moreover, the classical approach of Selvini's systemic-family therapy has been extensively reformed by the inclusion, within the treatment, of the individual variable represented by the position of the anorexic subject, not entirely attributable to the strategic framework of the transactions of the family system. In an analytical approach, not related to the classical forms of a psychoanalytical hermeneutics of meaning, but focused on the singular real of jouissance, the anorexic subject is never alone in the position of designated victim but rather subjectively involved in the choice of this position; nevertheless, they themselves develop a libidinal link toward their own symptom that goes beyond the dialectical requirements, of power and counter-power, internal to the family system. It is in this irreducible core underlying anorexia, this refusal as an internal jouissance to the anorexic position, that the cure meets its most extreme and intractable obstacle.

Beyond phenomenological characterizations: a structural formula for the family of the anorexic

In the light of what we have just said, it is important to confront the problem of the anorexic patient's family by taking into account the centrality of jouissance underlying their symptom. The thesis we put forward is that there may be a structural homology between the structure of the anorexic symptom and the structure of the family bond where it occurred. In other words, as in anorexia nervosa the symptom is deficient in its symbolic functioning of metaphor and shows itself in its status of narcissistic jouissance, in the same way, in the family of the anorexic, we witness the failure of the function of the family link operating a symbolic treatment of jouissance. In other words, in the different family systems of anorexics, we witness in differentiated forms what we could call the failure of the family as a discourse (Cosenza, 2007, pp. 14–16), that is to say as a regulation device humanizing the real of the drive. This implies that in these family forms, the bond is composed of a symbolically weak internal tissue and filled with an essentially narcissistic-specular material, as is most often the case in the family systems of patients who develop contemporary symptoms. At the center is not the regulating asymmetry of symbolic law but the deadly, confusing and boundless symmetry of narcissistic specularization.

The Selvini Palazzoli school has described in detail the specific characteristics of the family system of anorexic patients, identifying their variations and the pluralization of their forms which have occurred in recent decades, especially with the great diffusion of bulimia from the 1980s. Beyond the significant variations in the phenomenology of family forms, which clearly shows the difference between the hyper-controlling sacrificial trait of the family systems of the anorexic of the 1950s and 1960s compared to the more unregulated functioning of the last decades, one structural trait seems to remain constant and to function as a common thread: the tendency to make One in the family bond, without the Other. By this formula we mean that the family of the anorexic has difficulty in functioning as a symbolic device that prohibits, regulates and at the same time makes the subject's relationship to jouissance tolerable and bearable, producing as a consequence a deficit of symbolic separation on the part of its members, in particular of the daughter or son who becomes anorexic. But the parents themselves reveal, in their clinical histories, their own subjective difficulty in being able to separate themselves from the demands of their parents, especially from the mother who often continues to exercise, until death, a function of authority over her daughters and sons.

This is precisely the classic thesis supported by Selvini Palazzoli when she was still a Kleinian psychoanalyst in her 1963 treatise *L'anoressia mentale*: the thesis of the "superegoic matriarchy" in the family of the anorexic patient, where the central place of power is occupied by the maternal grandmother.

In this sense, it is a family that is One in the bond since it envelops its members in a dysregulated bond that does not allow the encounter with the law of the Other, a condition of separation. In this context, we must read, in my opinion, the so-called archaism of the anorexic's family where, in contradistinction to contemporary couples, the frequency of divorce is proportionally low. In a more subtle way, making an already dead, devitalized and devitalizing bond survive, beyond the requirement to correspond to a now outdated conformism, is the mark of the same enjoyment found in the anorexic position projected on the unifying cement of the family.

The partnership between the daughter's (or son's) symptom and the parents' anxiety

In this sense, it is necessary to rethink the subjective rectification as a displacement of the experience of anxiety: from the anguish of the anorexic's Other (above all their parents) to the emergence of the anguish of the anorexic subject herself. Indeed, at the beginning and during a long journey of clinical work in cases of anorexia nervosa, we are generally dealing with a partnership between the parents' anguish and the girl's symptom. This obviously implies that we have to think about working with anorexia while at the same time operating on the parents' anxiety that they pour out on her. We are thus led to rethink our clinic with the family, to refound it around the pivot of the real experience of anxiety. The anorexic, in fact, presents a symptom without anguish and the parents an anguish without symptom. The clinical work of rectification should aim at reducing the anxiety of the parents about their daughter's condition by making them work, if possible, on the symptomatic dimension of the family link. At the same time, it should aim at reintroducing the subjective space of anguish in the anorexic in order to chip away at the malignant egosyntony of the symptom. This is also the line of orientation that can be drawn from Polacco Williams' experience at the Tavistock, which focuses, in the relationship to anguish, on the key to access to eating symptoms and their treatment (Polacco Williams, 1999, p. 80). These are presented as a treatment for the daughter of the parents' anguish and as a symptom of the failure of their function as a symbolic container for the daughter's anguish. In this sense, Polacco Williams speaks, following Bion, of a reversal of the relationship between container and content in the eating disorder clinic: not only do the parents fail to contain the daughter's anguish, but they go so far as to project their anguish onto the daughter, who responds to it by constructing the eating symptom. For this reason, the double operation that must be carried out in our work is (a) to contain the parents' anguish, by offering them a symbolic space for speech; (b) to allow the daughter to be able to find her own relationship to anguish as a condition for a real request for a treatment.

Only when the anguish is anchored in the real does the request for a treatment acquire for the subject the value of a "true" demand for change. Otherwise it assumes the empty form of a desubjectivized demand, as it is often encountered, in particular in the phase of the preliminary interviews, where, in reality, the patient becomes the spokesperson of the parents' demand, without any real involvement in the treatment.

T1	*T2*
Parents' anxiety	*Patient's anxiety*
Patient's symptom	*Parents' symptom*

Beyond the symptom/demand binomial: starting from the real of anxiety

This way of conceptualizing and practicing the operation of rectification, in the relationship between the anorexic subject and the parental Other, represents an objective surpassing of a more classical approach to the problem, anchored in the symbolic dimension of the demand. Here the pivotal point is the reversal of the relationship between symptom and demand, which is found inverted in the parents and in the anorexic daughter (or son): in the former, the asymptomatic demand for help is matched by a symptom without demand in the latter. The clinical problem was posed, at this level, in terms of activating a demand in the daughter and symptomatizing the parents' position around the state of the family bond (Barbuto, Pace, 1998, pp. 250–268; Pace, 2010). The variation that I propose here is to posit in the first place the encounter with the real of anguish as the logical time that makes possible the subject's passage to an effective demand. In reality, therefore, it is not an alternative model, compared to the one centered on the symptom/demand binomial, but a more radical model, constructed from the real structure of the symptom indicating the factor that makes possible the subject's passage to an effective demand: the encounter with anguish.

The dynamic path of effective preliminary work, capable of rectifying the relationship between the anorexic subject and her parents in the non-psychotic forms, generally follows this path:

Parents
Anxiety→ Demand→ Symptom

Anorexic daughter or son
Symptom →Anxiety→ Demand

Preliminary work and a new theory and praxis of subjective rectification

Transforming the real of the symptom: from the nirvanic-egosyntonic to the uncanny-egodystonic status

What we are trying to introduce here is, in other words, the idea of re-founding, at its root, the clinic of anorexia from the real dimension of the symptom. And this operation must be practiced with the patient from their first steps in the treatment, from the preliminary interviews and, in particular, at the point which, in the treatment, represents the key: the idea of subjective rectification. It is classically configured as a passage made possible by the analyst in the subject's discourse: from the complaint of his own condition to the recognition of his unconscious responsibility for the very condition he complains about (Lacan, 2006, pp. 176–185). This is the operation carried out by Freud with Dora, rightly named by Lacan as "subjective rectification". This operation is integrally founded on the paradigm of the symptom as a metaphor of the subject and finds, in hysteria, a fertile ground for its production. The beginnings with our anorexic patients, even when we are faced with subjects who reveal themselves to be neurotic, only more and more rarely allow, in the preliminaries, an operation of rectification of this kind that is effective. This is precisely because, beyond the underlying structure, it is the nirvanic-egosyntonic dimension of the symptom as real that prevails and hinders symbolization. The subject presents themselves as wrapped up in the mesh of symptomatic jouissance and impervious to elaboration. At the beginning of the treatment, in fact, the real of the symptom presents itself as an obstacle to symbolization, as a refusal of symbolization. For this reason, the subjective rectification must be refounded around the real of the symptom, as a passage in the subject from the nirvanic-egosyntonic dimension to the uncanny (*Unheimlich*) egodystonic dimension of the symptom. This passage leads to the production in the subject of an anguish effect that breaks the homeostasis of self-destructive jouissance and introduces a real division in the subject at the level of affect:

Subjective rectification: production of an anguish effect.

To think of subjective rectification from the production in the subject of an effect of anguish is something completely different from thinking of it from an effect of recognition in the discomfort of which one complains. The effect of anguish is not, in fact, an effect of symbolic recognition but a real upheaval without solution, anchored in the body, which makes the subject jump out of the condition of silent and mortifying homeostasis where they had fallen asleep, waking him up as in a nightmare. Clinical experience teaches us this, moreover. In anorexia, it is when the subject breaks their honeymoon with the symptom to start to feel anguish that something can really start to change. As Charcot, the first to indicate hospitalization as the only therapeutic way to treat anorexics in the acute phase, already remarked, it is in this situation that anorexics can resume eating.

This is the effect that occurs, for example, when, for the first time, the anorexic subject manages to meet his or her own skeletal image in the mirror, or, more precisely, his or her own anguished gaze. A living and desperate look in a skeletal body that is almost dead. It is the appearance in the mirror of the real of one's own gaze, detached from the coating of the image, that causes anguish to the anorexic by revealing the troubling dimension contained in this repeated experience that is so central to his/her existence: looking at him/herself repeatedly in the mirror.

In the clinic of anorexia, the subjective rectification, thus conceived and practiced, consists, as Dewambrechies indicates, in an operation of restitution to the subject of the relationship to his/her own anxiety (Dewambrechies La Sagna, 2006, p. 70).

The gap between body and speech and their intersection: the point of anxiety as a bridge to desire

The clinical centrality of the experience of anguish is shown in all its magnitude when we find ourselves, in treatment, confronted with a typical situation with our patients that I could define by the formula: the gap between the body and the word. This situation describes a recurrent condition, in the treatments, where the subject seems to be engaged in a work of symbolization while the symptom, instead of being reduced or lightened, becomes radicalized. This is a paradoxical situation, obviously symptomatic, which should make us question what is really happening with the patient. I remember Fiorenza, a girl I followed for a few years, who presented this kind of position for a long time. About herself, Fiorenza said that she was doing excellent psychotherapeutic work but that the body remained frozen, not even allowing itself to be touched, and that this suited her perfectly. In reality, this situation becomes paradigmatic of what happens when the experience of anguish does not intervene to weld, in the subject, the relationship between their word and their body. It is precisely the anguish, in fact, that is the point of intersection in the subject between the experience of the body and the experience of speech. When the latter fails to emerge in the cure, the treatment is basically running on empty, without encountering the real of the subject's suffering.

This encounter in the treatment with the real of the subject's anguish is decisive since, without passing through this traumatic encounter, the subject has no chance of recovering a relationship with desire and of changing his/her position in the relationship with the Other and with jouissance. This becomes clear when the treatment is pushed to the point of cracking, reducing, dissolving the symptomatic dimension of the eating disorder. What do we encounter in our patients when this happens? I would say a double level of experience. On the one hand, anguish returns in the form of an extreme amplification of the affective dimension in its troubling aspects. In particular, with regard to the relationship with the other sex. This makes them suffer much more than before and they often say how much they regret their previous anesthetized condition, even though they feel that they cannot go back. On the other hand, this experience of anguish is for them an experience of desire that calls them to decide for themselves how to face the encounter with the desire for the Other. In this sense, the reduction of the anorexic symptom implies precisely, for the subject, the anguish of a renewed exposure of the body to the desiring gaze of the Other, which puts the subject's desire, his or her saying yes or no to what he or she encounters, back into play.

What rectification for psychoses? One form: rectification of the Other

In anorexic symptomatologies in psychotic subjects, the rectification operation cannot take the path of a subjectivation of anguish in relation to something for which the patient can consider him/herself responsible. Anguish does not open the door to desire and its possible assumption to the psychotic, remaining only anguish linked to the threat embodied by the Other and to their will to enjoy them without limits. Depending on the subject, the Other will assume an abandonment, sadistic, or persecutory form, but in all cases it will give life, in the patient's moments of difficulty, to a kind of fusion between the Other and his jouissance expressing itself, at the height of its invasive power, in the elementary phenomenon of acoustic hallucination.

However, if it is possible to speak of an operation of rectification, in the work with psychotic anorexics, it will be more a rectification of the psychotic's Other than a subjective rectification. By this expression, "rectification of the Other", we want to define the clinical maneuver by which we achieve, in the psychotic subject, a detachment between the field of the Other and the emergence of the invasion of jouissance. This maneuver proves to be essential to break the patient's rise of psychotic anguish and to defuse the paranoid certainty that the Other is persecuting him/her and that it wants to enjoy him/her. In the case of psychotic anorexia, this often takes the form of an Other who wants to force the patient to eat (who orders her "you must eat!") by force or deception (the classic delusions of poisoning and the more contemporary forms of food contamination are part of these cases). The most expected response in these cases is an extreme reinforcement of the rigidity of food restriction and a psychotic refusal of food.

What is effective here is to clear the field of the Other, by showing the patient that there is no will to enjoy themselves and by explaining to him/her that, in this area, not only they, but all of us, are subject to the rules of communal life and the conventionally established laws of the state; that it is the task and role of the carers to keep them alive, and that it is important for them to eat and so on. Emptying the field of the Other of the "flood" of jouissance, showing the subject that in the Other it is possible to find a reliable point of anchorage, all of this makes it possible to begin and continue work with the psychotic subject suffering from anorexia.

Scansions in the process of the treatment

The clinical experience with anorexic patients seems to allow us to isolate five fundamental scansions which organize an analytically oriented treatment and lead to its conclusion. It is possible to identify all these passages, in a sub-jectivized form, only in those cures where the analytical treatment has been pushed to its extreme consequences. This generally occurs in non-psychotic forms of anorexia in subjects who have accepted an analytically oriented treatment and not necessarily in its classical form linked to an individual treatment during the whole therapeutic course. In many cases, it must be emphasized that an important part of the treatment was carried out within the therapeutic device of the monosymptomatic, analytically led small group, or within a residential institution such as the therapeutic community, before continuing and ending within the framework of an individual analysis in its most advanced phase.

First scansion: loss of the imaginary control of the symptom

The first shift occurs when the patient experiences a loss of the imaginary mastery they themselves think they have to have over their own body through their symptom. This phenomenon introduces a discontinuity in the con-tinuum of their experience of pathology: anorexia ceases to present itself to the subject as an egosyntonic condition, as a form of jouissance with which to identify in an overwhelming way. The symptom as a factor of jouissance shows the subject, in a more obvious way, now, its face of jouissance beyond the pleasure principle and the fact that it is its slave and not its master. This is the end of the honeymoon with the pathology of food which, at this point, can rise to the status of a true symptom.

In the first place, this food pathology can become a symptom in the medical sense, that is, a signal of illness that affects the body as an organism. At this level, the subject can articulate a request for help addressed to the doctor to help him restore a condition of balance in their own organism. However, the problem that this request encounters is caused, in clinical experience, by three factors that weaken its effectiveness, to the point of invalidating it:

- de-subjectivized "compliance": when the subject agrees to be treated, their acceptance is generally more the effect of wishing to satisfy the request of their family or the nursing staff than the effect of a real assumption of the decision to overcome their own pathological condition;
- the ambivalence of the request: the subject, in fact, literally asks to be treated but generally keeps a project of *restitutio ad integrum* of the symptom in its plenitude and egosyntonic efficiency (Cosenza, 2001, pp. 227–249);
- the invasive character of jouissance: the subject asks medical science for a rebalancing of the physiological conditions of the body but, if, and as soon as, he/she has obtained them – as appears in an exemplary way in anorexia as well as in the clinic of obesity – he/she works irresistibly to invalidate the results, by returning to the bodily conditions preceding the intervention – nutritional, surgical, etc. – of medicine.

The eating pathology transforms its status of symptom when the subject manages to recognize that it is precisely his/her relationship to anorexia that is animated by this ambivalence and that what happens to them, each time they irresistibly hinder or invalidate the course of treatment requested by themselves, remains enigmatic for them. At this point, the subject witnesses the transformation into a psychoanalytic symptom of the pathology that previously seemed to challenge, through its demand, only the question of medicine. This premise is essential to orient us toward the logic that accelerates the preliminary phase of the treatment and, in particular, the work of the preliminary interviews. In fact, the most recurrent starting situation in this field of contemporary psychopathology is that of subjects who do not recognize suffering in their condition and who, therefore, do not ask for anything that goes in the direction of a change. It is the others around them who, on the other hand, recognize the evidence, at least bodily, of this condition and who push them toward a treatment that these subjects refuse. The preliminary interviews tend to lead the person with the disease to recognize its existence, in order to be able to ask for a treatment that involves it. To achieve this transformation, it is essential that two scans occur during the preliminary work.

From egosyntony to egodystony: the time of anxiety

As we have already underlined, in the clinic of anorexia, it is essential to achieve subjective rectification which, in the first instance, does not pass through the symbolic way of recognition but through the real way of anguish. It is a question, in fact, of restoring to the anorexic subject the relationship with his anguish that he has scotomized in the egosyntony of his own condition. In this first rectification, we are called upon to calm the anguish of the anorexic's Other (the family, the nursing staff) alarmed by their condition of risk, by bringing them out of their state of omnipotent and narcissistic imperturbability. This passage clashes with the economy of satisfaction without loss of the subject in anorexia, since it pushes toward the loss of the egosyntonic enjoyment of the illness. This is what happens in an obvious way during the phases of acute manifestation of the symptom, which place the patient in danger of death. The decision to hospitalize the patient in these situations, if acted upon appropriately, can reintroduce anguish in the subject by the emergence of a limit to the exercise of their jouissance.

In obesity, the effect of anguish produced by the request for a treatment is often linked to a malfunction of the organism's machine which reveals to the subject the impossibility of doing, in reality, things with the body to which they were accustomed (sitting on a chair, putting on a particular garment, having sexual intercourse, etc.) or is linked to the appearance of a collateral disease and its disabling effects. In these conditions, a request to the doctor usually occurs in patients, to restore a condition of the body that is not disabling for the subject.

From the request for help to the analytical request: the time of the symptom as enigma and the activation of the transference

While the appearance of anguish allows the subject to get out of an inertial and mortifying egosyntony, by the transformation of the real status of his symptom from nirvanic to uncanny (*unheimlich*), the foundations of the treatment are only laid in the modality of the treatment of anguish. An analytically oriented approach will act in the sense of a quantitative reduction of anguish but not in the sense of its disappearance, anguish being the potentially transformative factor of the subject's position. After having made the appearance of anguish possible, the properly analytical operation to be accomplished on it is twofold.

On the one hand, it is certainly necessary to reduce its threshold level but, on the other hand, it is necessary to act so that the subject, starting from anguish, transforms their share of anguish into a structured analytical symptom, that is, into a suffering traversed by an enigma to be articulated symbolically. Indeed, the dystonic-uncanny *(unheimlich)* appearance of anguish wakes up the subject who has fallen asleep in the nirvanic-egosyntonic sleep of anorexia, upsetting them as if waking them up from a nightmare. It is therefore essential, in order to avoid the patient becoming frightened by the appearance of anguish, to act promptly to contain the anguish (without eliminating it) in its manifestation and allow the subject to link it to the symptom. While, therefore, the first stage of the preliminary work is: from the honeymoon to the appearance of anguish; the second stage is: from anguish to the construction of an analytical symptom. This passage coincides, in the subject's discourse, with the transformation of their request: from a request for help, the response to which is entirely in the hands of the Other, to an analytical request in which the patient becomes responsible for their response to the enigma of their suffering, passing from the position of patient to the position of analysand.

The dynamic condition that allows this qualitative transformation of the demand is provoked by the activation of the transference, the opening of which is already an important result in the clinical work with anorexic patients. It is not only a question of an imaginary investment in the figure of the therapist, which must nevertheless be activated to a certain extent. It is rather the fact that the subject, during the treatment, begins to question their symptom as something enigmatic whose value escapes them.

It is at this moment of the treatment that the egosyntony of the anorexic patient is pierced by the encounter with "a hole in knowledge" (*trou dans le savoir*) that opens onto the enigma of the subject. If the anorexic, as Lacan indicates in The Seminar, Book XXI, does not want to know anything about the unconscious, the encounter with a hole in knowledge is what can change something in their position.

This phenomenon, when it actually occurs, testifies to the activation of a transference that is not only imaginary but symbolic, in the sense that Lacan formulated the structure of transference as subject-supposed-knowledge. Reaching this point, in the work with an anorexic subject, means having already led them to make a radical passage of transformation of his position. The effective production of this result takes place in a significant temporal arc of the treatment process, which can even last several years and which is not usually reduced to a few rare preliminary interviews, as happens, on the other hand, in the classic analytical treatment of a neurotic subject.

Second scansion: reactivation of signifying alienation (or recovery of the power of speech)

Reopening of the unconscious: from empty speech to evocative speech

This passage allows the subject's discourse to reopen to the evocative capacity of speech, by moving beyond the anonymous monotony of an anesthetized and repetitive reference to the food object, to the weight of the body, to the thin or fat image. It is the power of the word that is reinstalled, in this passage of the treatment, by producing the effect of a reopening of the subject's unconscious. In this passage, the subject discovers that he or she is in no way master of his or her body and even less of his or her word, which says and leaves its sign beyond the intentions of the speaker. Anorexic suffering no longer only assumes the form of a fetishistic blindness, positioned outside the discourse toward the food object, but it begins to include within itself a symbolization of this irresistible push. A process of historicization of the subject in its position is triggered, chapters of its own history can begin to be written, the formations of the unconscious (dreams, lapses, missed acts) begin to reach the subject again as enigmatic events in which it is involved. The powerful refusal of the symbolic dimension of the experience, which invades both the anorexic and the obese subject, leaves, at this moment of the treatment, a space of slow opening to the work of symbolization.

Control of the Other/signifying alienation

During the treatment, the anorexic, whatever the treatment modality that engages them – individual session, small group or the experience of the therapeutic community – generally relates to the Other as if they were not where they are but in a non-existent place, nowhere, in fact. This is the defensive modality, set up by the anorexic to make themselves untouchable by the action of the word: not being there, being there only as a dead body. The obese subject chooses the opposite strategy in order not to be touched by the word of the Other: the misrecognition of their symbolic status, by reducing the discourse that takes place in the session to a level of the hyper-concretism of the "here and now" erasing the uncanny dialectical significance (*unheimlich*) of the phenomenon of absence and presence. These opposing strategies are, however, aimed at a single goal, namely the control of the Other, which is another way of saying the refusal of the Other as unpredictable, as an encounter with the difference that the Other embodies. These strategies are brought into question when the treatment gives rise to a link, in the transference, where the absence and the presence (of the therapist, of the subject themselves, of the other patients of the group or of the community) acquire a value that enters the discourse and challenges the subject to say something about it. For example, this typically happens when a patient is absent from a group, especially if the absence is repeated and not previously announced to the group itself. The spontaneous response of the patients, if the group is not symbolically based, tends to take the direction of denial of the absence in various forms. In anorexia, the denial of absence often takes the form of the reduction of absence to non-existence: the absent Other is subjected to erasure in the patient's discourse. In obesity, the denial of absence more easily takes the form of its trivialization: B did not come because they probably went elsewhere. In this way, the obese subject extinguishes, as soon as it appears, the activation of a symbolic link with the group and the therapist, to avoid paying the price of the special investment that the activation of an effective transference link entails.

Anorexic strategies for controlling the Other: from stereotypy to semantic redundancy

This constant demand to tame the Other, while keeping oneself at a distance, exercising an obsessive control of one's movements, neutralizing the effects of the encounter with it, explains well the difficulty of the anorexic subject – just as in the obesity clinic – in assuming the consequences of the effects of their existence's signifying alienation. This assumption, which in classical analytic terms has to do with the experience of symbolic castration, entails the impossibility for the subject to exercise control over the Other, which, exactly the opposite, imposes its own constitutive laws on the subject.

The clinical experience with anorexic patients testifies to the importance, in working with them, of being aware of this work of defensive deactivation of the effects of transformation, introduced into the subject's life by the activation of the functioning of the signifying chain. If we refer to the level of the anorexic's relationship to speech, we witness different modalities of deactivation. In the initial phases of treatment, this generally takes the form of a fundamental stereotypy of the subject's discourse, of a desubjectivized language organized around an extremely limited semantic barrier, relating to food, the body and weight. The discourse of the anorexic takes the form of a continuous rumination within this closed circuit.

However, during the treatment, the demand for control of the Other never disappears on the part of the anorexic, who will reproduce the dynamic, even in the more advanced phases of the treatment, through a metamorphosis of the forms of deactivation of the real effects of signifying alienation. A typical mechanism that the anorexic puts in place, to neutralize the effects of re-opening the evocative dimension of speech, is represented by the abuse of the symbolization process, which has the substantial effect of invalidating it by emptying it. This mechanism, which we would call semantic redundancy, is put into action by the patients, once they have learned the lesson of psychotherapy. They think that they are thus giving back to the therapist, in the form of more or less original elaborations, what they imagine he/she wants to hear them say, and in so doing they reactivate the typical trait of complacency toward the Other, the centrality of which is known in anorexia nervosa, even before the first manifestations of the illness. This is a drift that must be prevented during the treatment, by appealing above all to the analytical principle according to which it is not necessary to add meaning but rather to eliminate the "too much meaning" with which the patient has pathogenically filled themselves in the course of their history. On this point, an analytic treatment, too anchored to a semantic-interpretative functioning, presents a risk of collusion, in fact, with this secondary defense mechanism in anorexic patients, and it may prove, as Hilde Bruch already underlined, not only inefficient but also deleterious.

Ways circumventing anorexic control: presenting surprise, giving space to anxiety

Until the moment when the carer is totally under the control of the anorexic and their movements are completely predictable, it is difficult for a transformation to take place during the treatment. With the necessary attention, especially in psychotic forms, and taking into account the patient's degree of tolerance to change at that moment, it is necessary to be able to introduce movements, scansions and highlights into the treatment in order to introduce surprise into the context of the treatment. The position of the subject at the peak of anorexia is, in fact, characterized by an anesthetic egosyntonic narcosis where indifference is the dominant affective tone. However, this immobile position can be sustained during the treatment, provided that the therapist is kept paralyzed in a reassuring mothering position where the patient feeds on the therapist's interpretations and feeds him/her in turn by making their own interpretations in line with his/hers. It is important, in the treatment of anorexia, to ensure that the therapist's being-there in the treatment does not coincide with the paralysis of their action and with the absolute predictability of their position. In Lacanian analytic practice, this requirement is facilitated, in certain respects, by the function of the variable-time session and by the character of the session, synchronized not with standard time but with the temporality of the signifying chain of the subject's discourse and its productions. This makes it possible, in the treatment, to enhance the surprise effect, internal to the patient's own discourse, without saturating it by the interpretative route but by giving it a tempo by the act that defines the end of the session. This operation leaves the interpretation to the patient themselves, who will be able to say something about it at the next session, or even at the door when they take their leave. Nevertheless, we must always bear in mind that the production of the surprise effect in the treatment can never be reduced to a technical problem and that the essential thing is the position of the analyst and their place in the patient's transference: only if the transference is efficiently structured can the scansion of the session efficiently produce the surprise effect in the subject, by introducing something enigmatic into the heart of their discourse. Otherwise, the scansion itself can be reduced to a form of ritualization of the intervention of the carer, empty and predictable by the patient, without any transformative efficiency.

Putting the enigma back at the heart of the anorexic subject's experience coincides with the partial failure or, on the positive side, with a more elastic reformulation of his strategy of control of the Other. The production of surprise and the appearance of anguish are the two main ways to produce in the subject the enigmatic effect that awakens them from the mortifying torpor of their anesthesia. As far as anguish is concerned, it is essential that, within the treatment, it remains on the patient's side and that it does not invade the position of the carer; this is not simple if we take into account the fact that the production of anguish in the Other is a central axis of the anorexic functioning. Basically, making oneself the object of the Other's anguish is the most radical way in which the anorexic exercises their control over those around them.

To be invaded by the patient's death anxiety thus means to settle, in the treatment, in the same position as the parents and to become, in fact, at this point, prey to the destructive omnipotence of the illness. It is essential that, where the therapist's anxiety for the patient has been activated, this is not consigned to the patient in the treatment, but rather carried into supervision or into the analyst's own analysis, in order to identify the point in the patient's discourse at which the analyst has specularly identified themselves. This maneuver allows the therapist to reposition him/herself and to keep separate the phantasmatic anguish that has troubled him/her from the real concern for the patient's condition. It is an operation that can make him/her more decisive and serene in his/her actions, for example in communicating to the patient and the family the need for hospitalization. The anguish of the carer, just like the reverse hypnosis that can affect many therapists in the treatment of anorexia, to the point of leading them to misunderstand the real seriousness of the patient's bodily conditions, is the factor that causes the greatest disturbance in the treatment, since it reactivates the fundamental impasse of the anorexic in their relationship to the parental Other: not only does the parent fail to make good the daughter's anguish, but they invade her with their own anguish.

When the anorexic encounters an Other who does not allow themselves to be distressed by them, the most threatening weapon they use to exert their control is deactivated and this can allow the opposite operation to take place in the treatment: that the experience of anguish manages to disturb them, to shake them up and to take them out of their mortifying indifference. This is precisely the operation of fundamental affective rectification of the anorexic subject's relations to the real, which we have indicated in the transformation of a nirvanic-egosyntonic position toward an uncanny (*unheimlich*)-egodystonic position.

Anxiety and the two meanings of "refusal of the Other" in anorexia nervosa

The entrance of the experience of anguish which, in the clinic of anorexia nervosa, generally takes the form of the anguish of disappearance, represents the event which, in the context of the treatment, introduces the occasion of an unprecedented symbolization on the part of the subject, which can uninstall them from their autistic isolation and allow the opening to the encounter with the Other. It is appropriate for the therapist to be ready for this recurrent moment in the treatment of anorexia nervosa, which can manifest itself in different typical ways: the patient's progressive and silent slimming down to the critical threshold, or their declared intention, at a given moment, to no longer wish to continue the therapy. The threat of disappearance, embodied in the gradual and silent consumption of the body or declared by the announcement of the interruption of the treatment, introduces an element of dramatic tension in the center of the treatment. Here we witness the appearance of anorexic refusal at the heart of the treatment.

It is essential that we therapists do not find ourselves, at this appointment with the anorexic patient, in the same position where, in similar circumstances, the patient's parents and all those who followed in their footsteps found themselves. First of all, this means, no doubt, not responding on our side with anguish. But there is something else: the anorexic sets up, by this maneuver, a refusal of the Other in the objective sense of the genitive: a refusal that is theirs vis-à-vis the Other. Here, they are the subject who refuses and the Other is the object they refuse. In this sense, the refusal represents an act of theirs, apart from the fact that it can take on the value of an acted fact or a passage to action. In this clinical situation, what proves to be essential is the way in which the Other, here embodied by the therapist, responds to the act of refusal carried out by the anorexic. Here, the other constant response, together with the anguished response, that the anorexic produces in the Other comes into play: the refusing response. The anorexic patient tends to become unbearable for the Other because of their immutable fixity and their confinement in the symptom. By this she/he provokes, in fact, the refusal of the Other. It is crucial that the therapist does not respond to the anorexic's refusal with their own refusal. That is to say, that he/she does not also embody, in their own response, the position of the refusing Other that the anorexic subject has encountered in their history. As several authors have pointed out, it is not a question, for example, of a parental couple not having provided their daughter with attentive care: on the contrary. What the clinical stories reveal, however, is an extreme difficulty for the daughter to bear the signs of disapproval and disappointment on the part of the parents and also a difficulty for the parents to give space to a singular desire of the daughter, different from their own and situated beyond their narcissistic horizon of investment. The parental response to the anorexic girl is traversed by a fundamental confusion that leads them to a misunderstanding about her appeal, as both Bruch's teaching (on the cognitive side) and Lacan's reading (on the affect side) underline. In other words, it is a question of a response that does not manage to tune in to the girl's subjective core, to the real demand from which her request stems, thus failing to recognize her own place.

It is on this basis that the undifferentiated sense of powerlessness, the paralyzing sense of ineffectiveness that pervades all thought and activity of the anorexic subject, which the indiscriminate nature of the refusal, according to Bruch, desperately tries to conceal, is built (Bruch, 1978, p. 298). Avoiding a response to their refusal, that is, avoiding the embodiment of the refusing Other, becomes an essential maneuver to try to defuse and bypass the autistic closure of the anorexic subject in the treatment, thus avoiding what becomes, to the highest degree, their position of symptomatic jouissance par excellence: being the waste, the refusal of the Other, can occur here, too. On this point, the structural diagnosis becomes revealing in the reading of the function of the patient's refusal and can orient the intervention. In hysterical anorexia, what predominates is the function of refusal as a demand aiming to provoke in the Other a recognition at the level of desire. In the forms of so-called anorexia vera, the patient often acts out the refusal, in order to find confirmed, in the Other's response of refusal, the condition of jouissance represented by the fact that it is they who embody the Other's refusal. In the first case, what prevails is thus refusal as provocation (and production) of desire, whereas, in the second, it is refusal as provocation (and production) of refusal.

Third scansion: isolation of the key signifiers of alienation

Signifying alienation and the lethal effect of speech on the body: isolation of the traumatic statements

The transition to the recognition of signifying alienation is necessary in the treatment, in particular when the lethal effect that certain key phrases appear, generally pronounced during the subject's childhood or puberty, and which appear at a given moment in the treatment, to have had on him and notably in his relationship with the body. These are sentences pronounced by central figures in the subject's life, normally the mother or father, by other family members (the centrality of the grandmother, especially the mother's mother, is often highlighted) or by adult figures outside the family but hyper-invested (the teacher, the swimming instructor, the priest, etc.). These sentences reached the patient in the form of an imperative judgment or reprobation that ended up leaving its mark on their drive orientation (Cosenza, 2010, pp. 25–34; 2015, pp. 93–100). In the passage from childhood to the period of prepuberty and puberty, the relationship with siblings and friendships with girls of the same age, which often create narcissistic-specular couples (the relationship with the so-called "best friend") whose rupture is often the conjuncture of the triggering of the anorexia, acquires no less importance (Recalcati, 2002, pp. 93–94). During the treatment, the patients often recount situations in which the encounter at school with the judgment on themselves or on their bodies by their peers left an indelible mark.

Several times we noted, in the account of apparently completely serene childhoods, the encounter with a point of anxiety (Lacan, 2004, pp. 265–279; Naveau, 2005, pp. 37–44) that had remained ingrained in the patient as a child: a transfer or a family move, announced only at the moment it occurred, or formulated as the greatest surprise, had a traumatic effect on them. Suddenly, their world was changed, their friendships were interrupted, a devastating break was introduced into their life, without it being possible for them to carry out the slightest subjectivation.

Clinical experience leads us to affirm that the subject who has developed an eating disorder has generally encountered, in the course of their previous history, normally during childhood but also in pre-adolescence, traumatic statements concerning their body or their relationship to food, which have had a psychic inscription effect in their subsequent life. The traumatic statement is inscribed in the body, becoming a drive program for the subject, a superegoic commandment from which they are unable to escape. While a real event of violence, abuse or physical maltreatment has not necessarily functioned in a traumatic way for the subject, in the clinical histories and in the analytical paths, we see emerge, at a given moment in the discourse of the patients, the formulation of trauma-statements that have left a lethal mark on them. And, in any case, even a traumatic event, such as a violence suffered, or even a bereavement, only acquires its psychic weight in relation to what has been said or not said – and how it has been said or not said – by the subject or to the subject (on the part of the family and especially significant persons). At its root, the experience of trauma is the encounter with something real that has left a sign and is still waiting to be enunciated by the subject who has suffered it.

In any case, it is precisely thanks to the appearance of these trauma-statements during the treatment that the subject in anorexia can recognize, in a radical way, the lethal effect on him of signifying alienation and the power of speech on the body and jouissance. The appearance of the traumatic statement in the discourse coincides with the recognition of the power of speech to affect the real of the body, even when it is accompanied by the affective reactivation of this traumatic effect. If, therefore, at the beginning of the treatment, the anorexic embodies the emblem of the therapeutic inefficiency of speech from the point of view of the incidence on the body, at the moment when this unravelling of the treatment occurs, they experience to the maximum the effect of speech through the cut that it has made in their drive life, in precise scansions of their existence that have marked its course. This re-emergence allows speech to regain its own power within the treatment and to succeed in isolating, in the signifying history of the subject that we have evoked here, those nuclei of nonsense around which it has been structured.

Return effects of the superegoic ideals on the anorexia

This unravelling allows the patient to experience emotionally in the treatment the weight, in their life, not only of the statements with traumatic content but also, and perhaps above all, of the ideal statements transmitted by the parents and functioning as orders that must be embodied in the experience of their daughters or sons. The effect of this is evident if we look at the lives of anorexic patients before the onset of the illness: we generally find an excess of adhesive adequacy of the little girl or boy to the ideals transmitted by the parents, which takes the form of the typical perfectionism preceding the onset of the illness. It is important to keep in mind that the anorexic refusal, which is clearly identifiable when the disease sets in, is nothing but the other side of the coin of perfectionist complacency toward the ideal transmitted by the Other, a complacency pushed to this extreme limit that we often find in the stories of most of these patients. An indiscriminate yes to the demand of the Other, which reaches the subject in the form of an order to be carried out, is followed, with the onset of anorexia, by an indiscriminate no of anorexic negativism. In the logic of the anorexic experience, the predominant factor is the rigid and scission dichotomy that leads to its extreme consequences, the moral Manichaeism characterizing the adolescent's relationship to the Other and to the ideal dimension, without having access to any way out. The passage to the neurotic recognition of one's own ambivalence toward the Other and the ideal, which occurs in the subject after crossing the crossroads of adolescence, is an unravelling that the patient recoils from. In the end, at the moment of the onset of anorexia, the patient ends up embodying the macabre and paradoxical core of their own deranged assumption of the parental ideal. The girl's anorexia often represents a macabre caricature of parental ideals. Frequently, for example, anorexic girls build the scaffolding of their existence around an ideal of autonomy and independence, but they end up playing this ideal as a card against the link to the Other, thus condemning themselves to isolation in the phases of the declared illness. The supposed autonomy thus shows its true face in anorexia by turning into a refusal.

The alienating vel "eat or die" and the anorexic response

Anorexia is presented, in fact and not rarely in the patients' discourse, as a challenge to the biological laws of self-preservation of life. Apart from those rare cases where the refusal to eat embodies a real suicidal tendency, anorexic subjects generally keep their paradoxical attachment to life, so well illustrated by Selvini Palazzoli in the "sthenic claw" of the anorexic. The hyperactivity that characterizes them, ideally driven by the obsessive thought of reducing calories, presents in fact the characteristics aimed at pushing to the limit the tension between the life of the organism and the laws of nature. In this sense, while the impulsive destiny of the anorexic goes in the direction of a deferred suicide, linked to the collapse of the organism, their intentionality is not normally suicidal. To be able to live without eating, without taking anything from the Other, is the logical paradox where their position is defined. For this reason, the anorexic, faced with the structural crossroads presentifying castration in the experience of the living being, "eat or die", decides to follow neither direction, not recognizing themselves in this law. Biology teaches us that, in fact, this principle cannot be ignored and that not choosing between eating and dying is, in effect, choosing death. But the anorexic does not give in to the constraining evidence of this law, which she/he tries, to some extent, to replace with another one of their own, according to which life is independent of the food given by the Other.

In our opinion, this is the clearest point of manifestation, in the clinic of anorexia nervosa, of the lack of symbolic inscription of the law and of the difficulty, typical of the anorexic, in bearing the effect of loss of jouissance that this inscription entails. Their link to life presents itself, in fact, in the form of a link to a mythical dimension of the living, uncontaminated by the regulating intervention of the signifier on the body. It is the link to this dimension that reactivates the mythical experience of full satisfaction in the relationship with the primary object, which functions, in fact, for the anorexic as an alternative law to the legal regime of symbolic castration. In this sense, in our reading, the anorexic is not in a position of renunciation of life. Rather, she/he is in the paradoxical position, if we take into account the deprivations she/he actually imposes on themselves, of not wanting to lose anything of the enjoyment of life, which represents an impossible experience for the subject. On this point, the thesis of the young Lacan of the *Family Complexes*, according to which anorexia nervosa, as much as drug addiction, would be the reactivation of an experience of mythical fusion with the maternal object, is welded to the key thesis of the last Lacan. The anorexic's solution to the bifurcation between eating and dying is that of finding an object to eat, the only one possible, which does not imply for themselves the passage to the dynamics of exchange, of the gift of the Other and of demand; in short, that does not imply the passage under the law of symbolic castration. For this reason, Lacan will support the thesis according to which the anorexic feeds on a special object that keeps them, finally, in an undivided relation to the domain of the living, while preserving themselves from the loss of jouissance: this is what he calls, precisely, the "nothing" object.

An unravelling in hysterical anorexics: extraction of the sign of love from the field of the Other

From the homogeneity to the ambivalence of the Other

An important unravelling, in the advanced treatment of anorexia, particularly in its hysterical-neurotic forms, is represented, once the power of speech has been reactivated and the door to one's own signifying history has been reopened, by a transformative effect that cracks the controlling and superegoic rigidity of the subject: the relationship to the Other and to the object (including food) begins to emerge from a linear schematism of inclusion and exclusion, of good and bad, to open up to an ambivalent tone. This passage allows the subject to accomplish an operation previously unheard of for them. As they have been able, in the course of the treatment, to reappropriate the relationship to anguish and the relationship to the word operating on the body in a lethal way, it is now possible for them to find, in the field of their history, the traces of the desire of the Other that were truly inscribed but that the subject, immersed in their symptom, was unable or unwilling to see.

This is a passage that destabilizes the anorexic at this moment of the therapeutic process, since it produces a crack in the solidity of their refusal position. The fact of finding in their own history the trace of the gift as a free act and as a sign of love especially for themselves introduces, in the relationship to the Other, a heterogeneous element that modifies its status. The Other is no longer, for them, integrally reducible to the locus of a refusal in its singularity, and is no longer articulated completely in the form of a demand for satisfaction addressed to the daughter or son by the narcissistic ideals of the parents. While the field of the Other begins to become, for the anorexic subject, a heterogeneous place opening its doors to the experience of ambivalence, this is not without effects on the subject themselves, who is re-convened, at this moment, at the crossroads between the acceptance or refusal of the gift that comes to him from the Other. Faced with this bifurcation, the question of the anorexic opens up again: the subject is called upon to decide to accept something from the Other and, therefore, to depend on him as the emitter of the gift that comes to him and not as the formulator of a superegoic demand that he must obey.

The question of love in anorexia nervosa

Faced with this bifurcation, the anorexic subject again experiences the encounter with anguish, this time in the form of an event that divides him or her in front of the appearance of the sign of the desire of the Other. In these circumstances, it is clear that what functions as a traumatic factor in anorexia nervosa is not only the sign of refusal on the part of the Other, but also and to the same extent, the encounter with the desire and satisfaction of the Other who says yes. This encounter, in fact, undermines at the root the system of control of the Other that the anorexic subject has built up through the construction of their own symptom. This can produce destabilizing and worrying effects of decompensation, especially in psychotic forms of anorexia where paranoid responses can be triggered (the desiring Other is put in the position of persecutor) or, on the contrary, in anorexic-bulimic forms where there are erotomanic responses (where the subject develops the indisputable certainty of being the object loved by the Other). In certain more melancholic-depressive forms of anorexia, what can be reactivated in the subject in this conjuncture is an abandonment anxiety that reactivates in them the experience of being let down by the Other.

In non-psychotic forms of anorexia nervosa, the encounter with a partner's desire introduces anguish into the subjective experience, in the form of a division between fear and desire. The affective turbulence becomes extreme and the subject is often nostalgic for the mortifying and passionless aridity of the declared phase of anorexia, of their isolation with their symptom, compared to the radical suffering they experience now, where the passions are, contrary to what happened before, amplified to the highest degree in their emotional scope. This explains two clinically recurrent phenomena in the clinic of anorexia. First, either the anorexic patient is alone in their illness (possible previous boy/girlfriends have moved away as the illness has taken over their life), surrounded by the anguish of the family – and this is the most frequent condition; or she/he has a link with a partner who for her/him is not an eroticized and therefore libidinally invested object, but rather a point of support, a de-eroticized partner in an anaclitic function. It is a safe haven to lean on, not the object of the patient's desire but the object of their demand for care. Not a partner who can contrast the reality of the symptom, but a partner who, for the patient, fits functionally into the symptomatic system of anorexia nervosa. The more the anorexic subject progresses in the treatment, the more this position is questioned; it is not by chance that, generally speaking, the rupture of the link with the support partner is a consequence of the progressive exit from anorexia, with the search for a partner of desire.

The passage, provoked by the treatment, from the condition of a sick subject to be treated to the condition of a desiring subject, typically introduces the patient into a condition thus summarized by the patients who have arrived at this point in the treatment: I would like to go back, but from now on I cannot. In their words, the crossing of a point of no return that the treatment has produced emerges, in relation to which the regressive maneuver of reactivating the symptomatic response no longer functions as before, since its libidinal scope has been reduced or emptied. The anorexia is no longer enjoyed by the patient as before. In spite of this, the subject engages in love life in an attempt to build bonds that she/he often causes to die at birth. The fort-da movement with food is replaced by a fort-da with the partner whose encounter is both sought and avoided. It is in a dialectic of devouring and refusing that the relationship of the anorexic subject to the partner is structured. It often appears, in the words of the patients but especially of their partners, that the most unbearable thing in the relationship with anorexics or bulimics is the anguish that they pour out on their partner of the moment. To feel controlled, devoured (or, on the contrary, refused), always insufficient to respond to their demand for love without limits, produces in many men an anguished fugue effect. This can also happen within the treatment, in the transference relationship, if the analyst does not take into account that he/she too embodies for the patient the object of devouring and refusing, and that they can for themselves as a perhaps unique opportunity to meet someone who actively remains in their place in their relationship with them, whatever happens, without devouring or refusing themselves.

A terminal point in the analytic treatment of anorexia: extracting the object nothing from the drive body

True anorexia and localized or partial foreclosure

The anorexic position can be defined as a response of the subject, arising in a second phase, to the inoperative action of the symbolic on their body, without the effective loss of jouissance having been possible. Soria speaks of it as a partial or total failure, underlying anorexia-bulimia, of the instantiation of the father as a signifier in the subject's life. The total failure of the embodiment of the father, in the clinic of anorexia, opens the way to the psychotic forms with anorexic symptomatology where the foreclosure of the Name-of-the-Father is structural. The clinical forms closest to what we can fit into the classical framework of anorexia vera, recently revived by Dewambrechies La Sagna, open us to the perspective of a signifying embodiment not non-existent but rendered inoperative around a key point. This is why we can speak in this regard, not of a structural foreclosure but, rather, of a localized or partial foreclosure of a position of the subject not structurally outside discourse, as happens in psychoses, but "*de facto* out-of-discourse". An obvious manifestation of this is the subject's aberrant relationship to food. The relationship of the anorexic, as well as the bulimic and the obese person, to food is in an outside-discourse relationship. Attending one of their meals, as we have done in therapeutic communities, is the best way to realize this.

Finally, what we have tried to do in this research is to trace the itinerary of the treatment of anorexia nervosa as a process in which this point outside of discourse, present at the heart of the symptom, is renewed around the problem of the subject in its relationship to the self-image, to the field of the Other and to the jouissance of the drive. Only in the light of this reconnection can the subject's aberrant eating behavior find its specific clinical *raison d'être*.

Encystment and embodiment

To the partial failure of signifying embodiment corresponds, in eating psychopathologies, an excess of embodiment on the phantasmatic level and a compulsive deregulation on the level of the act, both in the sense of too much (bulimia, obesity) and too little (anorexia). Indeed, the more the anorexic subject is immersed in the restrictive symptom, the more the embodiment phantasmatizations (devouring/being devoured) and the relative anguish take over. The effect of a debility of signifying embodiment, as Lacan understands it, is an excess of phantasmatic embodiment. This is the form of embodiment on the imaginary plane whose centrality in eating pathologies Karl Abraham has shown.

The terminal phase of the treatments of anorexic patients shows a recurrent transformation process: the more the subject becomes capable of completing the signifying embodiment process, which remained unaccomplished, the more a reduction of the embodiment fantasies occurs and the more this has the effect of repositioning the exercise of the eating function. This is why clinical experience teaches us that the subject's eating disorder cannot be treated effectively without modifying their position in relation to the Other and to jouissance, that is to say, his relationship to language and to the real of their body. The analytic treatment of anorexics bears witness to this defect of signifying embodiment, in the form of trauma-statements, or superegoic signifiers of parental narcissistic ideals that have been inscribed in the subject's body without having been embodied. In other words, these statements have left an indelible mark on the subject's life, without ever having been subjectivized by them, retaining a fundamental and sinister strangeness in relation to their decision. In this sense, it seems to me that we can speak, more properly, of signifying encystment in the experience of the anorexic, as an alternative to an effective process of symbolic embodiment. The fact that an encystment has occurred instead of a symbolic embodiment has, among other things, a fundamental effect: whereas signifying embodiment has the fundamental effect of cutting off the mythical full jouissance in which the subject is originally immersed, in order to transform it into a partial jouissance that can be staggered, encystment, for its part, does not manage to accomplish this fundamental operation. The signifier is thus inscribed in the body, encysted, grafted, without the subject embodying it and appropriating it. The main result is to keep, in the subject's body, a point of full jouissance, uncontaminated by the regulating action of the Other, which the subject in anorexia does not renounce and around which he constructs their own position. This point of uncontaminated jouissance, which has remained intact in the subject's body, Lacan tried to define, through the formulation of the function of the object "nothing", as the core of the anorexic's jouissance.

Trajectory of the treatment: from the fantasy of embodiment to the lack of signifying embodiment

The hypothesis that we put forward in this regard is that, in anorexia nervosa, the centrality of the devouring fantasy (devouring the Other/being devoured by the Other) is only the effect of a signifying embodiment that is absent (in psychotic forms) or deficient (true anorexia). In other words, signifying alienation is not assumed by the subject as a symbolic law constituting it, but achieves its operativity, in a partial way, in the form of an encystment of the signifier in the body or a grafting, in the body, of something foreign, leaving intact the primary jouissance that inhabits it. For this reason, the strategic course of the analytical treatment of anorexia aims at making the subject meet in their discourse, beyond the imaginary phantasmatizations revolving around the scene of devouring (devouring the Other/being devoured by the Other), with the nuclei of nonsense that structure it. These nuclei mark the trace of the signifying encystment in the history of the subject and testify to the defect in the process of signifying embodiment that constituted it. This passage occurs in the course of the analyses, generally in the form of a disturbing but at the same time revealing surprise effect. The threat represented by the Other is no longer situated in front of the patient, before their eyes, in the figures of the key characters of their life, but they themselves discover it as being behind their back, in the empty spaces of their discourse, in the points where speech freezes, their body recedes, where their desire atrophies in order to be dragged along by the thrust of an unspeakable and totalizing jouissance that recalls them to themselves.

Beyond the parasitism of nothing

The treatments of anorexic subjects, once they have reached their major point of accomplishment, produce the effect of breaking down the primary jouissance that inhabits the body and of transforming it into a jouissance in loss that is partial, which no longer paralyzes their life but which finds a residual location and becomes bearable. The patient learns to recognize it and finds a way to tame it, without having to suffer its effects in an imperative and devastating way. This result, much more accessible to a neurotic subject during the treatment, is the outcome, in cases of anorexia nervosa, of long and very hard work during which, at a given moment of the treatment, the subject is no longer satisfied with getting better but wants to know, completely, what happened to him/her to make him/her choose the anorexic solution. In this unravelling, analysis marks the passage from the status of therapeutic treatment to the radical subjective search for the roots of the subject's being, thus producing the effects of transformation. This cannot be achieved through analysis, practiced as a hermeneutic of the primary meaning, by an analyst who would have installed themselves, from the beginning, in the position of one who knows and interprets. In this respect, the critical lesson of Bruch and Selvini Palazzoli represents an inescapable point of no return in the relationship between psychoanalysis and anorexia.

According to our experience, analysis becomes effective if it aims to push the subject to isolate, within the framework of his/her discourse, the non-sense real around which the anorexic symptom is constructed and, in the times and modalities that are necessary, to empty this construction of the jouissance that supports it.

References

American Psychiatric Association (2022), *Diagnostic and Statistical Manual of Mental Disorders. Fifth Edition Text Revision. DSM-5-TR*. Washington DC: American Psychiatric Association Publishing.

Barbuto, M., Pace, P. (1998), Logiche del funzionamento e del trattamento della famiglia di soggetti anoressico-bulimici, Recalcati, M. (Dir.), *Il corpo ostaggio: clinica psicoanalitica dell'anoressia-bulimia*. Roma: Borla, pp. 250–268.

Bruch, H. (1978), *Les yeux et le ventre: l'obèse, l'anorexique*. Paris: Payot; (1973) *Eating Disorders: Obesity, Anorexia Nervosa, and the Person within*. New York: Basic Books.

Cosenza, D. (2001), La comunità terapeutica come luogo della cura, Colombo, L. and others, *La cura della malattia mentale. Vol. II. Il trattamento*. Milano: Bruno Mondadori, pp. 227–249.

Cosenza, D. (2007), Les liens familiaux dans la cliniques des pathologies de l'alimentation, *La lettre mensuelle*, no. 263, pp. 14–16, décembre.

Cosenza, D. (2010), El silencio y la voz en la anorexia mental, Gavlosky J., Cors Ulloa, R. (Dir.), *Polifonías en psicoanálisis*. Caracas: Pomaire, pp. 25–34.

Cosenza, D. (2015), Silence and the Voice in Anorexia Nervosa, *European Journal of Psychoanalysis*, vol. 2(1–2), pp. 93–100.

Dewambrechies La Sagna, C. (2006), L'anorexie vraie de la jeune fille, *La Cause freudienne*, no. 63, pp. 57–70.

Eidelberg, A. and others (2003), *Anorexia y bulimia: síntomas actuals de lo femenino*. Buenos Aires: Del Bucle.

Lacan, J. (2006), *Presentation on Transference, Écrits. The First Complete Edition in English*. New York/London: Norton & Company, pp. 176–185; *Intervention sur le transfert (1951). Écrits* (1966). Paris: Éditions du Seuil, pp. 215–226.

Lacan, J. (2004), *Le Séminaire. Livre X. L'angoisse*, 1962–1963. Paris: Le Seuil.

Ménard, A. (1992), Structure signifiante de l'anorexie mentale, *Actes de l'ECF*, vol. 2, pp. 3–7, février.

Naveau, P. (2005), L'angoisse dans l'anorexie féminine, *La Cause freudienne*, no. 59, pp. 37–44, février.

Pace, P. (2010), *Un dolore infame: genitori e anoressia*. Milano: Bruno Mondadori.

Polacco Williams, G. (1999), *Paesaggi interni e corpi estranei: disordini alimentari e altre patologie*. Milano: Bruno Mondadori.

Recalcati, M. (2002), *Clinica del vuoto, anoressie, dipendenze, psicosi*. Milano: Franco Angeli.

Selvini Palazzoli, M. and others (1998), *Ragazze anoressiche e bulimiche*. Milano: Cortina.

Conclusion

Having reached the concluding considerations of this work, it seems important to us to indicate some developments and research perspectives that are opening up, in our opinion, as a consequence of the path taken so far. We limit ourselves to indicating three directions to be followed in the years to come in order to deepen the work, developed over the last twenty years and systematized in this research, on the psychoanalytical clinic of anorexia nervosa.

First of all, one line of research that we have focused on in this work, and which we feel is essential to explore further, concerns anorexia nervosa in its relationship to contemporary adolescence. In chapter 9, we tried to articulate the anorexic question from the coordinates relating to the junction point that adolescence represents, as it is formulated in the perspective of Lacan's psychoanalysis, notably in the light of the reading of his text: *Preface* to Wedekind's *Spring Awakening*. In this text, written by Lacan in 1974, which expresses the consequences to which his last teaching in psychoanalysis leads, it seemed to us that we could identify the outline of a new theory of the process of adolescence, formulated in the light of the coordinates proper to the contemporary period. It seemed important to us to explicitly relate these two fertile sides of Lacan's teaching, his theory of anorexia nervosa and his conceptualization of contemporary adolescence, which have not been suffi-ciently articulated between them. The importance of this relationship emerges all the more in the light of clinical evidence that identifies in the time of adolescence the conjuncture of the privileged beginnings of anorexia nervosa and, in contemporary adolescence, the historical period of the greatest dif-fusion of the anorexic symptom. These considerations lead us to rethink the classical relationships between psychopathology and development of the subject and to try not to limit ourselves to considering anorexia nervosa, as well as the beginnings of juvenile addictions, only as failures in the process of puberty symptomatization. At the same time, it is also possible to question these new silent symptomatic formations, these symptoms without enigma and without demand for the subject who bears them, as extreme embodi-ments of a transformation which today invests, in a more general way, the passage of the young person facing the drive awakening which crosses their

DOI: 10.4324/9781003318439-12

body as well as the modalities of incarnation of this passage. In other words, this is the hypothesis that must be articulated here and put to the test in future research: contemporary anorexia nervosa leads us to question the status of the new symbolic order, different from the one that predominated in the classical period of the history of psychoanalysis, and to rethink its forms of constitution in the process of adolescent becoming. In this perspective, anorexia is no longer presented only as a position of refusal of the Other, but also as an extreme gateway that contributes to illuminating the impasse and the specificity of the current condition of the subject in adolescence. This is the lesson of methodology that Freud taught us and that Lacan revived: to make the stone of scandal a stone of comparison on which to found a new clinic.

Given that the structural question remains, as always for the adolescent, that of finding a singular way of assuming the drive that inhabits him/her and that the passage of puberty has awakened, the problem that opens up here is how to shed light on the forms of realization that this delicate operation assumes, in the young person, in the framework of the contemporary Other. The search for a subjective limit that allows the subject's drive to find a symbolic anchor in the ego ideal and an orientation framework in the structuring of a fundamental fantasy; what forms could it assume in the era of the Other that does not exist? Anorexia nervosa can help us, from its position of extreme frontier, to interrogate in a positive way the new physiognomy of the Other, not to read the clinical manifestations of contemporary adolescence through the lenses of the Other of Freud's time but, rather, in the light of the current forms of the malaise in Civilization. Within this framework, some thematic lines seem to impose themselves in the reading of contemporary adolescence, among which, undoubtedly, the function of the body as a place of inscription of a limit that tends to be written on the borders between the imaginary and the real, in the form of a practice of jouissance visible and identifiable by the gaze of the Other. The extreme diffusion of the practice of tattooing and piercing among contemporary adolescents is an ordinary manifestation of this, just as, at the same time, in the clinic, the positions of the beginnings of drug addiction and anorexia-bulimia are an extreme manifestation. Could we speak of a contemporary tendency of the subject in adolescence to externalize the limit on the surface of the body, and of a greater difficulty in "internalizing" it through the weakening of the symbolic law? More generally, for the adolescent, the question of how to "make a father" where the function of the father has wavered and how to find a way to inscribe oneself in the field of the Other open up here (Freda, 2009, pp. 11–15).

The so-called new symptoms beginning in adolescence could well be configured for many young people as active attempts to carry out this kind of operation.

The second question that seems to us essential to deepen is strictly linked to the first research perspective on contemporary adolescence and anorexia nervosa: the problem of anorexic jouissance in its relation to the problem of sexuation and to that of the question of femininity. In our work, we have tried to give reference coordinates and reading hypotheses which, however, need to be elaborated in a more articulated way. We will have to devote a place to a specific framework for the problem of anorexia in adolescent and adult boys, a decidedly rarer phenomenon, which we have not examined here. The answer to the eternal question "Why women?", at the heart of the clinic of anorexia nervosa (and also of bulimia) because of its massive presence in young girls and, more generally, in women, requires that we do not stop at sociological explanations linked to the position of the image of the woman in postmodern society. It seemed to us more fruitful to frame the question from the psychoanalytical coordinates of the relationship of the woman to her body, in the triple dimension of the body image, of the symbolic articulation on which it is based and of the real jouissance that supports it. In the passage of puberty, this relationship is put to the test in its overall hold by the effects of the transformations that invest the knotting in the body of the three Lacanian registers of the real, the symbolic and the imaginary.

We have sought a line of reading of the question of jouissance in anorexia nervosa – which will merit further investigation in a future research – from the perspective opened by Lacan in The Seminar, Book XX, *Encore*, through the formulas of sexuation and the identification on the feminine side of two different modalities of jouissance: phallic jouissance and what Lacan calls the other jouissance, or supplementary jouissance beyond the phallus (Lacan, 1975, pp. 94–95). The fundamental hypothesis, supported in the light of the few authors who have really dared to approach the theme of anorexia from this perspective and among whom we can mention Geneviève Morel (1997, pp. 33–36; 1999, pp. 15–21) and the group of the ICBA of Buenos Aires (notably Nieves Soria) (Eidelberg and others, 2003), is that the girl's jouissance, in the anorexic response, takes the path of the limitless by the effect of a failure in the structuring of phallic jouissance which ends up directing the subject toward an aberrant drift of feminine jouissance. This drift invests above all the girl's body as an object subjected to an implacable and forcible control of weight and image, the key to which – horror for unconscious knowledge – is indicated by Lacan in The Seminar, Book XXI, as we saw in Chapter 4. In this perspective, it is of great interest for us to try to frame the girl's anorexia nervosa within the current debate on the "clinic of excess" as typical of the feminine, especially within the specific coordinates of the contemporary malaise in Civilization. These coordinates, in fact, amplify and place in tension the dimension of excess, constitutive of the feminine (Francesconi, 2007, pp. 72–86; Eldar, 2009; Sobral, 2011) and which, generally, takes the way of deprivation, not only in anorexia nervosa but also in the new depressive forms and in melancholy, by the push to excess proper to the contemporary social discourse and by the imperative of enjoyment, proper to the discourse of the capitalist. The contribution that the Lacanian perspective can develop on this point seems to us decisive, as it is a wide-ranging theme which, around the theme of anorexia nervosa, allows for a different framing of the problem and helps to reposition the question from the problem of sexuation, thus differentiating itself from the perspective spread especially in the Anglo-American feminist literature of gender studies (Eidelberg ans others, 2003; Mambrini, 2010).

Finally, the third line of research concerns anorexia as a response of the subject who finds in the refusal of food a stabilizing solution to the problem, which they are unable to face, of sexual non-relation.

In this perspective, anorexia nervosa can be studied in its differential relationship with other psychopathologies that invest the food-object as a neuralgic and constant element of their symptomatic manifestation: first of all bulimia and also the pathologies of hyper-eating, that is, obesity in its different forms, from Binge Eating Disorder to the hyperphagic variant of psychogenic obesity. This line of research, in which we have been involved for several years, due to our institutional work with subjects suffering from psychogenic eating disorders, can make possible, in our opinion and in the light of the psychoanalytical coordinates of the Lacanian orientation, an alternative framework to the phenomenological-descriptive reading proposed by the existing international psychiatric classifications.

This means for us the need to rethink the foundations of the field of eating psychopathologies, questioned in the light of the position of the subject who is the bearer of them, of the function of desire that puts them in relation to the Other, and of the mode of jouissance that marks them in their being.

Certainly, this perspective faces a preliminary problem, of a textual type, in relation to Lacan. In fact, while we constantly find reference to anorexia throughout his teaching, it is quite different in the case of bulimia, and the reference becomes practically non-existent in his discourse when it comes to obesity as a clinical category. Moving in this direction will therefore imply an effort to elaborate a Lacanian theory of the obese subject, in the absence of an explicit teaching of Lacan in this respect.

With the exception of a few rare contributions, working on obesity means not being able to rely on reference to Lacanian authors. This does not apply to the field of anorexia and its relationship to bulimia, which benefits from a vast Lacanian literature.

The analytic contributions on obesity are in fact rather sparse (Recalcati, 2002, pp. 205–225; Cosenza, 2006, pp. 227–254) and at most based on little clinical material. It seems to us that these studies suffer in part from genuine and proper prejudices that do not allow researchers to get to the heart of the subjective issue of obesity.

Moreover, obesity is still today a field where the epistemological diatribe between organogenesis and psychogenesis, resolved for anorexia at the Gottingen Symposium in 1965, is still widely debated, and where contributions from psychopathology and in particular from psychoanalysis are rather rare. A medical-nutritional definition of the pathology prevails, as well as a neo-behavioral, and currently mainly surgical, approach to its treatment. The very rare contributions of a psychoanalytical nature do not go beyond the indications provided by Freud, and in particular by Abraham, on the pathologies of nervous hunger, which the German psychoanalyst traces back to the same matrix of alcoholic pathologies and dependence, within the framework of a fixation on the very first evolutionary stage of libidinal development, the oral cannibalistic stage.

Subsequently, it was above all Bruch's founding work that developed, from the 1940s onwards, the field of psychopathologies of eating behavior as a unitary whole, and to elaborate, from the perspective of Ego-Psychology, a new paradigm for reading anorexia and obesity, centered on a narcissistic deficit and on an early dysfunction of the mother-child interaction, in the process of primary learning of response to stimulation. While it is true that Bruch's work has the merit of basing, on the one hand, the clinic of eating psychopathologies on the structure of the subject's personality and of articulating it in the light of a vast and prolonged clinical experience, on the other hand, its limitation, dealt with in Chapter II, consists in bringing it back within a problem of an essentially narcissistic nature. And in her discourse, this applies equally to anorexia and obesity. Our hypothesis is that the Lacanian approach to the clinic of eating psychopathologies allows us to find a founding point around the knot of the refusal of the Other and its differential articulation, which can take into account both the structure of the subject and the particular solution found by the latter around the deregulated relationship with the food substance.

The fundamental hypothesis that we will try to demonstrate is that the field of food psychopathologies is represented as a clinic of the object nothing, which takes a concrete form (unlike, for example, drug addiction and other so-called new forms of the symptom) through the subject's differential recourse to food substances as a modality of enjoyment beyond the pleasure principle.

References

Cosenza, D. (2006), L'obesità nelle nuove forme del sintomo, Cosenza, D, Recalcati, R., Villa, A., *Civiltà e disagio. Forme contemporanee della psicopatologia*. Milano: Bruno Mondadori, pp. 227–254.

Eidelberg, A. and others (2003), *Anorexia y bulimia: sintomas actuales de lo femenino*. Buenos Aires: Del Bucle.

Eldar, S. (Dir.) (2009), *Mujeres, una por una*. Madrid: Gredos.

Francesconi, P. (Dir.) (2007), *Una per una. Psicoanalisi e femminilità*. Roma: Borla.

Freda, F. H. (2009), L'adolescent freudien, *Mental. Revue international de Psychanalyse*, no. 23, décembre 2009, pp. 11–15.

Lacan, J. (1975), *Le Séminaire de Jacques Lacan, Livre XX, Encore*, 1972–1973. Paris: Éditions du Seuil.

Mambrini, L. (2010), *Lacan e il femminismo contemporaneo*. Macerata: Quodlibet.

Morel, G. (1997), Des symptômes et des femmes: boulimie et féminité, *La Lettre Mensuelle*, no 16, septembre 1997, pp. 33–36.

Morel, G. (1999), Féminité contre identité, *Feuillets psychanalytiques du Courtil*, no. 17, mars 1999, pp. 15–21.

Recalcati, M. (2002), *Clinica del vuoto. Anoressia, dipendenze, psicosi*, Milano: FrancoAngeli.

Sobral, G. (2011), *Madres, anorexia y feminidad.* Buenos Aires: Edicions Seminario.

Index